The Revision Guide to Core Clinical Medicine

Part 2

The Revision Guide to Core Clinical Medicine

Part 2

Dr Ankit Chadha
University of Cambridge, UK

Reviewed by

Dr Faisal Karim and Dr Abhirami Gautham

Illustrated by

Dr Talia Patel

World Scientific

NEW JERSEY · LONDON · SINGAPORE · BEIJING · SHANGHAI · HONG KONG · TAIPEI · CHENNAI · TOKYO

Published by

World Scientific Publishing Europe Ltd.

57 Shelton Street, Covent Garden, London WC2H 9HE

Head office: 5 Toh Tuck Link, Singapore 596224

USA office: 27 Warren Street, Suite 401-402, Hackensack, NJ 07601

Library of Congress Control Number: 2026933053

British Library Cataloguing-in-Publication Data
A catalogue record for this book is available from the British Library.

THE REVISION GUIDE TO CORE CLINICAL MEDICINE
Part 2

ISBN 978-1-80061-874-9 (hardcover)
ISBN 978-1-80061-878-7 (paperback)
ISBN 978-1-80061-875-6 (ebook for institutions)
ISBN 978-1-80061-876-3 (ebook for individuals)

For any available supplementary material, please visit
https://www.worldscientific.com/worldscibooks/10.1142/Q0552#t=suppl

Preface

Building on the success of my first book, *The Revision Guide to Core Clinical Medicine*, I am delighted to present *The Revision Guide to Core Clinical Medicine – **Part 2***.

Since the release of my first book, which I created to support fellow medical students and future doctors, I have been overwhelmed by the demand and positive feedback received. Part 2 covers the remaining 6 specialties – dermatology, gynaecology, haematology, obstetrics, paediatrics and psychiatry (as well as a bonus chapter on electrolytes) and completed the full medical syllabus to help you ace your exams.

Having graduated with a first-class degree in medicine from the University of Cambridge, I have experienced firsthand the demands and difficulties associated with medical school. I can recall the struggles faced by medical students, constantly searching for bits of information from various sources to grasp the extensive range of conditions, drug names, and key clinical knowledge required as a junior doctor. This often means long hours studying for exams, interspersed with time on the wards to acquire essential clinical skills.

Motivated by my desire to support fellow medical students and future doctors, I have written *The Revision Guide to Core Clinical Medicine* Parts 1 and 2, which cover the entire UK medical syllabus. This all-encompassing yet succinct resource caters to the needs of medical students, providing a thorough understanding of the subject matter while emphasising key information for exam achievement.

Instead of requiring various books for the different specialties and topics like pharmacology, this all-inclusive revision guide series contains all the necessary information in one convenient source. It aims to assist medical students by saving both money and time while also potentially reducing levels of anxiety and burnout.

About the Author

Dr Ankit Chadha
MB BChir (Cantab), MRCP, University of Cambridge, Mount Vernon Hospital

Dr Chadha is a specialist registrar in clinical oncology currently working at Mount Vernon Hospital, London. He is a member of the Royal College of Physicians and graduated with a distinction from the University of Cambridge and has a first-class intercalated degree in psychology.

He secured an academic foundation post in gynae-oncology conducting research at Hammersmith Hospital, London. His work in this field has been recognised by the British Gynaecological Cancer Society, who awarded him with an entry-level scholarship. In addition to his clinical and academic work, he is the founder of an online medical education portal for students and has received a foundation merit award for his teaching programme.

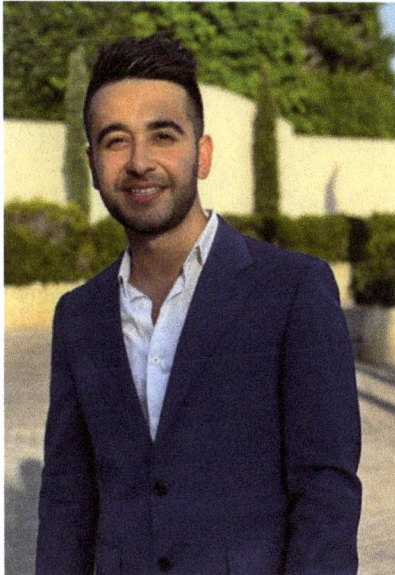

About the Illustrator

Dr Talia Patel
BMBS (Hons), BMedSci (Hons), University of Nottingham, Royal Derby Hospital

Dr Talia Patel graduated with honours from the University of Nottingham, where she obtained a first-class degree in Medical Sciences. She is currently undertaking a specialised foundation post in medical education, conducting research at the University Hospitals of Derby and Burton.

Combining her interests in medicine and art, Talia has illustrated this revision guide as a way to bring core clinical concepts to life. A visual learner herself, she has long relied on illustration to enhance her own studies. She now hopes that the visual elements in this book will provide fellow students and trainees with an engaging and supportive learning tool.

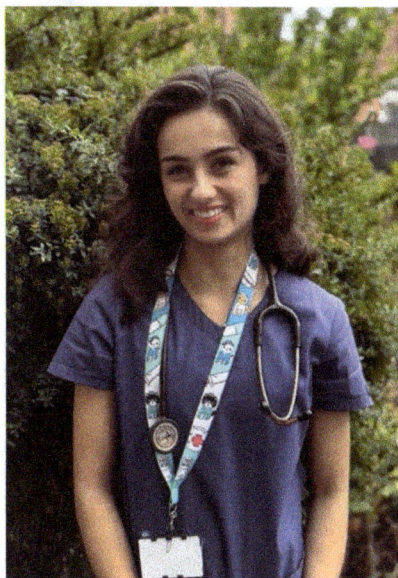

Acknowledgements

Lead Reviewers

Mr Faisal Karim
MBBS, BSc (Hons), MRCOG, The Royal Marsden Hospital

Mr Faisal Karim is an obstetrics and gynaecology registrar currently based at The Royal Marsden Hospital. He trained at the GKT School of Medical Education, King's College London, before embarking on specialty training in South London. He is currently completing his MD research, a collaboration between The Royal Marsden Hospital, The Institute of Cancer Research and Barts Cancer Institute. His research focuses on how the application of hyperthermic intraperitoneal chemotherapy impacts ovarian cancer on a cellular level.

Dr Abhirami Gautham
MBChB, MRCP (UK), MSc (Oxon), PGCert (Distinction), Northwick Park Hospital

Dr Abhirami Gautham is a gastroenterology registrar in North West London with clinical interests in hepatopancreatobiliary (HPB) medicine and interventional endoscopy. She studied medicine at the University of Manchester and went on to complete an MSc in Evidence-Based Health Care at the University of Oxford, receiving the Outstanding Dissertation Prize for her research on artificial intelligence in colonoscopy for ulcerative colitis. Her work has been presented internationally and published in *Gastrointestinal Endoscopy*. Alongside her clinical training, she holds a Postgraduate Certificate in Education for Health Professionals with Distinction and was awarded the Dean's Prize for innovation in teaching. She is committed to integrating research, education, and service development into clinical practice to drive improvements in patient care and outcomes.

Illustrator

Dr Talia Patel
BMBS (Hons), BMedSci (Hons), University of Nottingham, Royal Derby Hospital

Dr Talia Patel is also author of the Electrolytes chapter.

Chapter Reviewers

Dr Libin Mathew (Dermatology)
MBBS, MRCP (UK), St John's Institute of Dermatology

Dr Faisal Karim (Gynaecology and Obstetrics)
MBBS, BSc (Hons), MRCOG, The Royal Marsden Hospital

Dr Abhirami Gautham (Haematology)
MBChB, MRCP (UK), MSc (Oxon), PGCert (Distinction), Northwick Park Hospital

Dr Andres Almario (Paediatrics)
MD, MSc, Consultant in Paediatric Respiratory Medicine, Evelina London Children's Hospital

Dr Sachin Patel (Psychiatry)
MBChB, BMedSci, MRCPsych, Liaison Psychiatry, Imperial College Healthcare Trust

Other Reviewers

Dr Janvi Lalchandani
MBBS, Obstetrics and Gynaecology, Imperial College Healthcare Trust

Dr Aya Hammad
MBBS (Hons), University of York, Royal Devon and Exeter Hospital

Saoban Safavi
Plovdiv Medical University

Contents

Haematology

Obstetrics..177

Paediatrics..263

Psychiatry **385**

Disclaimer

The treatment recommendations outlined in this revised guide are primarily based around NICE guidelines which are used in the UK. This may result in differing diagnostics, medications, and disease management protocols among countries. For accuracy, we suggest verifying the details in this book with your local hospital's protocols and national guidelines. Our team of experienced specialists has thoroughly reviewed the clinical data in this book, and it reflects the latest information as of its publication date. However, we recognise the constantly evolving field of medicine and acknowledge that there may be revised guidelines since this guide was released.

Professionals and researchers are urged to use their expertise and knowledge when utilising any information, methods, compounds, or experiments mentioned in this text. In doing so, they should prioritise their safety as well as the safety of others for whom they have professional obligations. It is recommended that readers refer to the most up-to-date instructions provided by either (i) the featured procedures or (ii) the manufacturer of each drug or pharmaceutical product before administering it, to confirm the appropriate dosage or formula, method and duration of administration, and any contraindications. The responsibility falls on professionals to use their experience and understanding of patients to make diagnoses, determine dosages, and devise the best course of treatment for each patient while taking all necessary safety measures. To the fullest extent of the law, neither the Publisher nor the authors, contributors, or editors can be held liable for any harm or damage to persons or property due to actions taken or not taken based on information presented in this book.

Dermatology

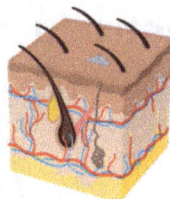

Introduction

The skin functions as a protective barrier, regulating body temperature and providing somatosensation. It consists of the epidermis, dermis and subcutaneous tissue.

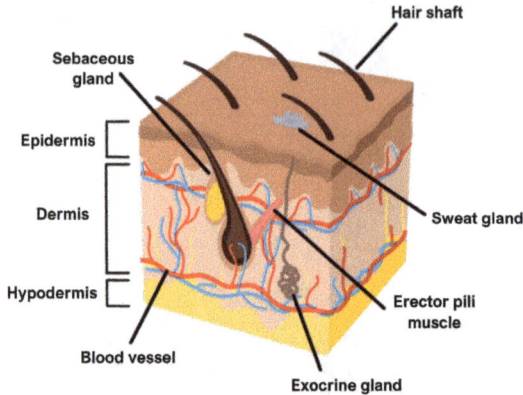

The epidermis is divided into 4 layers:

- Stratum corneum (Children can present with a variety horny layer) – this is composed of dead keratinocytes
- Stratum granulosum (granular layer) – keratinocytes produce granules
- Stratum spinosum (prickly layer) – this layer is characterised by desmosomes between keratinocytes
- Stratum basale (basal layer) – this is the proliferative layer which contains regenerative stem cells

To describe skin lesions accurately, it is important to refer to the 7 S's, which provide a detailed and complete dermatological description.

Site
- Location on the body
- Distribution relative to each other
- Symmetrical or unilateral

Shade
- Pigmented (hypo/hyper)
- Colour e.g. erythematous, black etc.

Style
- Macule/patch, papule/plaque etc.

Size (mm or cm)

Shape
- Horizontal or vertical (cross-section)
- Teardrop, annular, circular

Surface
- Smooth/rough, scaly/flaky
- Dry or moist

Sides
- Well defined or indistinct borders

There are specific terms used to describe various types of skin rashes and lesions.

Macules and patches

These refer to flat, impalpable areas of skin without elevation or depression.
- They have a change in surface colour, but do not have any textural difference from the surrounding skin.
- A macule is < 0.5 cm.
- A patch is > 0.5 cm.

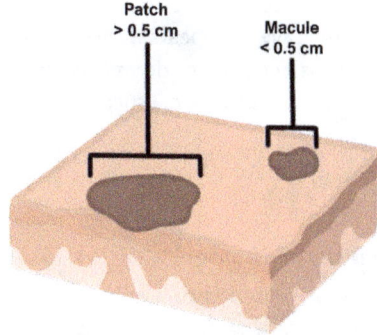

Patch
> 0.5 cm

Macule
< 0.5 cm

Papules and plaques

These are well circumscribed, solid elevations of skin.
- They do not have any fluid underneath.
- They are palpable and can be skin-coloured or pigmented.
- A papule is < 0.5 cm.
- A plaque is > 0.5 cm.

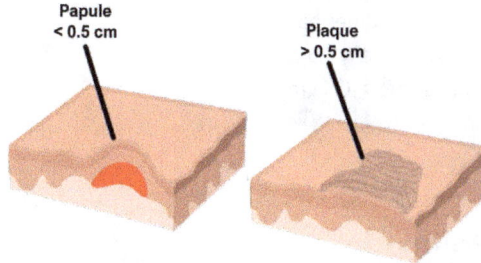

Papule
< 0.5 cm

Plaque
> 0.5 cm

Nodule

This is an elevated, circumscribed lesion, which is similar to a papule, but centred deeper in the dermis.
- Nodules are > 0.5 cm.

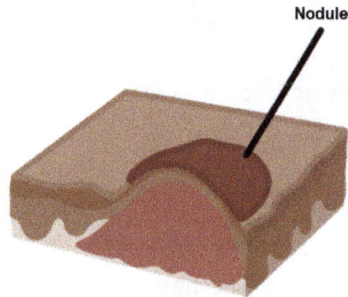

Nodule

Cyst

This is a hollow mass that is surrounded by an epithelium-lined wall.
- It is well demarcated from the adjacent tissue and can contain fluid.

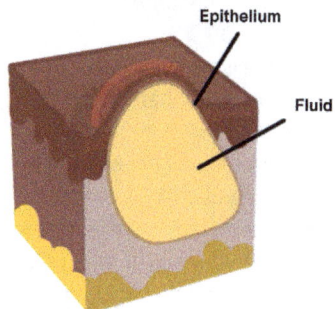

Epithelium

Fluid

Wheal

This is a raised red or skin coloured lesion that typically disappears within 24 hours.
- It is characterised by dermal oedema due to histamine release e.g. urticaria.

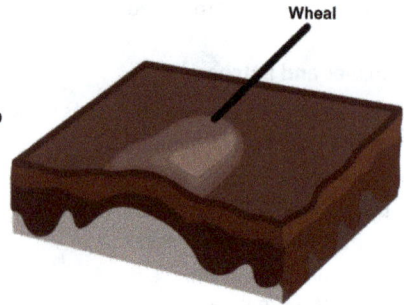

Vesicles and bullae

These are raised, circumscribed lesions which contain clear or serous fluid (sometimes haemorrhagic).
- Vesicles are < 0.5 cm.
- Bullae are > 0.5 cm.

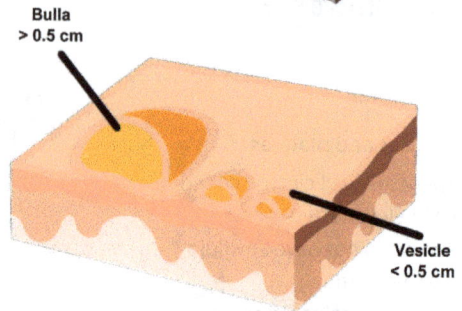

Pustules

These are raised, circumscribed lesions filled with purulent fluid.
- They can be sterile or infectious.
- They are < 0.5 cm.

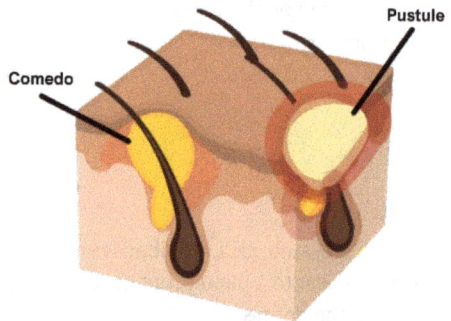

Fissures, erosions and ulcers

These lesions differ by the extent to which they penetrate the layers of the skin.
- A fissure is a crack which extends through the epidermis to the dermis.
- An erosion refers to partial or complete loss of the epidermis.
- Ulcers are deeper lesions, characterised by full thickness loss of the epidermis and at least part of the superficial dermis.

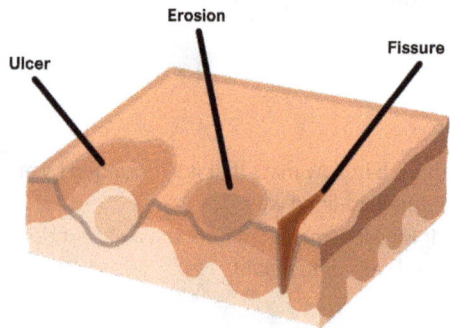

Eczema (Dermatitis)

Eczema or dermatitis (interchangeable terms) is an inflammatory skin condition which is typically characterised by a rash which is red, scaly and itchy.
- It is usually divided into exogenous and endogenous types.

- **Atopic eczema (atopic dermatitis)**

This is the most common type of eczema which affects about a fifth of children under 5 as well as about 10% of adults.
- It is an immunologically mediated inflammatory skin reaction, mediated by an increase in T_h2 cells, which leads to increased IgE levels, resulting in inflammation.

Causes

- Combination of genetic predisposition and environmental triggers
- It is associated with loss of function variants of the filaggrin gene, which is important for epidermal barrier function
- This leads to increased allergen and irritant penetration of the skin and microbial colonisation, which results in inflammation

Risk factors

- Atopy – associated with a family history of atopic conditions. Patients often get eczema first, then asthma and rhinitis ("the atopic march")
- Diet – eczema is exacerbated in some infants due to things such as eggs, cow's milk, nuts, soy, and wheat protein

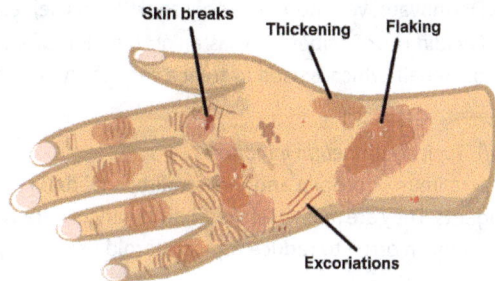

Skin breaks | Thickening | Flaking | Excoriations

Symptoms

- Erythematous (appears brown/hyperpigmented in skin of colour), scaly patches with lichenification (thickening) and excoriation marks (scratch marks)
- In babies, lesions are more concentrated around the face and the torso
- As children grow older, lesions are more likely to be found in the flexor surfaces, including the elbows, behind the knees, neck, wrists and ankles

Management

i) Emollients

This refers to moisturising treatment which softens the skin, soothes discomfort, rehydrates and restores barrier function

- These come in the form of gels, lotions, creams and ointments
- They vary in terms of greasiness, with greasier products containing more paraffin
- Examples of emollients include Hydromol and Diprobase
- Emollients should be applied at least twice a day to the affected areas
- They should be applied 15–30 minutes before or after topical steroid application
- You can also prescribe a soap substitute emollient to use in the shower or bath instead of standard shower gels/soaps as can dry skin further

ii) Topical steroids

1 fingertip unit (FTU) treats an area twice that of adult human hand. Steroids are usually prescribed in weaning regimes to stop rebound flare:

- Hydrocortisone (mild strength) – this is available over the counter in the UK
- Eumovate (moderate) – typically used on the face, useful for mild eczema on body
- Betnovate and Elocon (potent) – typically used on the body
- Dermovate (very potent) – only short-term use, reserved for severe eczema on body
- Fucidin H or Fucibet – this is a combination of a topical steroid with fucidin (an anti-bacterial), which is used to treat a secondary skin infection

iii) Topical calcineurin inhibitors

Tacrolimus (Protopic) and Pimecrolimus (Elidel) can be used as steroid sparing topical agents. They are most useful as maintenance therapy in patients with moderate to severe eczema in order to reduce topical steroid use

iv) Phototherapy

This is used in moderate to severe eczema

v) Systemic immunosuppressants

These include drugs like methotrexate and ciclosporin

vi) Biologic drugs

These include monoclonal antibodies like dupilumab and JAK-inhibitors e.g. barictinib, abrocitinib

- **Eczema herpeticum**

This is a potential complication of atopic dermatitis which occurs due to a superimposed viral infection, due to herpes simplex virus 1 or 2.
- It can be a dermatological emergency.

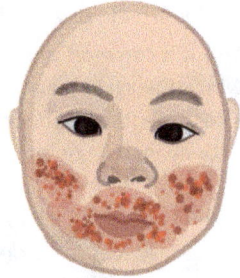

Symptoms

- Papulovesicles and punched out erosions
- This gives widespread crusted lesions which can be purulent
- It can be associated with systemic upset with fever and enlarged lymph nodes
- If untreated, especially in those at risk such as immunocompromised patients, it can progress to affect the eyes, brain and lungs

Key tests

- It is a clinical diagnosis
- Can take viral swabs for PCR sequencing but it is important not to delay treatment whilst waiting for the results

Management

- Mild/localised cases can be treated with oral acyclovir
- In severe/immunocompromised cases, admit to hospital for IV acyclovir
- If there is eye involvement, ophthalmology should be involved

- **Discoid eczema**

A type of eczema characterised by the presence of round erythematous patches.
- It is seen in all ages, but more common in adults, usually seen on the arms and legs.

Symptoms

- Round (coin shaped) or oval scaly erythematous patches/plaques
- Rash starts off as a group of red spots
- These merge together to form a round patch which is very itchy

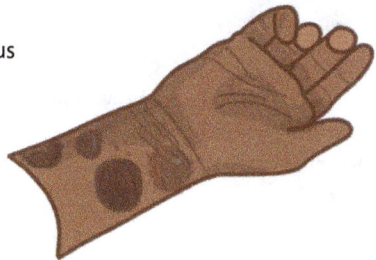

Management

- Similar to atopic eczema with topical emollients and steroids
- Escalation to phototherapy and immunosuppressants in refractory disease

- **Seborrheic eczema/dermatitis**

This is a common, chronic type of dermatitis that primarily affects parts of the body which are rich in sebum, such as the scalp and face. It affects both infants and adults.
- It is thought to be due to an abnormal response to the yeast Malassezia (usually a skin commensal organism), which can lead to inflammation of the skin.

○ **Infants**

It is usually seen in children younger than 3 months.
- Produces lesions with a yellowish-scale on the scalp (cradle-cap) and eyebrows.
- It can also affect skin folds such as the neck, axilla and groin giving a pink patchy rash which is not very itchy, so the baby is unlikely to be perturbed by the rash.

Management
- Emollient alone in mild cases
- If more severe, short course of combination steroid-antifungal creams

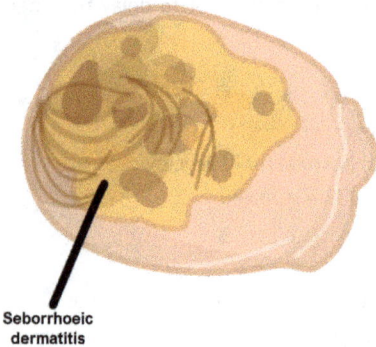

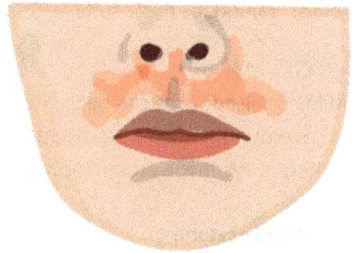

Seborrhoeic
dermatitis

○ **Adults**

This usually starts in the late teens but can be seen at any age.
- It affects the scalp, eyebrows and cutaneous folds such as the naso-labial fold and ear creases, but can also be seen centrally on the chest.
- It is characterised by pink thin scaly patches and plaques and usually follows a chronic, relapsing course.

Management
- For acute flares on face and torso, topical steroid-antifungal combination (e.g. daktacort) for short periods (up to two weeks)
- For the scalp, medicated anti-fungal shampoo can be used (ketoconazole)

- **Contact dermatitis**

This is inflammation of the skin which occurs due to direct contact with an agent.
- It is the most common occupational skin disorder, often seen in populations of cleaners, food workers and hairdressers who wear gloves or work with chemicals.
- It is divided into irritant or allergic subtypes.
- The irritant type is the most common and is due to a non-allergic reaction to various chemicals, often seen in the hands due to direct contact in a glove distribution.
- The allergic type is mediated by a type IV hypersensitivity reaction, often at the margins of the hairlines due to an allergy to chemicals in hair dyes.

Symptoms
- Erythema and itchiness, with drying/flaking of the skin
- In severe cases can cause vesicles and blisters
- Repeated exposure leads to lichenification (thickening) of the skin with fissures

Erythema

Lichenification

Key tests
- Patch testing can be used to identify the allergen

Management
- For allergic dermatitis, mainstay of management is avoidance of exposure to the allergen identified by patch testing. Avoid irritants if possible
- Hand protection with gloves, emollient and soap substitutes
- Topical steroids may also be used to calm down the inflammation

- **Dyshidrotic eczema (pompholyx)**

This condition is characterised by the presence of vesicles, which may form blisters on the fingers, palms and soles of the feet.
- There is no known cause, but it is associated with a history of atopy, allergic/irritant dermatitis and increased humidity (sweating).

Symptoms
- Starts with an intense burning itch followed by skin coloured or pink crops of vesicles which can blister
- These last up to 3 weeks before they dry and heal

Pompholyx

Management
- Potent topical corticosteroids are highly effective

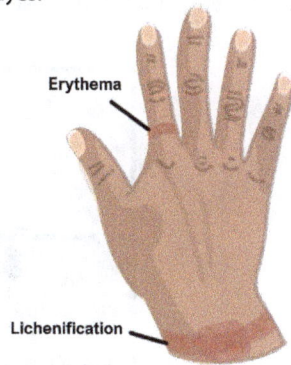

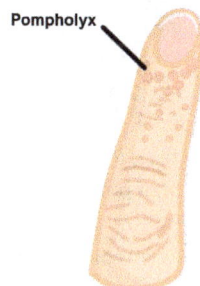

Inflammatory Skin Conditions

- **Acne vulgaris**

This refers to a chronic inflammatory condition of the pilosebaceous unit.

- It is thought to be related to increased sebum production due to androgens and abnormal follicular keratinisation.
- This causes excess keratin production which block follicles making comedones.
- In people with acne, there is a higher concentration of the anaerobic bacteria Cutibacterium which colonise the plugs and may induce inflammation.

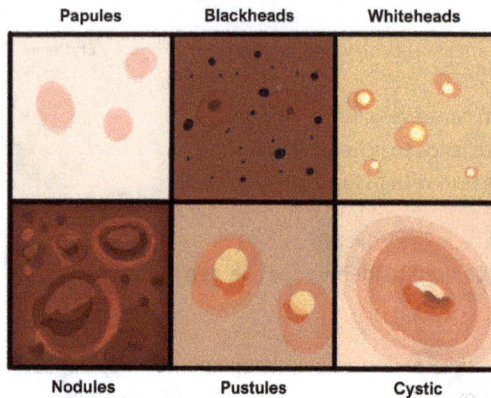

Papules	Blackheads	Whiteheads
Nodules	Pustules	Cystic

Symptoms

- Red spots with pustules on face, cheeks, neck and upper trunk
- Open comedones – blackheads
- Closed comedones – whiteheads

Management

- 1st line topical therapy is benzoyl peroxide (antimicrobial) and topical retinoids (anti-comedonal) either used alone or in combination
- If lack of response, use oral antibiotics – tetracyclines (unless pregnant or under 12) with or without a topical retinoid
- In women, can use combined oral contraceptive pill (avoid progesterone-only pill)

If no response at 3 months, refer to dermatology for consideration of **oral isotretinoin**

- This is a vitamin A derivative which is the most effective treatment but there is a long list of potential side effects, most commonly dry skin
- It requires monitoring of liver function and lipids
- It is important to monitor for depression and suicide risk
- It is also teratogenic, and patients should be on contraception if at risk of pregnancy

Acne variants

- Acne fulminans – this refers to a severe sudden onset of nodulocystic acne with ulceration and systemic symptoms (arthralgia and fever). It should be managed with prednisolone either alone initially or with low-dose isotretinoin.

- Acne conglobate – this refers to a severe sudden onset of nodulocystic acne without systemic symptoms.

● **Rosacea**

This is a chronic skin disorder of unclear cause in adults which characteristically affects the nose, cheeks and forehead.
- It usually occurs between the ages of 30–60.
- It is more common in fair skinned individuals.

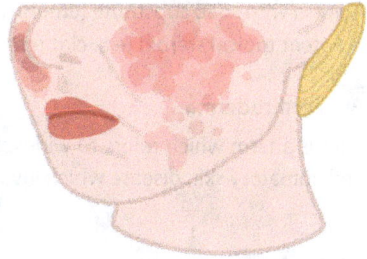

Symptoms
- Starts with flushing leading to persistent redness
- Papules/pustule formation and prominent blood vessels (telangiectasia)
- Can lead to rhinophyma – bulbous nose with skin thickening and prominent pores

Management
- Conservative measures – regular sunscreen, avoid factors which may cause flushing such as alcohol, spicy foods and hot drinks
- Topical metronidazole, ivermectin or azelaic acid
- Tetracycline antibiotics (doxycycline, lymecycline) can be used
- If still persistent, can trial low dose isotretinoin
- Laser therapy for persistent telangiectasia and facial erythema

● **Lichen sclerosus**

This is a chronic condition that usually affects the genital and anal areas.
- It is much more common in women and associated with increased risk of vulval SCC.
- In males it affects the penis, causing balanitis xerotica obliterans (BXO). This is thought to be related to post-micturition dribbling and occlusion under the foreskin.
- This is also associated with an increased risk of SCC.

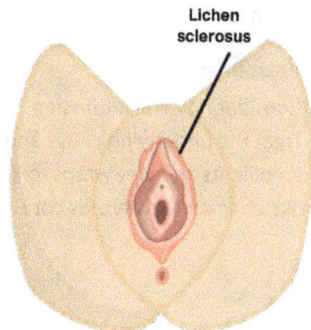

Lichen sclerosus

Symptoms

- White, itchy, atrophic patches around vulval and perianal skin "figure-of-eight"
- Gives rise to erosions, tearing and ulceration
- Urination can cause stinging, and patients often experience dyspareunia

Key tests

- Clinical diagnosis but biopsy if failure of response to treatment or suspicion of cancer

Management

- Wash with soap substitute (emulsifying ointment), use emollients to relieve dryness
- Potent topical steroid (e.g. clobetasol propionate 0.05% – dermovate)

- **Erythroderma**

This is a term which refers to widespread reddening of the skin with scaling due to an inflammatory skin disease which involves > 90% of the body surface area.

Causes

- Inflammatory skin disease (eczema, psoriasis)
- Cutaneous T-cell lymphoma
- Bullous skin disease
- Infections
- Idiopathic
- Genetic causes
- Drugs e.g. penicillins, sulphonamides, anticonvulsants

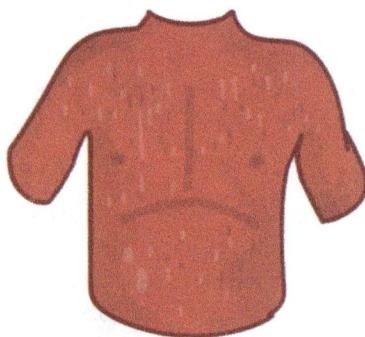

Symptoms

- Skin appears red, warm, oedematous, scaly with itchy/tightness sensation
- Patients are systemically unwell (and may have lymphadenopathy)
- It can lead to secondary infection, fluid loss and hypovolaemic shock

Management

- Consider hospital admission
- Treat the underlying cause and stop any potential drug culprits
- Emollients and wet-wraps to keep skin moist +/- topical steroids
- Systemic corticosteroids considered (usually avoided if secondary to psoriasis)

- **Psoriasis**

This is a disease which refers to a T-cell mediated disorder with abnormal keratinocyte proliferation. It is divided into a few subtypes.

- In patients with psoriasis, you may also get nail changes (pitting, onycholysis) as well as an overlap with psoriatic arthritis (seen in 5–30% of patients with psoriasis).
- It can be exacerbated by various factors: alcohol, drugs (NSAIDs, lithium, beta-blockers, ACEi) and trauma.

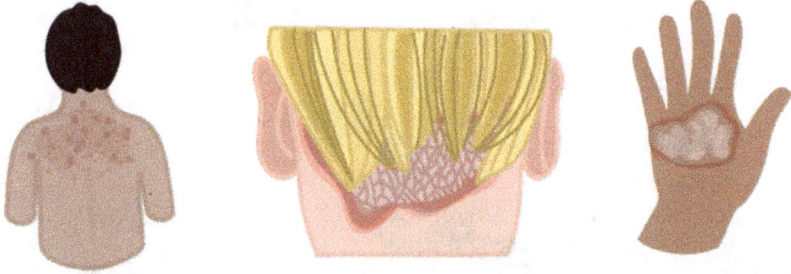

○ **Plaque**

This is the most common type charactered by well-defined red/salmon colour patches and plaques with a silvery scale.

- These are usually seen on the extensor surfaces and the head (can be generalised).

○ **Flexural**

This involves smooth well-defined plaques which are seen in body folds and genitals.

○ **Guttate**

This type is defined by teardrop red lesions on the trunk and extremities. It is often preceded by streptococcal infection and usually self-resolves after a few months.

○ **Generalised pustular**

This refers to sheets of pustules superimposed on inflamed skin.

Management

- 1st line topical therapy – topical corticosteroid in combination with topical vitamin D analogue (calcitriol/calcipotriol) for 4 weeks alternating with topical vitamin D analogue alone for 4 weeks
- If extensive or lack of control with topical therapy, phototherapy (narrowband UVB) or systemic immunosuppressive agents e.g. oral methotrexate or ciclosporin
- For refractory disease, drugs include biologics, apremilast (PDE IV inhibitor)

- **Urticaria and angioedema**

This refers to a type 1 hypersensitivity reaction mediated by histamine release.
- Histamine increases the permeability of small capillaries and venules resulting in fluid shift to the extracellular space and pruritus, causing localised swelling.
- Acute urticaria (< 6 weeks) is caused by infections, foods, drugs, bee stings etc.
- Chronic (> 6 weeks) is usually idiopathic (consider autoimmune vs autoallergic).

Symptoms

- Urticaria refers to swelling of the superficial dermis
- Itchy red wheals which appear all over the body
- The key history point is a rash lasts < 24 hours
- Angioedema refers to a deeper swelling of the dermis, more localised. It typically causes swelling of the face (tongue and lips), hands and feet

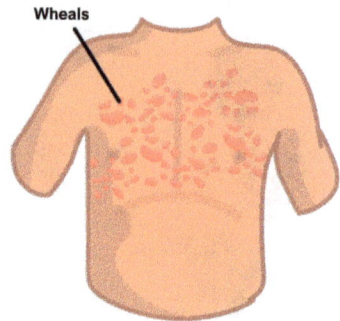

Wheals

Management

- Avoid the causative substance. Involve anaesthetics if there are airway concerns
- Antihistamines are first-line (take up to four times a day)
- If persistent can trial steroids or biological agents (e.g. omalizumab)

- **Hereditary angioedema**

This is an autosomal dominant condition which occurs due to a deficiency in complement 1 inhibitor (C1-INH), which regulates the kallikrein system, which is responsible for the synthesis of bradykinin, a vasodilator.
- This causes excessive bradykinin release which causes oedema and inflammation.

Symptoms

- Spontaneous attacks which begin in childhood and worsen in adolescence
- Angioedema is worse for the first day then subsides and affects limbs and abdomen
- Approx one third get an early red rash (erythema marginatum) before the attacks

Key tests

- Blood tests show low C4 and C1-INH, with normal C1 and C3 levels

Management

- If acute, give IV C1-inhibitor, kallikrein inhibitor or a BDKRRB2 antagonist
- For prophylaxis – purified plasma-derived human C1 esterase inhibitor concentrate

Skin Infections

Bacterial infections

- **Bacterial folliculitis**

This refers to infection and inflammation of one of more hair follicles, which can occur anywhere where there are hair follicles on the body.
- The most common pathogen is the bacterium Staphylococcus aureus.
- Pseudomonas aeruginosa is associated with hot-tub folliculitis, which gets its name from patients acquiring it from hot tubs that were not cleaned properly before use.

Symptoms
- Red follicular papules with pustules located around the hair follicles

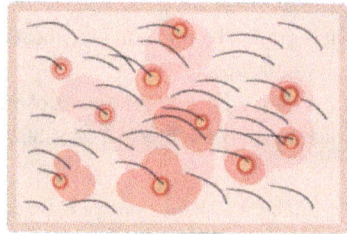

Management
- Topical antiseptic wash
- May require topical antibiotics (e.g. mupirocin or fusidic acid)

- **Impetigo**

This is a superficial bacterial infection due to S. aureus or S. pyogenes.
- It is most commonly seen in children, usually in warmer months, and affects the face.
- It is contagious, spread by direct contact, but can also spread indirectly through contaminated clothing and other items.

Symptoms
- Non-bullous vesicles on an erythematous base that easily rupture
- Exudate causes golden-brown crust
- Apart from the visual lesions, it is relatively asymptomatic (non-painful, non-itchy)

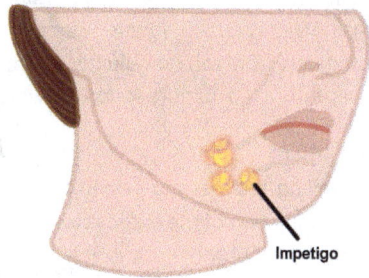

Impetigo

Management
- If localised, 1st line is hydrogen peroxide cream or fusidic acid cream
- If widespread, oral antibiotics (e.g. oral flucloxacillin) can be used
- Children should be excluded from school for 2 days after starting antibiotics

- **Cellulitis**

This is used to describe inflammation of the loose connective tissue under she skin, which usually co-exists with erysipelas.
- Common pathogens are Gram positive organisms such as S. pyogenes or S. aureus.

Symptoms

- Usually seen on lower limbs affecting one leg
- Gives acute onset red, tender swollen skin
- Skin is typically warm and may weep
- May have associated systemic upset e.g. fever

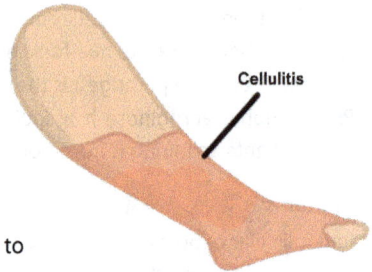

Cellulitis

Management

- It is graded by the Eron Classification according to systemic upset
- If < class 2 (systemically well), can be managed with oral antibiotics (flucloxacillin)
- If ≥ class 3, patient is < 1-year-old, or facial cellulitis, then IV antibiotics are preferred

Erysipelas is an acute infection, usually due to S. pyogenes which is very similar.
- This typically affects tissues more superficial to cellulitis and the rash is more raised and well demarcated.

- **Periorbital cellulitis**

This is an infection of the soft tissues in front of the orbital septum (eyelid, skin).
- It can be caused by breaks in the skin around the eye allowing bacterial entry.
- Patients usually have a history of sinusitis or URTI, most commonly secondary to Gram positive bacteria S. aureus, S. epidermidis and streptococci.
- It differs from orbital cellulitis, which is infection of the soft tissues behind the orbital septum, a much more serious infection which is treated with intravenous antibiotics.

Symptoms

- Swelling, redness and pain in one eye
- Inflammation of the eyelids can cause a partial or complete ptosis
- Systemic symptoms e.g. fever, malaise
- No loss of vision, proptosis (bulging of the eye), ophthalmoplegia (these are features of orbital cellulitis)

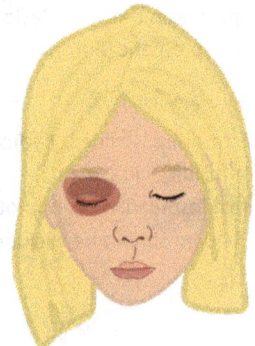

Key tests
- Blood tests show raised infection markers (CRP, WCC)
- If any suspicion of orbital cellulitis, diagnostic imaging is a contrast CT of the orbit

Management
- 1st line is antibiotics e.g. co-amoxiclav (if untreated, can lead to orbital cellulitis)

- **Necrotising fasciitis**

This refers to a bacterial infection of the subcutaneous tissue and fascia which covers muscles. The bacteria release toxins which cause thrombosis of blood vessels.
- This leads to necrosis of the tissue and fascia.
- If this is not treated promptly it can be fatal.

There are several types of necrotising fasciitis:
- Type 1 – this is the commonest type due to a mixture of aerobic and anaerobic bacteria. It is usually seen in elderly patients with comorbidities (diabetes)
- Type 2 – due to haemolytic group A Streptococcus e.g. S. pyogenes, MRSA
- Type 3 – due to Clostridium perfringens leading to gas gangrene

Symptoms
- These can develop within 24 hours of minor injury
- Gives a rapidly worsening cellulitis with signs of necrosis
- The pain is very severe and out of proportion to physical signs
- The lesion spreads almost like it is eating away the skin and can lead to septic shock

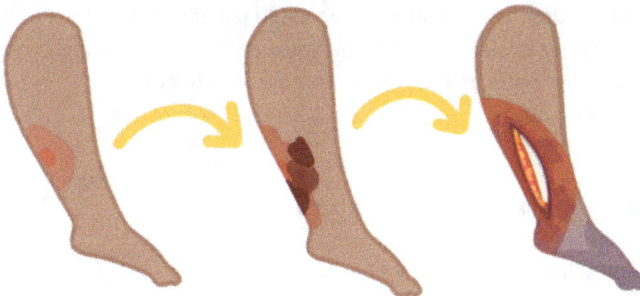

Management
- Sepsis 6 protocol, treat with IV fluids and IV antibiotics
- Surgical debridement is required to remove all necrotic tissue (usually repeated multiple times for a few days)

Viral infections

- **Viral warts (verruca)**

This is a viral infection of keratinocytes, due to the human papilloma virus (HPV).
- HPV causes excess keratin (a hard protein) to develop in the epidermis.
- The extra keratin produces the rough, hard texture of a wart.
- The warts are usually found on the hands and feet and notoriously have a high risk of recurrence.

Symptoms
- Can be solitary or multiple skin-coloured lesions, which have a rough surface
- Variations include warts with finger like projections

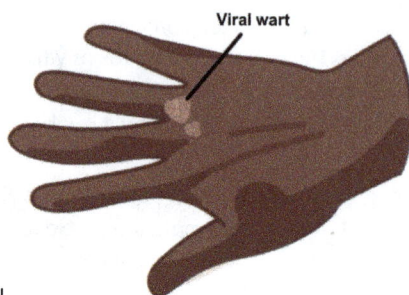

Viral wart

Management
- Many resolve spontaneously
- Treatment is required if painful, functional disablement or cosmetic deformity
- 1st line is salicylic acid with paring and occlusion
- Alternative treatments include cryotherapy at 1–3 weekly intervals, electrosurgery, curettage & cautery and pulsed dye laser

- **Molluscum contagiosum**

This is an infection which is due to the poxvirus Molluscipoxvirus.
- It is most commonly seen in children aged younger than 10.
- It can become widespread in immunosuppressed patients (e.g. HIV infection).
- Transmission occurs by skin-to-skin contact, sexual contact as well as via contaminated surfaces. It can also occur as a secondary complication to eczema.
- Lesions usually do not arise on the palms of hands or sole of feet.

Symptoms
- Clusters of round pink-white papules around 1–6 mm diameter
- These have a shiny, waxy appearance with a central pit (umbilication)
- Predilection for skin folds, lateral trunk, thighs and genitals

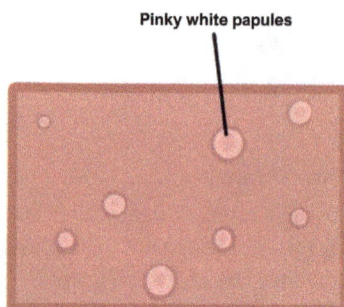

Pinky white papules

Management

- It is a self-limiting condition that usually resolves within 2 years
- Topical agents such as potassium hydroxide, imiquimod, podophyllotoxin can trigger irritation and as such worsen inflammation
- Physical treatments include cryotherapy (can leave white scars) or curettage
- Treat background eczema with topical steroid and emollients to reduce the risk of dissemination with scratching

Fungal infections

• Pityriasis versicolor

This is a skin condition which is caused by the yeast Malassezia furfur, resulting in discoloured patches typically found on the torso and the back.
- Hypopigmentation occurs due to a chemical that impairs melanocyte functioning.
- It most often affects young adults and is seen more commonly in hot humid climates.

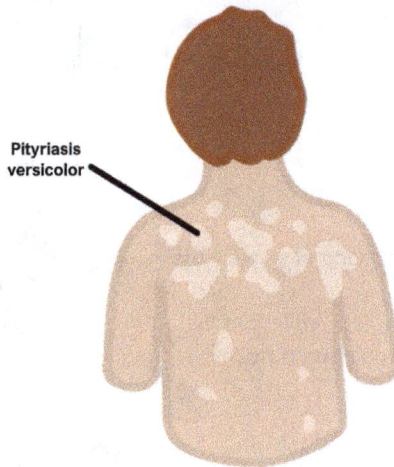

Pityriasis versicolor

Symptoms

- Hypopigmented, pink or brown patches most commonly on the trunk
- It is usually asymptomatic
- The patches can start scaly, but the scale becomes more subtle over time
- Scaling can be made prominent by firm scraping

Management

- Topical antifungal shampoo (ketoconazole) is first line, but has a recurrence risk
- Oral therapy rarely used but consider itraconazole in extensive or recalcitrant cases

- **Dermatophytosis**

This describes a superficial fungal infection which usually affects the hair, skin or nails.
- Colloquially, it is known as tinea or ringworm.
- The usual causative agent is the fungus Trichophyton rubrum or Trichophyton tonsurans, but other pathogens include Candida and Microsporum.

Key tests
- Clinical diagnosis
- If diagnostic doubt, you can take fungal scrapings from the patient

○ **Tinea capitis**

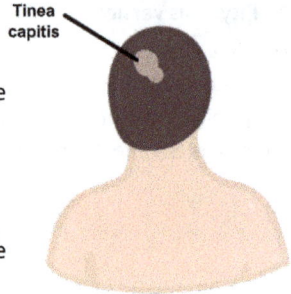
Tinea capitis

This is an infection of the scalp usually seen in children.
- It causes dry scaling (like dandruff) and black dots (where the hairs break off the scalp).
- It can give an inflamed spongey mass called a kerion.

Management
- Oral antifungals e.g. terbinafine is usually given first line in the UK
- Other antifungals include griseofulvin or itraconazole

○ **Tinea corporis**

This is a fungal infection found in parts of the body.
- It gives well-defined annular red lesions with sharp raised edges and can have pustules.

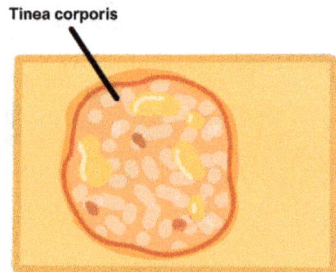
Tinea corporis

Management
- Topical antifungal agents are first line
- If unsuccessful, oral terbinafine or itraconazole

○ **Tinea pedis**

This is colloquially known as athlete's foot.
- It is very common and seen more in younger people.
- It results in itchy skin with peeling between toes.

Management
- Topical terbinafine

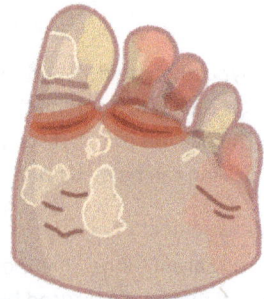
Athlete's foot

Parasitic infections

- **Scabies**

This is a condition caused by the mite Sarcoptes scabiei.

- Transmission occurs by direct contact and occasionally via objects such as clothing.
- The mite colonises the skin and lays eggs within the epidermis.
- This then leads to a type 4 hypersensitivity reaction to the eggs which can occur up to a month after the initial exposure.

Symptoms

- Pruritus, which is particularly worse at night
- Burrows – wavy, thread-like brown lines that can have a small papule (a black triangle at the end of the burrow which can be appreciated by dermoscopy)
- Typical locations are the finger web spaces, wrists, axillae and penis

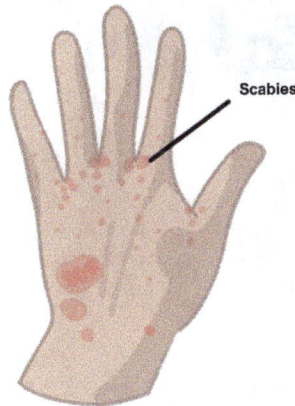

Scabies

Management

- Treat whole household contacts even if they are asymptomatic
- 1st line is repeated applications of permethrin cream 5%, alternative is malathion
- 2nd line is oral ivermectin
- Launder clothes and bedsheets at high temperature
- A post scabietic itch may persist for several weeks after treatment

- **Crusted scabies**

This is a more severe form of scabies, more commonly seen in immunosuppressed patients (e.g. HIV), where the lack of immune response allows the mite to multiply to great numbers leading to crusting of the skin.

Management: Combination therapy with topical permethrin and oral ivermectin

- **Head lice (Pediculosis capitis)**

This is a common condition caused by the parasite Pediculus humanus capitis which colonises the human scalp.
- Transmission occurs via direct head-to-head contact or sharing hats.
- It can spread quickly in children who play together.

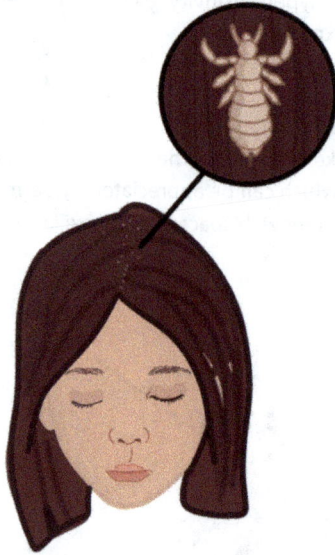

Symptoms

- Many individuals are asymptomatic
- Pruritus and scaling of head and neck
- Small brown or white eggs (nits) in your hair

Key tests

- Detection combing of wet or dry hair (wet hair is more accurate)

Management

- Children do not need to be excluded from attending school
- Wet combing with a louse detection comb to remove lice is recommended as first line in pregnant and breastfeeding women and children aged < 2 years old
- Physical insecticides (dimeticone, isopropyl myristate and cyclomethicone) can be used, which physically coat the lice and suffocate them
- Chemical insecticides include malathion
- All affected family members should be treated on the same day

Autoimmune Conditions

- **Bullous pemphigoid**

This is an autoimmune skin condition which causes subepidermal blisters.
- It occurs due to autoantibodies binding to components of hemi-desmosomes between the epidermis and dermis.
- IgG antibodies are directed against intracellular plaque proteins BP 180 and BP 230.
- It is more common in elderly patients > 70 years.
- It can be drug induced e.g. furosemide, DPP4 inhibitors.

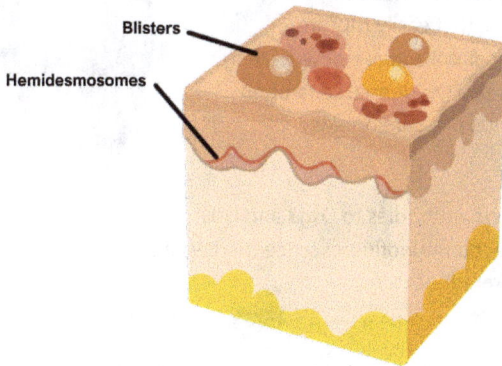

Symptoms

- Can start with pruritus with no obvious skin lesions (non-bullous phase)
- Tense blisters with an erythematous base which heal without scarring
- Blisters contain clear or cloudy yellowish fluid
- Urticated plaques
- Predilection for trunk and limbs (flexures), rarely affects the mouth and genital areas
- Nikolsky sign negative (epidermis does not separate following pressure on skin)

Key tests

- Skin biopsy of blister – shows subepidermal bulla with infiltrate of eosinophils
- Direct immunofluorescence (biopsy from skin next to blister i.e. perilesional) staining shows IgG and/or C3 antibodies along the basement membrane zone
- Blood tests – positive for antibodies against BP 180 and BP 230 and eosinophilia

Management

- Initial management involves very potent topical corticosteroids
- If severe may require oral corticosteroids (weaning course) with doxycycline
- Immunosuppressive agents e.g. azathioprine can be used as steroid sparing agents

- **Pemphigus vulgaris**

This is an autoimmune condition, which leads to the formation of superficial blisters.
- It affects all ethnic groups but is more common in Ashkenazi Jews, Iranian and Indian populations with a peak in incidence between the ages of 30–60.
- It is due to IgG autoantibodies against desmoglein 3, an epithelial cell adhesion molecule found near the bottom of the epidermis.

Symptoms

- Starts with oral ulceration (very common, other mucosal sites often affected)
- Later thin walled, flaccid blisters filled on an erythematous base that easily rupture
- Blisters are often painful and are slow-healing
- Nikolsky sign positive (epidermal separation following horizontal pressure on skin)

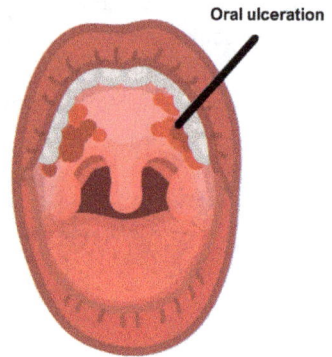

Oral ulceration

Key tests

- Blood tests – shows antibodies to Dsg3 and Dsg1
- Skin biopsy – direct immunofluorescence (perilesional) staining shows IgG antibodies and often C3 on keratinocytes

Management

- Initial management involves very potent topical corticosteroids
- If severe, systemic corticosteroids (weaning course) alongside immunosuppressive agents e.g. azathioprine/mycophenolate as steroid sparing agent

- **Alopecia areata**

This is a condition which leads to patches of hair loss on the scalp (most commonly), but can also affect the beard, eyebrows and eyelashes.
- It is thought to be an autoimmune mediated reaction which occurs due to a breach in the immune privilege of the hair follicles.

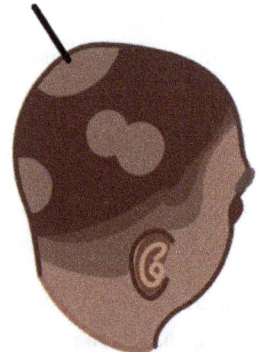

Well demarcated patch

Symptoms

- Circular patches of hair loss. This can progress to total loss of scalp hair (alopecia totalis) or loss of all hair on body (alopecia universalis)

Management

- If very mild disease with signs of re-growth, can consider watchful waiting
- If extensive or no signs of re-growth in mild disease, use potent or very potent topical steroids or intralesional steroid injections
- Occasionally systemic immunosuppression is given
- JAK inhibitors are due to become available in the UK for severe alopecia areata
- In 50–80% with mild disease, complete regrowth will occur within a year

- **Lichen planus**

This is an extremely pruritic rash, thought to be autoimmune in origin.
- It classically gives itchy planar, polygonal, purple papules which are most commonly found on the wrists, ankles and the lumbar region, but can be widespread.

Symptoms

- The 6 P's – pruritic, purple, polygonal, planar, papules and plaques
- Characteristic feature is white reticular lines on surface (Wickham striae)
- Approximately half of patients have mouth involvement, especially on the buccal mucosa with a white lacework pattern
- Lesions can affect the genitalia
- Koebner phenomenon, where new lesions appear at the site of minor injury

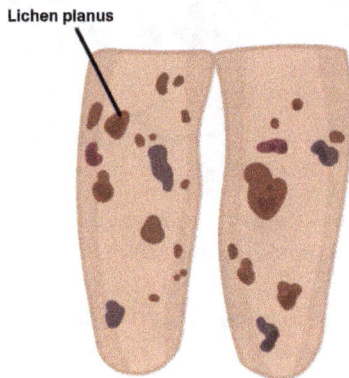

Lichen planus

Management

- Most cases resolve within 2 years without treatment
- The aim of treatment is to reduce pruritus and the time to resolution
- First-line treatment is very potent topical corticosteroids
- Oral corticosteroids are needed in widespread disease which can then be replaced by steroid sparing agents
- Oral disease may require oral steroid mouthwash to alleviate symptoms

Traumatic Conditions

- **Burns injury**

In a burn, there is local response with progressive tissue loss and release of inflammatory cytokines. Loss of capillary membrane integrity leads to fluid leaking into the interstitial space, leading to hypovolaemic shock.

- There is increased risk of bacterial infections (e.g. S. aureus), acute peptic stress ulcers, organ dysfunction, lung injury and sepsis.
- When treating a burn, it is essential to measure the extent and depth of the burn.

Extent

- This can be measured by Wallace's Rule of Nines
- Divide the body into units of surface area divisible by 9 (each is about 11% worth)
- Use this to estimate the total body surface area (TBSA) involved

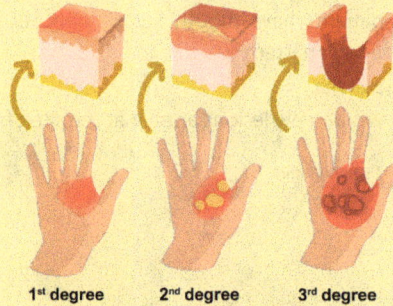

1st degree   2nd degree   3rd degree

Depth

- This measures the depth that the burn penetrates through the skin
- 1st degree – confined to the epidermis and likely to be red and tender. It usually does not require hospital assessment
- 2nd degree – this is where the burn penetrates the dermis either superficially or deep, which causes blisters and weeping
- 3rd degree – this is where the burn penetrates the full thickness of the skin. It causes loss of sensation to light touch and pin prick and will appear brown/black (leathery)

Management

- Burns injuries in the UK are typically by plastic surgery teams at specialist burns centres alongside an MDT
- Primary survey (airway, breathing and circulation) followed by secondary survey assessing for other injuries, and estimating total body surface affected

Immediate fluid resuscitation using crystalloid if total body surface area > 15% using the Parkland formula
- Total fluid in 24 hours = 4 ml × total burn surface area (%) × body weight (kg)
- 50% is given in first 8 hours, and the remaining 50% is given in the next 16 hours
- Give fluids till urine output 0.5–1 ml/kg/hr and then titrate to maintain urine output
- Further management involves topical antimicrobial creams and dressings
- Surgery – surgical debridement with autografting or temporary use of skin substitute

• **Pressure sores**

This refers to wounds that develop over bony prominences when continuous pressure or friction damages the skin.
- Constant pressure reduces blood flow causing cells to die and skin breakdown.

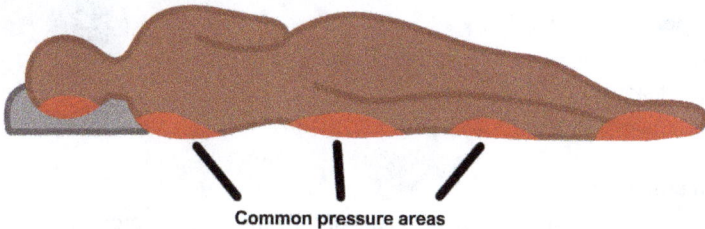

Common pressure areas

Risk factors
- Immobility (bed-ridden or after surgery)
- Malnourished, incontinent
- Reduced vascular perfusion e.g. diabetes, hypertension and smoking
- The Waterlow score is used to screen for patients at risk of pressure sores

Symptoms
- Varies from blanchable erythema to full thickness tissue loss typically over bony prominences (sacrum, hips, heels, elbows)

Management
- Pressure sores are managed by tissue viability teams but dermatology may be asked to review if there is diagnostic doubt whether there is any other cause of ulceration
- Pressure relief – increase patient mobility and regular turning of immobile patients
- Wound care – regular cleansing, debridement of slough, wound dressing with the choice of dressing based on the extent of the ulcer and degree of exudate present
- If evidence of secondary infection, treat with antibiotics

Benign and Malignant Lesions

Benign lesions

- **Seborrhoeic keratosis**

This is an extremely common benign epidermal proliferation of basaloid and squamous cells, which is more common in the elderly population.

- An eruptive onset of many lesions is known as the Leser-Trélat sign and is associated with GI carcinoma.

Symptoms

- Raised brown/black plaques, usually on trunk/face
- "Stuck on" warty appearance that can be variable

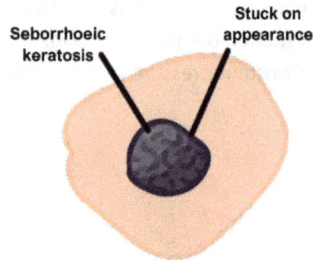

Management

- Completely benign with no malignant potential, so can be left alone
- They are removed if there is diagnostic uncertainty

- **Dermatofibroma**

This is an overgrowth of fibrous tissue in the dermis, made up of fibroblasts.

- It is thought to be a reactive process, which occurs secondary to minor trauma such as an insect bite. It is completely benign and does not become malignant.

Symptoms

- Firm nodule found usually on the legs and arms
- "Pea-like" texture on palpation
- Dimple sign – overlying skin dimples on pinching the lesion
- Usually < 1 cm and do not usually cause symptoms (but can be painful/itchy)

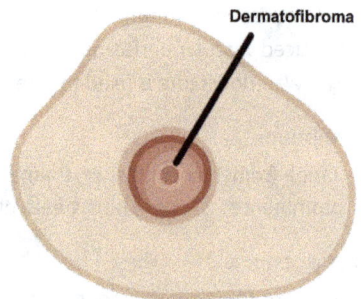

- **Sebaceous cyst**

This is a benign, non-cancerous lump under the skin filled with keratin and sebum.

- True cysts are composed of a complete epithelial lining whereas false cysts are without such a lining. The two most common true cysts are epidermoid and pilar cysts.
- An epidermoid cyst is where the lining looks like the epidermis.
- Pilar cysts originate from the outer sheath of hair follicles.

Symptoms
- Mobile masses usually seen on scalp, face, neck and trunk
- The centre of the lump can have a punctum
- Smooth and mobile lumps containing fluid or keratin (cheesy looking) which gives an offensive smell
- Rupture due to trauma or infection can cause redness, swelling and tenderness

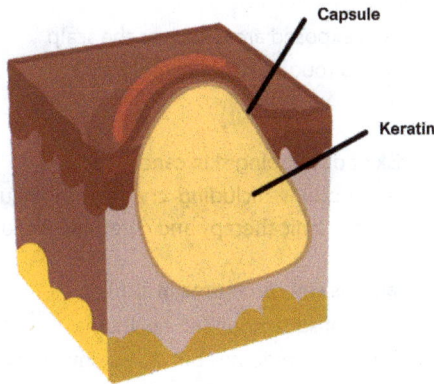

Capsule

Keratin

Management
- Oral antibiotics if infected
- Occasionally incision and drainage is required followed by surgical removal of the whole sac (or else they will recur)

● **Lipoma**

This is a benign proliferation of adipocytes, typically occurring in adults.
- They are asymptomatic unless they cause pressure on other structures.

Symptoms
- Smooth, mobile, non-tender lump, with a doughy consistency
- Can occur anywhere, but usually found on the arms, back of neck, torso and the thighs

Management
- Most require no treatment
- Surgical excision if symptomatic
- If they start to change size, become painful or are situated deeper in tissue, they are removed in order to rule out liposarcoma

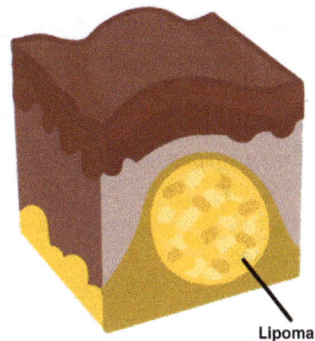

Lipoma

Pre-malignant lesions

- **Actinic keratosis**

This is a precancerous lesion which is due to abnormal skin proliferation, usually found on areas of sun-exposed skin.
- It has a low risk of transformation over a long period of time.

Actinic keratosis

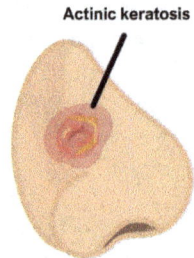

Symptoms

- Pink/red scaly lesion on sun exposed areas such as the scalp
- White/yellow scales causing a rough texture on palpation

Management

- It is treated due to the risk of developing skin cancer
- Wide variety of treatment options including cryotherapy (liquid nitrogen), topical 5-fluorouracil cream, photodynamic therapy and curettage & cautery

- **Bowen's disease (squamous cell carcinoma in situ)**

This is an early superficial type of squamous cell carcinoma.
- Squamous cells proliferate in the epidermis but do not invade into the dermis.
- It is often found in sun-exposed areas of skin such as the legs and hands.
- Risk factors include UV radiation, arsenic, HPV infection and immunosuppression.

Symptoms

- Irregular orange-red scaly plaques up to several centimetres

Management

- Treatment is similar to actinic keratosis. If superficial, cryotherapy (liquid nitrogen), topical 5-fluorouracil cream, photodynamic therapy
- Thicker lesions require curettage and cautery or excision

- **Keratoacanthoma**

This is a benign tumour typically occurring on sun-exposed skin.

Symptoms

- Dome-shaped nodule with a keratin filled crater centrally
- It grows rapidly initially, but usually regresses by itself

Keratoacanthoma

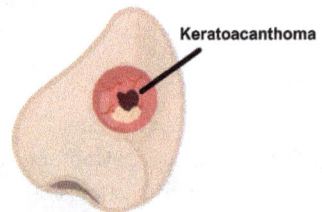

Management

- Surgical excision as it is difficult to clinically distinguish from a SCC

Malignant lesions

- **Squamous cell carcinoma (SCC)**

This is a malignant tumour of epidermal keratinocytes that invades the dermis.
- It grows slowly over weeks to months and has a low risk of metastasis.

Risk factors

- UV radiation
- Immunosuppression e.g. post-transplant, AIDS
- Marjolin ulcer is an SCC which develops within a scar or ulcer

Symptoms

- Erythematous, tender keratotic nodule which may ulcerate
- Favours sun exposed sites such as the face, lips, ears and limbs

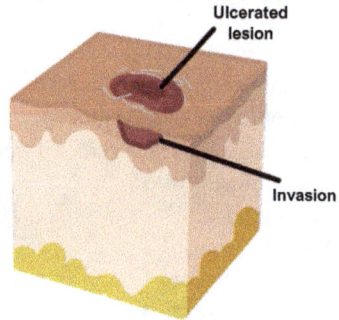

Management

- Surgical excision (Mohs micrographic surgery is used in high-risk sites)

- **Basal cell carcinoma (BCC)**

This is an abnormal proliferation of basal cells, a type of keratinocyte found at the bottom of the epidermis.
- It is the most common cutaneous malignancy, usually seen in the elderly.
- Metastasis is extremely rare as it usually grows slowly and invades locally.

Risk factors

- Sun damage, genetic syndromes such as xeroderma pigmentosum

Symptoms

- Skin coloured/pink (pearly) papule or nodule with rolled edges and telangiectasia
- Variants include superficial BCCs which look like pink patches or morphoeic which are scar-like
- It can bleed with recurrent scab formation

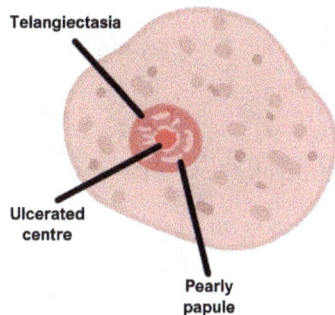

Management

- Surgical excision (Mohs micrographic surgery for high-risk lesions)

- **Malignant melanoma**

This refers to a malignant neoplasm of melanocytes.
- It can grow in 2 phases, with radial growth along epidermis and the superficial dermis and vertical growth into the deep dermis.
- The are associated with a BRAF mutation which leads to uncontrolled cell division.
- It usually metastasises to lymph nodes, lung, other parts of skin, bone and the brain.

Symptoms
- It can arise on otherwise normal looking skin or from a pre-existing mole
- ABCDE features raise clinical suspicion of melanoma:

Asymmetry
Borders irregular
Colour not uniform
Diameter > 6 mm
Evolution (change)

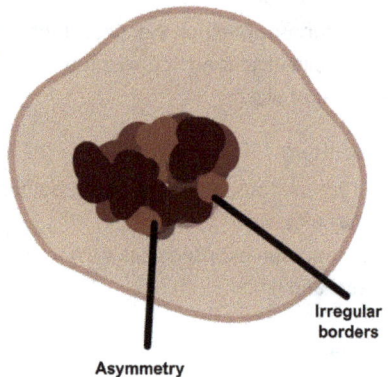

Irregular borders

Asymmetry

Types
- There are 4 main types of melanomas
- Superficial spreading – the most common subtype
- Nodular – second most common, typically presents as a large bleeding nodule
- Lentigo maligna – this is the precursor to lentigo maligna melanoma, which initially resembles a freckle which then becomes more atypical
- Acral lentiginous – a subtype seen in the palms of the hands, soles of the feet, or under the nails. This subtype is the most common in darker skinned populations

Key tests
- Excision biopsy of the whole lesion ideally to confirm diagnosis

Management
- Wide local excision (surgery) and sentinel lymph node biopsy (to stage melanoma)
- Immunotherapy and targeted therapies have significantly improved the prognosis in advanced melanoma stages
- The Breslow thickness (invasion depth of tumour) aides prognosis. If < 1 mm, almost all patients survive 5-years or more, whereas if metastatic, < 50% survive > 5 years

Disorders of Melanocytes

These conditions are marked by an intrinsic problem with melanocytes, the pigment producing cells in the skin.

- **Vitiligo**

This is an acquired condition which leads to the destruction of melanocytes causing depigmentation of the skin (leukoderma), with onset usually before the age of 30.
- The exact cause is unknown, but it is thought to be autoimmune in origin.
- In people with darker skin, areas of vitiligo are much more apparent and can have a significant psychological impact.
- It is associated with other autoimmune conditions such as type 1 diabetes, Addison's disease, thyroid disease and connective tissue disorders (SLE, rheumatoid arthritis).

Symptoms

- Distinct patches of depigmentation which commonly affects the face, neck, eyelids, fingertips and lips
- Koebner phenomenon occurs, the development of lesions at sites of injury
- Can affect hair follicles such as eyelashes and body hair too

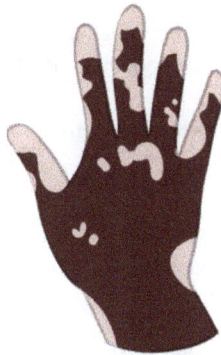

Management

- At present treatment is unsatisfactory with high rates of recurrence
- Conservative measures include cosmetic camouflage
- Medical management includes topical steroids and calcineurin inhibitors
- Phototherapy, particularly narrowband ultraviolet B (NB-UVB), can lead to at least a mild response in a majority of vitiligo patients
- Another option involves depigmentation of normal skin to attain more uniform skin pigmentation in patients with widespread vitiligo

- **Melasma**

This is an acquired hyperpigmentation disorder that primarily affects the face (cheeks, upper lip and forehead) but can occur on chest and forearms.
- Whilst the exact cause is unknown, it is associated with pregnancy and thought to be due to melanocyte dysfunction leading to more melanin production.
- Risk factors include the oral contraceptive pill and hormone replacement therapy.

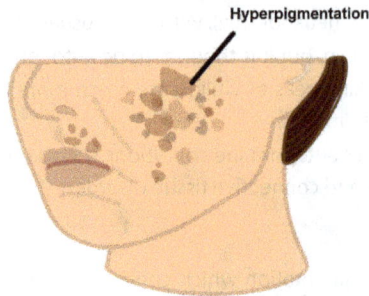

Hyperpigmentation

Symptoms

- Brown to grey-brown patches with irregular borders

Management

- Photoprotection very important
- Topical hydroquinone (depigmenting agent) either as monotherapy or in combination with retinoid and steroid
- Other treatments include topical azelaic acid, tranexamic acid and laser therapy

- **Albinism**

This is a condition which caused a congenital lack of pigmentation in the skin.
- It is due to an autosomal recessive mutation which causes a defect in the tyrosinase enzyme which impairs melanin production.
- The two main categories are oculocutaneous (eyes and skin) or ocular albinism.
- It is associated with an increased risk of developing skin cancer.

Symptoms

- White eyes/skin with high risk of sunburn/cancer

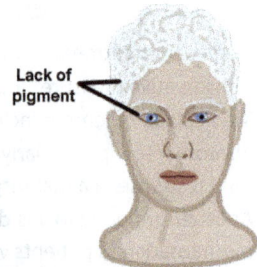

Lack of pigment

Management

- There is no cure, so conversative measures such as photoprotection is advised

Genetic Disorders

- **Neurofibromatosis (NF)**

This refers to a group of distinct genetic conditions in which benign tumours grow in the nervous system. They also often involve the skin or surrounding bone.

○ **Type 1 (NF1) – von Recklinghausen disease**

This is a complex multi-system disorder, caused by an autosomal dominant mutation in the NF-1 gene on chromosome 17.
- This mutation causes the loss of the protein neurofibromin in many cells.
- This disease has specific skin manifestations as well as other organ involvement.

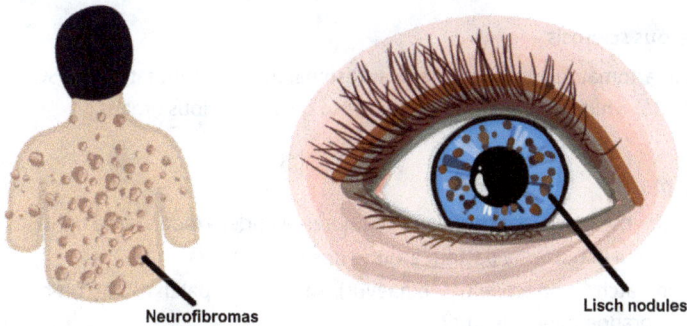

Neurofibromas

Lisch nodules

Skin symptoms
- ≥ 6 café au lait marks – these are uniformly pigmented brown macules > 5 mm in prepubertal and > 1.5 cm diameter in post-pubertal patients. They occur due to an increased collection of pigment producing melanocytes in the epidermis of the skin
- Freckles found in the axilla and groin region
- Two or more neurofibromas (skin coloured or pink nodules) or one plexiform neuro-fibroma (deeper nodules that can resemble a bag of worms)

Other symptoms
- Skeletal – scoliosis of the spine, senoid wing dysplasia
- Eye – Lisch nodules (dome shaped papules on iris surface), optic nerve glioma (slow growing tumour in or around the optic nerve)
- Endocrine – pheochromocytoma (adrenaline secreting tumour of chromaffin cells)
- Learning difficulties
- Cardiovascular – hypertension, due to renal artery stenosis
- Tumours – neurofibromas

Management: No cure, so an MDT approach is required to manage the symptoms

- **Neurofibromatosis type 2 (NF2)**

This is an autosomal dominant condition which is due to a genetic mutation on Chromosome 22. Unlike type 1, it does not usually present with skin manifestations.

Symptoms

- Bilateral acoustic neuromas – sensorineural hearing loss, tinnitus and vertigo
- Tumours are benign but can cause problems due to compression and raised ICP
- Associated with intracranial tumours such as schwannomas and meningiomas

Management

- Screening in affected families (hearing tests, MRI) after puberty
- Neurosurgery for acoustic neuromas

- **Tuberous sclerosis**

A rare hamartomatous disorder due to autosomal dominant mutation in TSC1 (Chr 9) or TSC2 (Chr 16) which causes benign tumours to grow in various organs.

Skin symptoms

- Hypopigmented "ash-leaf spots" which fluoresce under Wood's lamp light
- Angiofibroma in butterfly pattern around nose and cheeks
- Shagreen patch (connective tissue naevus), an elevated patch of skin on back, said to resemble orange peel or leather
- Ungual fibromas (firm flesh covered papules around or under nails)

Other symptoms

- Cardiac rhabdomyomas (benign tumours of muscle)
- Lung – benign tumours and lung cysts
- Kidneys – polycystic kidney disease and benign tumours
- Eye – hamartoma formation on the retina rarely causing visual distrubances
- CNS – epilepsy due to cortical tubers in the brain
- Associated with learning difficulties

Ash-leaf spot

Management

- No cure, so an MDT approach is required to manage the symptoms and complications

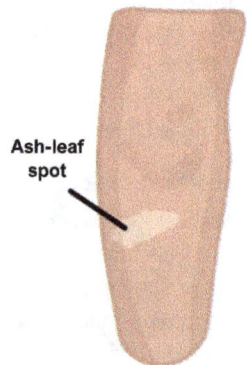

Systemic Skin Manifestations

There are skin many lesions which are associated with systemic conditions.

Diabetes

- **Diabetic dermopathy**

This is a type of skin lesion usually seen in people with diabetes mellitus, known as "shin spots".

- It is characterised by dull-red papules that progress to well-circumscribed, small, round, atrophic hyperpigmented skin lesions usually on the shins.
- It is thought to occur due to changes in the microvasculature and minor leakage of blood following minor trauma.
- It occurs in up to a third of diabetic patients.

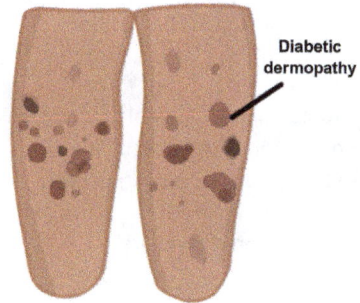

Diabetic dermopathy

- **Diabetic ulcers**

A painless neuropathic ulcer which occurs due to peripheral (diabetic) neuropathy.

- Patients lose sensation which causes overpressure on pressure points on the feet.
- This leads to microtrauma and tissue breakdown.
- Poor wound healing means that the tissue is not repaired causing ulcer formation.

Symptoms

- Ranges from superficial ulcer to deep tissue involvement, usually on the pressure points of the feet
- Associated with trophic changes (shiny skin, hair loss)
- Ulcers are painless due to reduced peripheral sensation
- If left untreated, they can become infected with complications including osteomyelitis, gangrene and amputation

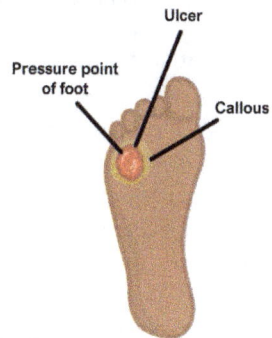

Ulcer

Pressure point of foot

Callous

Management

- Diabetic foot clinic with wound management and specialised cushioned footwear
- Optimise blood sugar control
- If signs of infection/osteomyelitis, treat with antibiotics (with involvement of surgical team to discuss debridement/amputation)

- **Necrobiosis lipoidica**

This is characterised by red/brown waxy plaques with an atrophic yellow centre that are slow growing and can ulcerate, typically occurring on the shins.
- It is seen in approximately 1% of patients with diabetes mellitus.
- Histology shows collagen degeneration with surrounding granulomatous inflammation.

Management
- Topical or intralesional corticosteroids (however these generally give disappointing results)
- PUVA (psoralen and ultraviolet A) light therapy

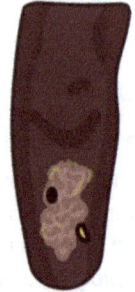

- **Granuloma annulare**

This refers to the presence of skin coloured or red papules which form a ring. It can occur in patients of any age.
- It can be seen anywhere on the body, but is more common over the backs of hands, knuckles and feet.
- Usually asymptomatic but can be itchy.

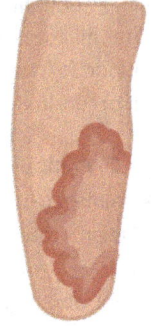

Once thought to be associated with diabetes, more recent evidence suggests the prevalence is not actually greater in diabetic patients. It is associated with several conditions including HIV, autoimmune thyroiditis and lipid abnormalities.

- **Acanthosis nigricans**

This is a skin condition characterised by thickening and darkening of the skin in certain areas.
- It particularly affects the axillae, groin and neck.
- It is a non-specific skin sign which is associated with a host of systemic conditions and malignancies:
- Diabetes mellitus
- Hypothyroidism
- Obesity
- GI cancer
- Oral contraceptive pill use

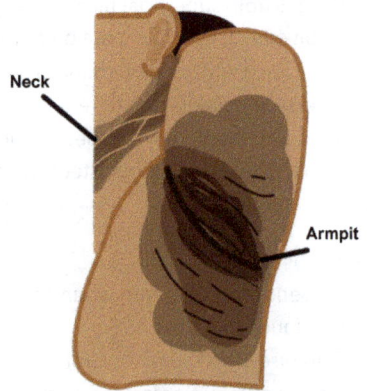

Inflammatory conditions

- **Dermatitis herpetiformis**

This is an autoimmune skin condition associated with coeliac disease, which occurs when IgA antibodies become deposited in the skin.

Symptoms

- Symmetrical itchy vesicular lesions on the skin which appear in groups
- The blisters often become eroded and crusted due to the itching
- Classically seen on extensor surfaces like the elbows, knees and buttocks

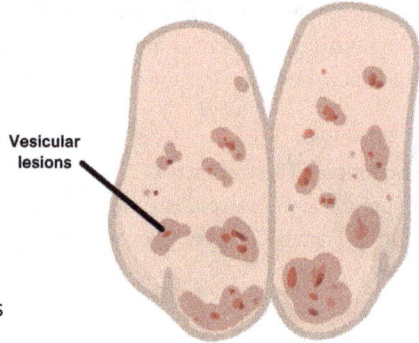

Vesicular lesions

Key tests

- Immunofluorescence of skin biopsy shows deposition of IgA in the dermis

Management

- Gluten-free diet is the mainstay of treatment
- Dapsone is an antibiotic which inhibits synthesis of dihydrofolic acid and helps to reduce the itch within days

- **Pyoderma gangrenosum**

An extremely painful ulcer that occurs typically on the lower limbs suddenly at site of minor injury. It is usually idiopathic but associated with several systemic conditions.
- It is not caused by a pathogen, but instead by improper functioning of neutrophils.

Associations

- Inflammatory bowel disease
- Autoimmune – rheumatoid arthritis, SLE
- Cancer – lymphoma, myeloid leukaemia
- Primary biliary cirrhosis

Pyoderma gangrenosum

Symptoms

- Starts as a small red pustule/papule which quickly breaks down into an ulcer
- This eventually leaves a deep ulcer with a characteristic violaceous border
- If left untreated, the ulcer may keep growing larger, persist or slowly heal

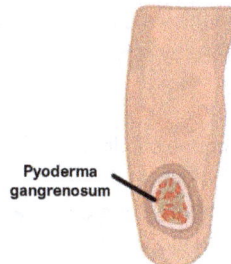

Management

- 1st line is steroids (oral prednisolone) and wound care
- Large ulcers may need combination of oral steroids, ciclosporin or biologic agents

• Erythema nodosum

An inflammatory disorder which affects the subcutaneous fat cells under the skin.
- This leads to the development of painful red nodules usually on the shins.
- It is more common in women than men and usually seen in ages from 20–40.

Associations

- Infection – TB, streptococci
- Autoimmune – sarcoidosis, IBD
- Drugs – amoxicillin, contraceptive pill
- Lymphoma
- Pregnancy

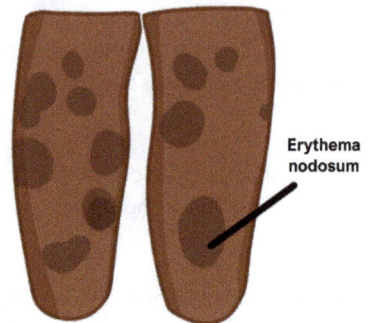

Erythema nodosum

Symptoms

- Erythematous tender nodules/plaques
  mainly on the shins and thighs
- They are initially red, but then go purple,
  brown or like a bruise before self-resolving
- The lesions do not form ulcers and heal without scarring

• Livedo reticularis

This refers to a lacey purplish mottled eruption of the skin following a vascular pattern, most commonly seen on the legs.
- It occurs due to slow arterial blood flow resulting in collection of hypo-oxygenated blood in the venules.
- It is caused by conditions which increase the risk of forming clots in small vessels.

Associations

- Autoimmune conditions – systemic lupus erythematous,
  rheumatoid arthritis
- Prothrombotic conditions – antiphospholipid syndrome,
  thrombophilia (e.g. Factor V Leiden), sickle cell anaemia
- Vasculitis – polyarteritis nodosa, ANCA-associated
  vasculitis

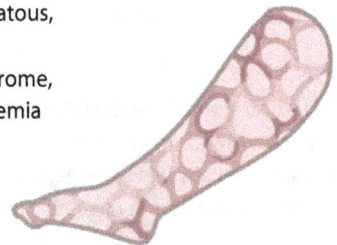

Drug Reactions

- **Drug exanthem**

This is the most common type of drug rash, which can occur after almost any drug, usually within a couple of weeks of taking it.
- Common culprits are penicillins, other antibiotics, NSAIDs and allopurinol.

Symptoms

- Morbilliform/maculopapular eruption
- This most commonly affects the trunk
- Can be itchy

Management

- Identification and cessation of culprit drug
- Simple emollients
- Topical coritcosteroids can help hasten resolution

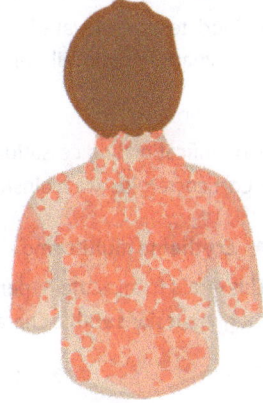

- **Acute generalized exanthematous pustulosis**

This is one of the more severe cutaneous adverse reactions (SCAR).
- It usually occurs within 2–5 days of starting the culprit drug.
- The most common culprits are antibiotics, terbinafine and hydroxychloroquine.

Symptoms

- Sheets of non-follicular pustules, which are usually first seen in the flexures
- Patients may have systemic symptoms such as fever

Management

- Identification and cessation of drug
- If limited, topical corticosteroids
- If widespread/systemic features, oral corticosteroids can be used

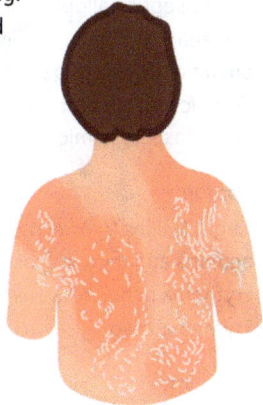

- **Drug reaction with eosinophilia and systemic symptoms (DRESS)**

This refers to drug exanthem with systemic features.
- It usually has a latency of 1–6 weeks between taking the drug and symptom onset.
- Common culprits include allopurinol, anti-epileptics, antibiotics and omeprazole.

Symptoms

- Widespread maculopapular/morbilliform rash and facial oedema
- Lymphadenopathy, fever
- Systemic features can include interstitial nephritis, pneumonitis, colitis, pericarditis

Key tests

- Blood tests – elevated eosinophils and deranged liver function (can be at risk of fulminant hepatic failure)

Management

- Identification and cessation of drug
- Corticosteroids are mainstay of treatment, if prolonged disease add in ciclosporin

- **Erythema multiforme**

This refers to an acute hypersensitivity reaction, usually due to drugs or infections.
- It gives lesions with a characteristic appearance and can also involve the mucosa.

Causes

Target lesion

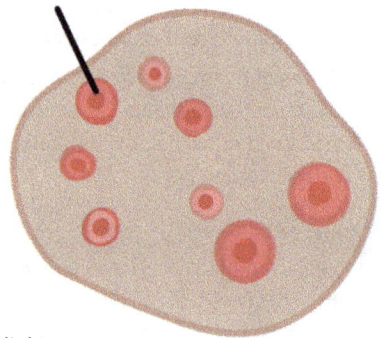

- In up to half of cases, no cause is found
- Most common cause is herpes simplex virus
- Drugs – penicillin, NSAIDs, sulphonamides, anti-epileptics, allopurinol
- Bacteria – Mycoplasma (gives an atypical pneumonia with target lesions)
- Chronic inflammatory states – malignancy, sarcoidosis, systemic lupus erythematosus

Symptoms

- Target lesions (central necrosis surrounded by lighter oedema and then ring of erythema) on the hands, feet and the torso
- Erythema minor – lesions with minimal mucosal involvement
- Erythema major – lesions with mucosal involvement, patients systemically unwell

Management

- Cessation of causative drug and systemic corticosteroids are mainstay of treatment
- Aciclovir if HSV suspected. If recurrent, patients can have long term prophylaxis

- **Stevens-Johnson syndrome/Toxic epidermal necrolysis**

This is a severe life-threatening mucocutaneous reaction which usually occurs 7–10 days after drug exposure, although a minority of cases can be triggered by infection.
- It is a cytotoxic immune reaction causing keratinocyte apoptosis which leads to necrosis and epidermal detachment.
- Stevens-Johnson is the term used to describe < 10% body surface area (BSA).
- The term toxic epidermal necrolysis (TEN) refers to lesions which cover > 30% BSA, with overlap 10–30%.
- The most common culprits are allopurinol, anti-epileptics and antibiotics.

Symptoms

- Prodromal illness e.g. fever with upper respiratory tract infection may precede the rash
- Dusky red macules that form large confluent areas with blistering and epidermal detachment
- Nikolsky sign positive – this is when gentle lateral pressure of skin results in detachment of the epidermis
- Mucosal involvement – blistering/ulceration of lips and intra-oral, inflammation of eyes and eyelids, genital blistering/erosions
- Systemic upset – tachycardia, hypotension and risk of hypovolaemia shock

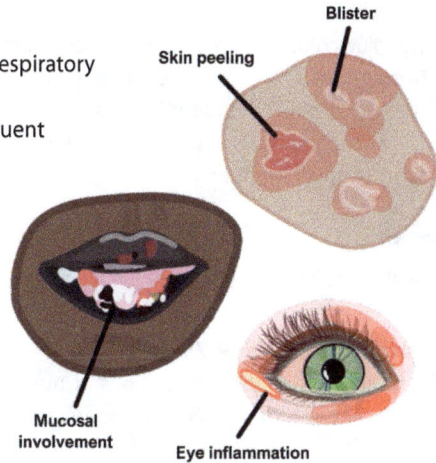

Blister

Skin peeling

Mucosal involvement

Eye inflammation

Management

- Stop the suspected drug culprit
- Supportive measures – fluid replacement, nutrition, analgesia, airway support
- Consider early catheter to prevent strictures
- Involve opthalmology from the beginning (risk of ocular scarring)
- MDT involvement – oral medicine, gynaecology, urology may also be required
- Care in side room
- Skin care is the most important – decompress blisters, care on frictionless sheets (Exudry), liberal and frequent emollient use (50% white soft parrafin with 50% liquid paraffin), non stick dressings over denuded areas, gentle skin cleaning
- There is limited evidence for active therapy – short coureses of corticosteroid, IV immunoglobulin or ciclosporin can be considered if early in the acute phase

Birth Marks

Children can present with a variety of birthmarks – these are usually asymptomatic but, in some cases, can give rise to secondary complications.

- **Congenital dermal melanocytosis (CDM)**

These are congenital marks, which occur most commonly in Asian children.

- These were formerly known as Mongolian blue spots.
- The blue colour occurs as dermal melanocytes become interrupted in their migration from the neural crest to epidermis in utero.
- They are completely asymptomatic, and often spontaneously disappear by in early childhood.

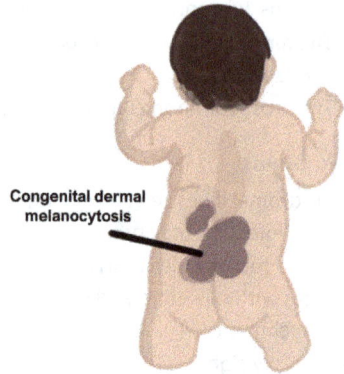

Congenital dermal melanocytosis

Symptoms

- Blue-grey macules, usually in the lumbosacral region

- **Congenital melanocytic naevi**

These are congenital proliferations of melanocytes that are present at birth or become apparent within the first year of life.

- They are classified as small (1.5 cm), medium (1.5–10 cm), large (11–20 cm) and giant (> 20 cm).

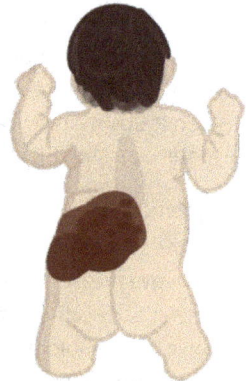

Symptoms

- Brown plaque which can be slightly bumpy +/- hairy

Complications

- Giant congenital melanocytic naevi (GCMN), are associated with complications:
- Neurocutaneuous melanosis – melanocyte proliferation into the CNS
- Melanoma – the malignancy risk of GCMN is up to 15% in giant lesions, especially those which have "satellite" lesions
- 70% of melanomas occur before puberty, and can be extra-cutaneous (involving the central nervous system)

Red birthmarks get their red colour as they involve the vascular system. They are split into two categories.

Vascular tumour

This refers to a benign or malignant tumour (abnormal growth) of the cells forming the arteries, veins and capillaries.

- **Infantile haemangioma**

A common benign vascular tumour usually seen in up to 10% of Caucasian infants.
- It may be evident shortly after birth and can rapidly grow in the first 3 months of life.
- It usually slows by 5 months of age.
- It is typically found on the face, scalp and back.
- It starts of as a premonitory patch (pale, few blood vessels) followed by a rapid proliferation phase. Over the next few years, it stabilises and involutes.

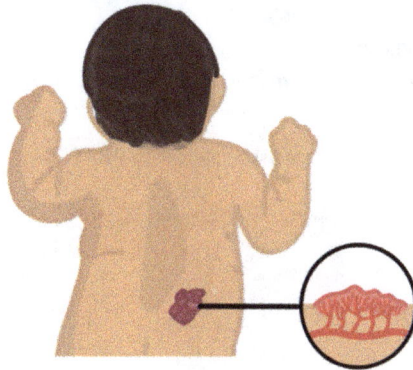

There are several different variants of infantile haemangiomas:
- Superficial – this affects the blood vessels in the uppermost layers of the skin, giving a red colour
- Deep – these cavernous haemangiomas affect blood vessels deeply set in the dermis, giving a more blue/purple colour
- Mixed – this is a mix of superficial and deep types

Symptoms
- Presents as red, raised, bumpy lesion on the skin
- One of the main complications is ulceration/bleeding
- It can also rarely obstruct the visual fields or airway

- **Segmental haemangioma**

This is a vascular tumour which is associated with a higher risk of complications.
- It usually occurs at a younger age and is often much larger.

Management

- Most haemangiomas spontaneously involute without complication
- Treatment is recommended for haemangiomas with specific risks including:
- Ulceration
- Airway obstruction
- Periocular haemangiomas – these can compromise the visual axis and the development of binocular vision
- Cosmetic concerns

1st line treatment is topical timolol for small lesions
- Other options include oral propranolol – this is thought due to induction of vasocon-striction and reduces pro-angiogenic factors
- Pulsed dye laser can be used
- Surgery is used in cases if medical management is unsuccessful

Facial segmental haemangiomas are associated with **PHACES syndrome**

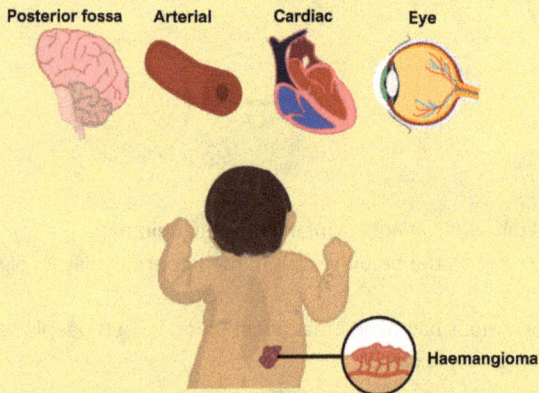

Posterior fossa   Arterial   Cardiac   Eye

Haemangioma

Posterior fossa abnormalities
Haemangiomas
Arterial abnormalities
Cardiac abnormalities
Eye abnormalities
Sternal notch/dim

Vascular malformation

This term refers to an error in the development of vascular embryological tissue.
- These are present at birth and grow slowly and proportionately with the child.

• Naevus simplex (stork bite)

A common benign capillary malformation seen in about 40% of Caucasian infants.
- It gives rise to pink marks which become more prominent with crying.

Symptoms

- A flat, pink macule which occurs on the forehead, eyelids and back of the neck
- Usually fades spontaneously within 2 years

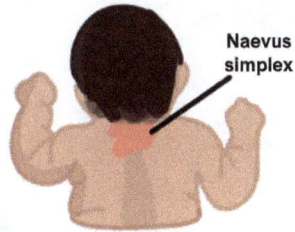

Naevus simplex

• Port wine stain

This is a type of permanent capillary malformation which is present at birth and grows proportionately with the child. It occurs anywhere including the face.

Symptoms

- Red/purple well-defined patch
- It often darkens and becomes bumpier with time

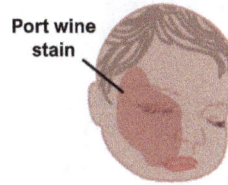

Port wine stain

Management

- There is no cure available but laser therapy can be used to reduce the colour

• Sturge-Weber syndrome (SWS)

This is a rare congenital neurological and skin disorder associated with a port wine stain on the forehead, due to a genetic mutation of the gene GNAQ.
- It causes overabundance of capillaries around the ophthalmic and maxillary distributions of cranial nerve V.

Symptoms

- Port wine stain – due to abnormal development of vascular tissue
- Seizures – due to angiomas involving the leptomeninges
- Glaucoma – due to vessel abnormality around the eyes

Management

- Treated with MDT approach to manage symptoms e.g. ophthalmology for glaucoma, anti-epileptics for seizures, pulsed dye laser for the cutaneous mark

Gynaecology

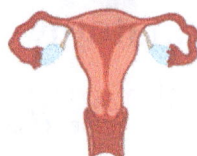

Anatomy of the Genital Tract

The female reproductive system lies posterior to the bladder and anterior to the rectum. It includes the uterus, ovaries, cervix, fallopian tubes and the vagina.

- **Ovaries**

The ovaries are the main female reproductive organs, which produce egg cells and the sex hormones oestrogen and progesterone.
- The ovaries lie lateral to the uterus close to the pelvic wall, located in shallow depressions known as the ovarian fossae.
- The right ovary lies close to caecum and the left near the sigmoid colon.
- Lymph drains to the para-aortic nodes.

Blood supply: Ovarian artery (direct from abdominal aorta)

Venous drainage: Ovarian vein, which drains into the IVC (right) and renal vein (left)

Nerve supply: Sympathetic supply from T10

- **Uterus**

The uterus (womb) is the organ responsible for the development of the embryo and foetus during pregnancy.
- It can be divided into 4 parts: the fundus (at the top), body, isthmus and cervix.

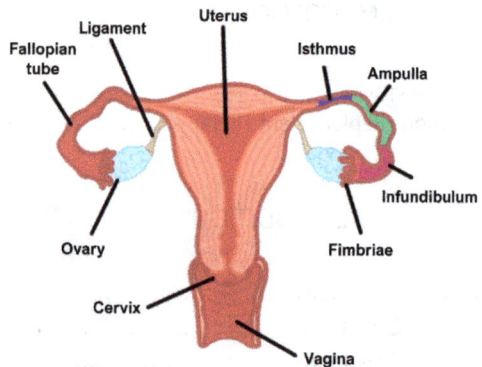

The uterus is divided into 3 tissue layers:
- Endometrium – this is the inner lining made of outer columnar epithelium with glands and inner connective tissue. This functional, superficial layer responds to reproductive hormones and is shed during menstruation.
- Myometrium – this is the smooth muscle layer which contracts during delivery.
- Outer serosa/perimetrium – this is the outer layer.

Blood supply: Dual supply from uterine artery (from internal iliac) and ovarian artery

Venous drainage: Uterine vein which drains into the internal iliac vein

Nerve supply: Sympathetic from T11-L2 causes contraction and vasoconstriction
- Parasympathetic supply from S2-S4 (pelvic splanchnic) gives vasodilation

Lymphatic drainage is to para-aortic nodes (fundal area) and the external and internal iliac (all other parts) lymph nodes.

The uterus is held in place by ligaments which attach it to pelvic structures.

Round ligament	Extends from the uterine body to the labia majora via the inguinal canal, assisting anteversion
Broad ligament	Attaches the sides of the uterus to the pelvic sidewalls
Cardinal ligament	Extends from the cervix to the pelvic sidewalls
Uterosacral ligaments	Extends from the uterus to the sacrum

- **Cervix**

This is the lowest part of the uterus composed of fibroelastic connective tissue.

- It has two openings: the internal os connects the cervix to the uterus and the external os connects the cervix to the vagina.
- The cervix produces mucus sealing off the uterus from the external environment, maintaining sterility of the upper female reproductive tract.
- This mucus varies in pH and thickness throughout the uterine cycle (under the influence of oestrogen and progesterone) to either facilitate or inhibit the passage of sperm into the uterus.
- The cervix also allows broken down endometrium to pass out the uterus to the vagina during menstruation.

The cervix is divided into 3 parts:

- Endocervix/endocervical canal – the innermost part of cervix between the internal and external os (opening of uterus), lined by simple columnar epithelium with mucous producing cells.

- Ectocervix – this is the part of cervix projecting into the vagina. Its opening is the external os which marks the transition to the endocervical canal. It is lined by squamous epithelium.

- Cervical transformation zone – this is the junction between the endo/ectocervix. Here there is a border between the inner columnar epithelium and distal squamous epithelium.

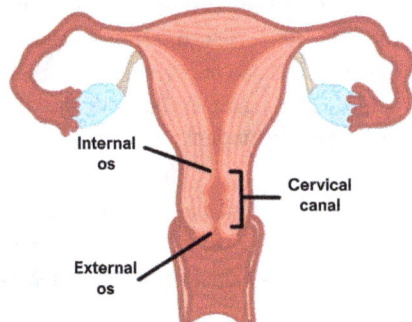

- **Fallopian tubes**

These tubes connect the ovaries with the uterus. Each tube is divided into 4 parts.
- From the ovary there is the fimbriae, the infundibulum, the ampulla and the isthmus.
- The isthmus is the narrowest part, and fertilisation usually occurs in the ampulla.
- The tubes are responsible for transporting ova from the ovaries to the uterus, but also sperm in the opposite direction. They are lined with cilia which are needed to transport cells to uterus and secrete nutrients.

Blood supply: Ovarian artery (lateral 2/3) and uterine artery

Nerve supply: Same as the uterus

- **Vagina**

This is an elastic muscular canal that connects the uterus to the outside world.
- It is lined by non-keratinized stratified squamous epithelium.
- It is supported by muscles and ligaments of the pelvic floor, which attach to the perineal body between the urogenital and anal triangles.
- If these become damaged, it increases the risk of rectal, bladder and uterine prolapse.
- The hymen is a membrane the partially covers or surrounds the vaginal opening.

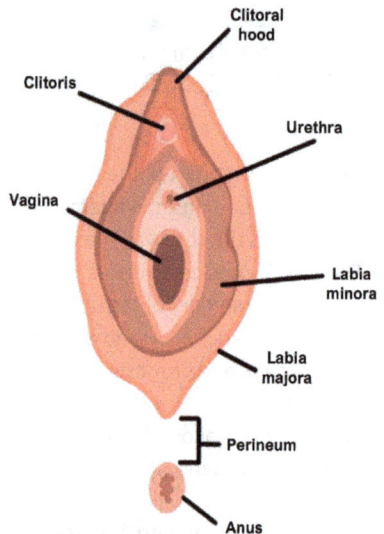

- **Vulva**

This is the outermost part of the female genitalia.
- It includes the opening of the vagina (vestibule) and the clitoris (main erogenous zone of the female).
- Bartholin's glands are two pea-sized glands located slightly lateral and posterior to the vaginal opening, which secrete an alkaline fluid for lubrication during sex.
- Oestrogen has an important role in the keratinisation and proliferation of the vulvar epithelium. It maintains thickness and prevents atrophy (atrophy in menopause is due to reduced oestrogen).

There are 2 sets of skin folds on the vulva:
- Labia majora – contain sweat and sebaceous glands, pubic hair, external skin folds
- Labia minora – hairless but contain sebaceous glands; lie within the labia majora

The Menstrual Cycle

This describes the approximate 28-day cycle which occurs in women around the ages of 12 to 51, which controls the synthesis and release of egg cells, the preparation and maintenance of the endometrium and associated hormonal changes.
- The cycle starts on the first day of the bleeding (menstruation) and ends prior to the next menstrual period.
- Ovulation occurs mid-cycle i.e. around day 14 of a 28-day cycle.

The changes that occur in the female reproductive system are coordinated by the hypothalamic-pituitary-ovarian axis.
- The hypothalamus produces gonadotrophin releasing hormone (GnRH) in a pulsatile fashion (if produced continuously, it does not have the effects described).
- This stimulates the anterior pituitary to secrete follicular stimulating hormone (FSH) and luteinising hormone (LH) which act on follicles within the ovaries.
- LH stimulates theca cells to produce androgens.
- FSH stimulates growth of follicles, the conversion of the androgens to oestrogen by granulosa cells and also stimulates inhibin production.

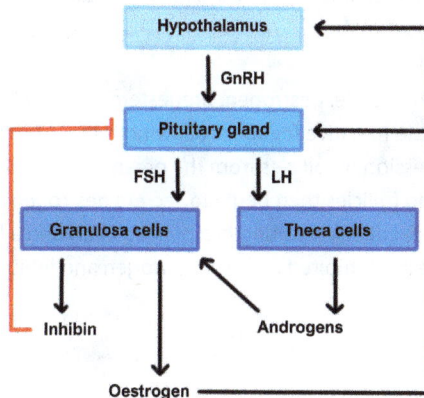

This axis is under the influence of positive and negative feedback

i) Negative feedback
- Slowly rising oestrogen inhibits LH and FSH secretion
- Progesterone inhibits LH and FSH secretion
- Inhibin inhibits FSH secretion selectively

ii) Positive feedback
- Rapidly rising oestrogen stimulates LH and FSH secretion

The ovarian cycle

In the ovaries, oocytes (egg cells) develop within follicles which contain 2 cell types:

- Theca cells – these express LH receptors and are stimulated to produce androgens.
- Granulosa cells – these express FSH receptors and are stimulated to convert the androgens made by theca cells to oestrogen.
- They also secrete inhibin which suppresses FSH production by negative feedback.

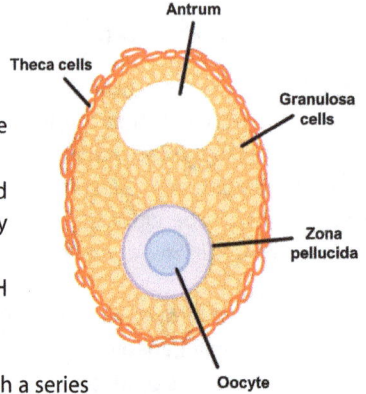

During the ovarian cycle, follicles progress through a series of development phases.

- They start as primordial follicles, then preantral and antral follicles. The follicles rupture during ovulation, and then become the corpus luteum and corpus albicans.
- Follicles progress to the preantral phase in the absence of exogenous hormones.
- However, to progress to the antral stage, follicles require the influence of FSH/LH.
- Follicles that are not stimulated by FSH/LH will undergo atresia.
- The ovarian cycle is divided into two phases, follicular (early and late) and luteal.

Early follicular phase

At the start of a menstrual cycle, oestrogen, progesterone and inhibin levels are low.

- As such, they exert little negative feedback allowing LH and FSH levels to rise.
- This allows the progression of follicles from the preantral to antral stage.
- In turn, the developing follicles then begin to secrete oestrogen and inhibin.
- These exert negative feedback resulting in a plateau in LH and a fall in FSH.
- FSH declines because it is inhibited by both oestrogen and inhibin.

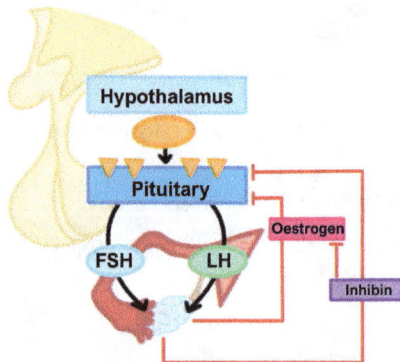

Late follicular phase

The levels of FSH are insufficient to maintain all the developing follicles.
- Therefore, a single dominant follicle is selected (the others undergo atresia).
- Selection of a dominant follicle leads to a rapid rise in oestrogen.
- This has a positive feedback effect, leading to a surge in LH.
- The LH surge triggers ovulation, rupture of the follicle with release of the oocyte into the fallopian tube. Follicular rupture results in a fall in oestrogen and LH.

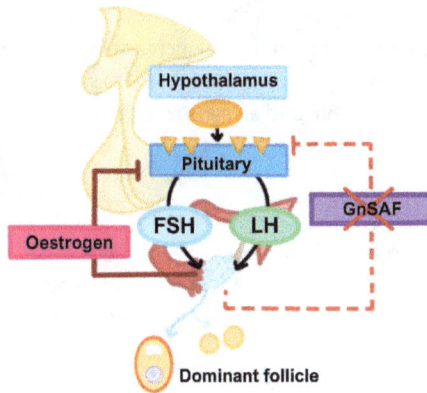

The luteal phase

The ruptured follicle develops into the corpus luteum.
- The corpus luteum secretes progesterone, oestrogen and inhibin.
- These exert negative feedback on LH/FSH secretion, resulting in low levels of LH and FSH throughout the luteal phase.
- The corpus luteum has a lifespan of about 14 days.

The next stage is dependent on whether fertilisation occurs or not.

i) If fertilisation does not occur
- The corpus luteum degenerates (luteolysis).
- Luteolysis leads to a decline in luteal progesterone, oestrogen and inhibin.
- This causes a rise in LH/FSH which begins the next cycle with menstruation.
- The corpus luteum does not fully disappear; it remains in the ovary as a mass of fibrous scar tissue known as the corpus albicans.

ii) If fertilisation occurs
- The embryo secretes hCG which stops luteolysis and maintains the corpus luteum.
- This results in continuous production of progesterone which prevents menstruation.
- The placenta eventually takes over the role of the corpus luteum (from 8 weeks).

The uterine cycle

Structural changes in the uterus also occur alongside those occurring in the ovary.
- These changes are also divided into phases.

Proliferative phase

This coincides with the follicular phase of the ovarian cycle.
- The main hormone responsible is oestrogen.
- This phase is characterised by changes that enhance the chance of fertilisation.
- The endometrium undergoes thickening, an increase in vascularity and development of simple tubular glands which secrete a fluid that aids sperm transport.
- The cervical mucus becomes thin and alkaline to enhance sperm penetration.

Secretory phase

This coincides with the luteal phase of the ovarian cycle and begins after ovulation.
- The main hormone responsible is progesterone.
- This phase is characterised by changes that prepare for implantation of an embryo.
- The endometrium thickens further and there is further development of glands to become branched and more complex.
- These secrete fluid that aids implantation of a fertilised ovum.
- The cervical mucus becomes thick and acidic to prevent more sperm penetration.

Menses

Menses marks the beginning of a new cycle, which involves the shedding of the uterine lining via the vagina.
- Menstrual bleeding usually lasts 2–7 days (average = 5 days).
- Blood loss is usually between 20–90 ml (equivalent of 1–5 teaspoons).
- The average length of a complete cycle is 28 days, but this can vary (the NHS considers a normal menstrual cycle lasting between 23 and 35 days).
- Ovulation usually occurs 12–16 days before a woman's next period.

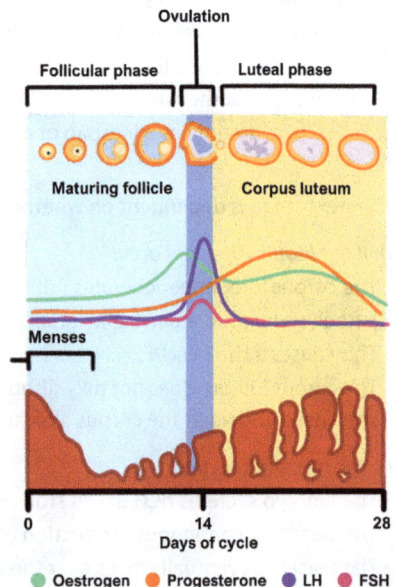

Ovulation

Follicular phase   Luteal phase

Maturing follicle   Corpus luteum

Menses

0   14   28
Days of cycle

● Oestrogen ● Progesterone ● LH ● FSH

Tests and Investigations

- **Swabs**

A superficial test which involves taking (usually multiple) swabs to screen for infection.
- They can be "double" (i.e. two) or "triple" swabs depending on the hospital.
- They are taken as high vaginal or endocervical swabs.
- The scrapings can be sent for culture of organisms or nucleic acid analysis amplification tests to determine the pathogen.

Type of swab	What it tests for?
Endocervical chlamydia swab	Chlamydia
Endocervical charcoal media swab	Gonorrhoea
High-vaginal charcoal media swab	Bacterial vaginosis, Trichomonas vaginalis, Candida and group B Streptococcus

- **Ultrasound scan**

This uses high frequency sound waves to visualise the pelvic structures and is usually performed in two ways.
- Trans-abdominal – this is used to visualise the uterus, ovaries and adnexal structures, urogenital tract (e.g. obstruction, retention) and assess foetal development in obstetrics.

- Transvaginal – this is best for viewing ovaries (enlarged due to cysts, tumours and follicular maturation), the uterus and measure endometrial thickness. It is used in gynaecology and early pregnancy.

- **Colposcopy**

This is a procedure used to visualise the cervix.
- A speculum is used to view the ectocervix.
- You can then apply compounds to identify pre-malignant or cancerous lesions.

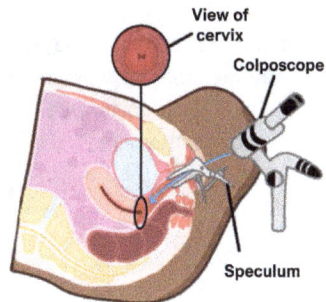

View of cervix
Colposcope
Speculum

Acetic acid stains white areas with high nuclear/cytoplasmic ratio i.e. abnormal changes in cells.
- If there are no white lesions, you can apply Lugol's iodine solution.
- This normally reacts with glycogen and turns brown (in normal tissue).
- Abnormal areas have less glycogen so turn yellow rather than brown.

- **Hysteroscopy**

The inspection of the uterus using a fibreoptic scope through the cervix.
- It is used to diagnose and treat uterine pathologies.

- **Mammogram**

This is the investigation which uses low energy X-rays to visualise the breast tissue.
- It is used to detect breast cancer, through detecting masses and calcifications.
- It has a false negative rate of > 10% and it can be difficult to spot small tumours.

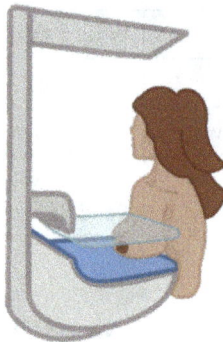

- **Hysterectomy**

This is the surgical removal of the uterus, of which there are various subtypes:

Radical hysterectomy – this refers to removal of uterus, cervix, fallopian tubes upper vagina and parametrium. It is usually indicated for cervical cancer.
- The lymph nodes and ovaries are also removed.

Total hysterectomy – the removal of the uterus, cervix and fallopian tubes +/- ovaries.

Subtotal hysterectomy – the removal of the uterus but leaving the cervix in situ.
- In pre-menopausal women, the ovaries can be preserved to maintain hormonal balance. The fallopian tubes are removed as recent research has shown that ovarian cancer originates here.

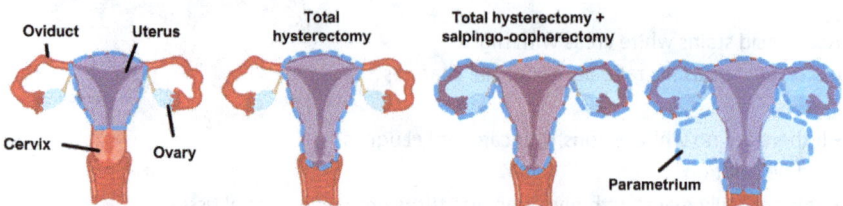

Contraception

There are many different forms of contraception. These include physical barriers, directly impeding the sperm from reaching the egg as well as hormonal methods.
- Contraception is not required in the first 21 days after childbirth.

Barrier methods

- **Male condom**

This is a latex/polyurethane/synthetic rubber sheath placed over the erect penis.

Advantages: Provides protection against STIs, no hormonal side effects

Disadvantages: Relatively low success rate with typical use

- **Female condom**

This is a polyurethane sheath that lines the vagina and covers the area just outside.

Advantages: Provides protection against STIs, no hormonal side effects

Disadvantages: Relatively low success rate with typical use

Note that oil-based products (for example, body lotions) damage latex or polyisoprene condoms and so should be avoided.

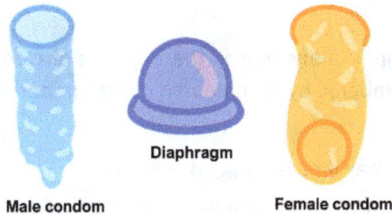

Diaphragm

Male condom   Female condom

- **Diaphragm/cap**

This is a flexible latex/silicone device placed in the vagina to cover the cervix.
- It is used with spermicide. Patients should be fitted to ensure they use the right size.
- After giving birth, women should wait 6 weeks before using diaphragm again as the uterus size changes during pregnancy.

Advantages: Can be inserted three hours prior to sex

Disadvantages: Relatively low success rate with typical use (71–88%)
- Does not protect against STIs
- Some women find it difficult to insert into the correct location to cover the cervix

Combined hormonal contraception

This type of contraception contains both oestrogen and progesterone.
- The oestrogen component prevents pregnancy by inhibiting and thickening the cervical mucus (more difficult for sperm to reach the egg).
- The progesterone thins the uterine lining (which reduces chance of implantation).

Advantages
- More effective than barrier methods and does not interrupt sexual intercourse
- Periods tend to be lighter, more regular and less painful
- Can improve acne, especially with third and fourth generation progestogens
- Helps to reduce the risk of endometrial, ovarian and colorectal cancer

Disadvantages
- Does not protect against STIs
- Can cause breast pain and mood changes
- Breakthrough, unexpected, vaginal bleeding can occur over the first few months
- Higher risk of DVT (increased if positive family history, high BMI +/- smoker)
- Higher risk of arterial thrombosis (increased if BMI, smoker, hypertension and migraines with aura)
- Small increased risk of breast and cervical cancers; this goes back to baseline after 10 years of stopping the pill
- Common medications can affect the efficacy of the pill (anti-epileptics, antiretrovirals, antibiotics)

There is a list of contraindications due to the high risk of cardiovascular disease and cancer. This can be remembered by the mnemonic **S**ome **I**mportant **V**otes **C**an't **B**e **D**one **B**y **M**ail.

Smoking > 15 cigarettes/day if patients aged > 35 yrs

Immobilisation – major surgery with prolonged immobilisation

VTE – history of thromboembolism or thrombogenic mutation

CVS disease – history of stroke or IHD or uncontrolled hypertension

Breast cancer – current active breast cancer

Diabetes – severe diabetes (with DM diagnosed > 20 yrs ago)

Breastfeeding < 6 weeks post-partum (can only be used after 6 weeks)

Migraine with aura

Women on combined oral contraceptives should be followed up at 3 months and annually after to monitor the following:
- BP and BMI
- Ask about development of migraines
- Monitoring of side effects
- Enquire about new contraindicating factors

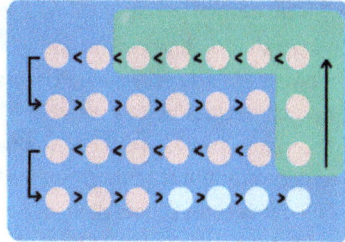

- **Combined oral contraceptive pill (COCP) – Ethinylestradiol + progestogen**

This is colloquially known as "the pill".
- This pill is usually taken once a day for 3 weeks followed by a pill free interval of 1 week (but there are variations to this).
- Women are protected during the pill-free week presuming the pill has been taken correctly and the next pack is commenced on time.

When giving the pill to patients, it is important to inform the patient of the following.

i) Initiation
- If started within first 5 days of menstrual cycle, no additional contraception needed.
- If started at other point in cycle, use barrier contraception or abstain for 7 days.
- The pill should be taken regularly around the same time of the day to be effective.

ii) Missed pills
- If 1 pill is missed, take the missed pill even if it means taking two pills in a day.
- No additional contraceptive measures are required if correct use in week 1 and 7 days prior to the pill free interval.

- If 2 days are missed, take the most recent missed pill and not the one before.
- They should also use barrier contraception for 7 days.
- If the missed pill occurs in week 3, advise the patient to omit the pill free interval and take two courses back-to-back.

iii) Vomiting/diarrhoea
- Vomiting with 2 hours or severe diarrhoea affects absorption of the pill.
- If vomiting occurs within 2 hours of taking pill, then take another pill.
- If vomiting persists > 24 hours, count each day as a missed pill.

- **Transdermal patch** – Ethinylestradiol + norelgestromin **(progestogen)**

This is a short acting contraceptive which lasts for 1 week.
- Women should apply the patch on the same day every week for 3 weeks and then have a patch free period of 1 week.
- The patch can be applied to sites including the upper outer arm, buttock, lower abdomen and it is advised to use a different site each time.
- The patch can become detached from the skin, cause skin irritation and there may be a delay in return to fertility.

- **Contraceptive vaginal ring** – Ethinylestradiol + etonogesterel **(progestogen)**

This is a flexible transparent ring which is self-inserted into vagina.
- A ring should be used for 21 days and followed by a ring free interval for 4 or 7 days.
- The ring can be expelled whilst removing a tampon or during sexual intercourse, so it is important to inform patients about this risk.
- Unlike the contraceptive pill, is not affected by diarrhoea and vomiting.
- However, it can cause a delay in return to normal fertility.

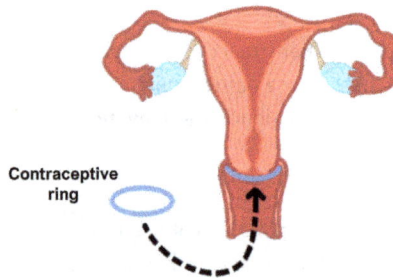

Contraceptive ring

Progesterone-only contraception

This class only contains a progestogen which works by inhibiting an egg's progress through the fallopian tubes, thickening cervical mucus and thinning the endometrium.
- Some progesterone-only contraception can also suppress ovulation in women.

Advantages
- More effective than barrier methods and can be used when the COCP is not suitable
- May reduce risk of endometrial cancer and can be used whilst breastfeeding

Disadvantages
- Not protective against STIs
- Increased risk of ovarian cysts and ectopic pregnancy
- Breast tenderness, periods can become heavier and painful for a few months

- **Progesterone-only pill (POP) – Levonorgestrel, norethisterone, desogestrel**

This is colloquially known as "the mini pill". Unlike the COCP, the POP is taken for 28 days consecutively with no pill-free interval.
- Its efficacy can be reduced by liver modifying drugs (as the hormone has to undergo first-pass metabolism).

When giving this pill to patients, it is important to inform the patient of the following:
i) Initiation
- If the pill is started within the first 5 days of the menstrual cycle, no additional contraception is needed.
- If the POP is started at other point in menstrual cycle, use barrier contraception or abstain from sex for the first 2 days.
- The pill should be taken regularly at the same time of the day to be most effective.

ii) Missed pill
- If 1 pill is missed, take the missed pill even if it means taking two pills in one day.
- Use barrier protection or abstain from intercourse for the next 48 hours.

iii) Vomiting/diarrhoea
- If vomiting occurs within 2 hours of taking the pill, then take another pill.
- If vomiting persists > 24 hours, count each day as a missed pill.

- **Progesterone-only injection – Medroxyprogesterone acetate, norethisterone**

This is a long-acting contraceptive which is taken every 8–13 weeks.
- It can take up to 1 year to return to normal fertility.
- It may also cause weight gain, lower bone density (this normalises after stopping the injection) and injection site reactions.
- Most frequently, periods stop completely. However, in some cases, it can cause irregular bleeding and/or bleeding which is heavier and longer.

- **Progesterone-only implant – Etonogestrel (Nexplanon)**

This is a long-acting contraceptive which is inserted into the upper arm and provides protection for 3 years.
- Fertility returns as soon as the implant is removed.
- The most common side effect is an erratic bleeding pattern.
- This method releases progestin directly into the bloodstream, circumventing the liver and avoiding first-pass metabolism.

Intrauterine contraceptives

These are devices which sit inside the uterus and are referred to as "the coil".
- They are long-lasting and one of the most effective contraception methods.

- **Copper intrauterine device (Cu-IUD)**

This is a small T-shaped device with strings of copper which lasts for 5 or 10 years depending on the type.
- It prevents the survival of sperm because copper is toxic to sperm.
- It also thickens the cervical mucus preventing sperm entry to the uterus.
- The device alters the lining of the endometrium, preventing implantation.
- When using the coil, it is effective immediately after insertion.

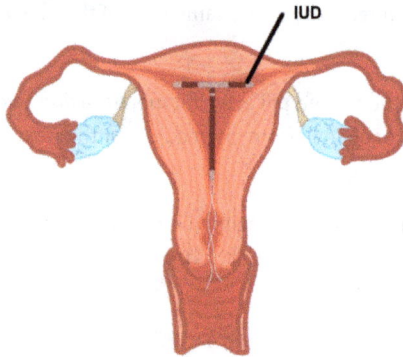

Advantages
- Very effective (> 99%)
- Provides long-term contraception (5 or 10 years)
- Normal fertility returns as soon as the coil is removed
- No interactions with other medicines
- Reduced risk of endometrial and cervical cancer and no hormonal side effects
- No systemic hormonal side effects

Disadvantages
- Does not protect against STIs and increases risk of pelvic inflammatory disease
- Increases the risk of ectopic pregnancy
- Causes irregular bleeding and periods can become heavier, longer and/or more painful (this may settle after a few months)
- Higher risk of infection secondary to its insertion
- Risk of expulsion from the uterus
- Risk of uterine perforation – causes pelvic pain, changes in periods, dyspareunia

- **Levonorgestrel-releasing intrauterine system (LNG-IUS)**

This is a long-acting reversible contraceptive which contains varying amounts of the progestogen levonorgestrel.
- It is a small, T-shaped plastic device which is inserted into the uterus.
- Levonorgestrel thins the endometrial lining, prevents fertilisation and thickens the cervical mucus.
- The IUS is effective 7 days after insertion.
- There are a variety of brands used such as the Mirena and Kyleena coil, which can be used for 5–10 years depending on the type.

Advantages
- Very effective (> 99%)
- Provides long-term contraception
- Normal fertility returns as soon as it is removed
- Can be used when the COCP is contraindicated and during breastfeeding
- Periods often stop (or become lighter) and may become less painful
- Protective against endometrial cancer, particular in women taking HRT

Disadvantages
- Does not protect against STIs and increases the risk of pelvic inflammatory disease
- Increases risk of ectopic pregnancy
- Increases risk of functional ovarian cysts (normally no treatment required)
- Progesterone side effects – acne, breast tenderness, headaches, irregular bleeding for 3–6 months post-insertion
- Risk of uterine perforation
- Infection secondary to its insertion
- Expulsion from the uterus

Women who have been fitted with an IUCD should check for the IUCD threads regularly and then seek medical attention if they cannot locate the threads.
- If the patient cannot feel the threads, make sure to exclude pregnancy.
- Perform a speculum examination: if threads can be visualised, refer for ultrasound.
- If the threads cannot be located, the coil may have been expelled from the uterus.

Irreversible contraceptive approaches

These are surgical approaches which are irreversible and have close to 100% pregnancy prevention rate.

- **Male sterilisation (vasectomy)**

This refers to a surgical procedure (under local anaesthetic) to permanently occlude the vas deferens, thus ensuring the sperm cannot enter the semen.
- This is done using an incision on the scrotum.
- To check the efficacy of the procedure, post-vasectomy semen analysis is needed to confirm azoospermia.
- This is done 12 weeks post-procedure, and other methods of contraception should be used in the meantime.

Advantages
- Very effective and permanent

Disadvantages
- Does not protect against STIs
- Not easily reversed
- Side effects include chronic post-vasectomy pain (CPVP)

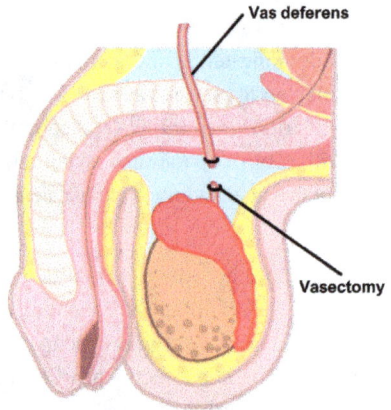

Vas deferens

Vasectomy

- **Female sterilisation**

This involves a surgical procedure (usually laparoscopic under general anaesthetic) to place clips on the fallopian tubes, occluding them to prevent fertilisation.
- Pregnancy must be excluded before the procedure.
- Post-procedure, other methods of contraception should be used until tests confirm tubal occlusion.

Advantages
- Very effective, does not interrupt sexual intercourse and permanent

Disadvantages
- Requires a surgical procedure and the risks which come with this
- Does not protect against STIs
- Irreversible
- Increased risk of ectopic pregnancy in the event of failure

Emergency contraception

There are 3 methods of emergency contraception currently available in the UK.

- **Levonorgestrel**

This is a progestogen taken as a single tablet with an unknown mechanism of action.
- It is given within 72 hours of unprotected sex, but it is ineffective after ovulation has occurred.

Side effects
- Nausea, vomiting, headaches
- Menstrual irregularities (delay, irregular bleeding, spotting)

- **Ulipristal acetate (EllaOne)**

This is a selective progesterone receptor modulator which is taken as a single tablet.
- If given before ovulation, it suppresses follicle development.
- If given after the LH surge has started, it can delay follicular rupture.
- It is given within 120 hours of unprotected sex, but it is ineffective after ovulation has occurred.

Side effects
- Nausea, vomiting, headaches
- Menstrual irregularities (delay, irregular bleeding, spotting)

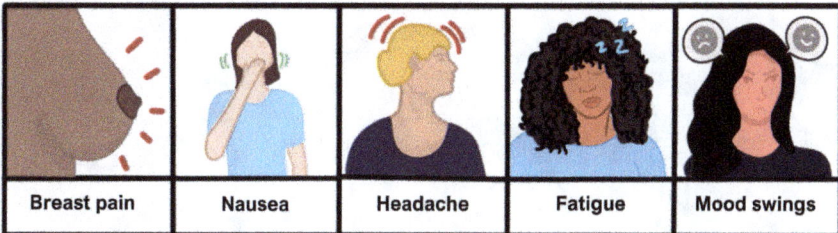

| Breast pain | Nausea | Headache | Fatigue | Mood swings |

- **Copper IUD**

The copper releasing intrauterine device can be used as emergency contraception.
- It needs to be inserted within 120 hours of unprotected sex or, if > 120 hours since unprotected sex and within 5 days of earliest expected date of ovulation.
- If given pre-fertilisation, copper is toxic to sperm and ovum so prevents fertilisation.
- If given post-fertilisation, it works by preventing implantation.

Hormone Replacement Therapy

HRT has been a revelation in the management of menopause in middle-aged women.
- The basic principle is to replace the oestrogen that falls during menopause.
- This alleviates symptoms and protects against complications like osteoporosis.
- When prescribing HRT, the two most important things to consider are whether the patient has her uterus in situ and if she is peri- or post-menopausal.

Risks of HRT
- Breast cancer – a small increased risk of breast cancer (if using both oestrogen and progesterone, related to the duration of HRT; risk reduces after stopping HRT)
- Thrombosis – increased risk of venous thromboembolism with tablet form HRT only
- Cardiovascular – increased risk of stroke with tablet form HRT in women > 60 yrs
- Side effects – breast tenderness, headaches, fluid retention

Contraindications
- Current or past breast cancer
- Any oestrogen sensitive cancer
- Undiagnosed vaginal bleeding
- Untreated endometrial hyperplasia

When taking HRT, options include oestrogen-only or combined HRT with oestrogen and progesterone. Here is a useful flowchart from the British Menopause Society.

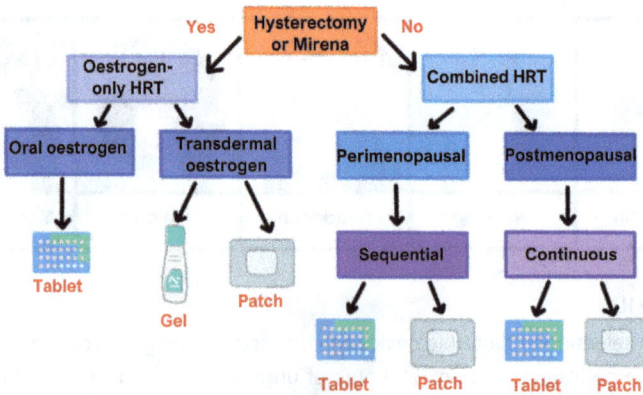

- **Oestrogen-only HRT – Oestradiol**

This form of hormone replacement therapy provides a direct replacement for the fall in oestrogen levels. It is available in several different forms.
- It can only be used in patients without a uterus, or a progesterone coil in situ due to the increased risk of endometrial cancer.

○ **Oral tablet**

These are tablets which are absorbed by the gut and enter the systemic circulation.

- They carry a small increased risk of VTE and so should be avoided in certain patient groups, e.g. high BMI, history of VTE.

○ **Oestrogen-only patch**

This is a patch which releases oestrogen into the skin.

- Unlike the tablets, this does not increase the risk of VTE or stroke.

Indications for transdermal use

- BMI > 30	- Poor symptom control with oral
- Previous or family history of VTE	- Gallbladder disease
- Variable BP control	- On drugs which alter liver enzymes
- Migraine	- GI disorder affecting absorption

○ **Vaginal gel**

This is a gel which can be applied over the vagina, used to prevent vaginal atrophy.

- There is minimal systemic absorption so it can be used in patients with a uterus.
- It is used in women with vaginal symptoms.

● **Combined HRT – Oestradiol + progestogen**

This form of HRT involves both oestrogen for replacement and progesterone for protective purposes. It is needed in women with their uterus in situ as the progesterone provides protection against endometrial cancer.

- It is given via combination tablets, combination patches or separate oestrogen and progesterone tablets.
- It can be given sequentially/cyclically or continuously.

○ **Sequential**

This is used for peri-menopausal women (those whose last period < 1 year ago).

- In this type of therapy, women will still have a bleed every month.
- In monthly HRT, women take the oestrogen tablet every day and the progestogen alongside it for the last 14 days of their menstrual cycle.

○ **Continuous**

This is used for post-menopausal women (those whose last period > 1 year ago).

- Women take combined oestrogen and progestogen every day without a break.

Ovarian Conditions

It is not uncommon to develop cystic masses on the ovaries.

- In premenopausal women, most ovarian masses are benign.
- On the other hand, postmenopausal women are at a higher risk of malignancy.
- There are both benign and malignant types of ovarian masses.

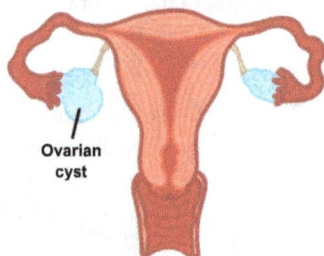

Ovarian
cyst

Benign

○ **Physiological/functional/simple cysts**

These are cysts which develop as part of the menstrual cycle. They are considered physiological and usually self-resolve over 2–3 menstrual cycles. They include:

- Follicular cyst – the dominant follicle does not release the egg and fills with fluid.
- Corpus luteum cyst – this occurs when the corpus luteum fails to breakdown after the egg is released; it may contain blood.

○ **Epithelial**

This is the most common type of benign ovarian tumour, including:

- Serous cystadenoma – this has a smooth outer surface and is filled with clear fluid. It is most common in women aged 40–60 yrs.
- Mucinous cystadenoma – this can be large and extend into the abdomen (it secretes mucus which can rarely cause pseudomyxoma peritonei).

○ **Germ cell tumours**

This is a proliferation of the germ cell layers, which are seen in younger women.

- Dermoid cysts/mature cystic teratomas – these are most commonly seen in women of reproductive age and may contain differentiated tissues (e.g. hair, teeth, fat).

○ **Endometrioma**

This is a cyst which develops in individuals with endometriosis.

- It is known as a "chocolate cyst" because of its brown appearance when it ruptures.

○ **Sex-cord stromal tumour**

This is a tumour that forms in the tissues that support the ovaries or testes.

- Fibroma – this is uncommon before the age of 30 years and is composed of spindled cells with collagenous stroma; it may present with Meig's syndrome (ovarian tumour, ascites and pleural effusion).

Malignant

○ **Epithelial**

This is the most common type representing 90% of primary ovarian cancers.

- High-grade serous – this likely originates from the fallopian tubes. Ovarian cancer is almost synonymous with high-grade serous ovarian cancer, even though there are other histological types.

○ **Germ cell tumours**

These are most commonly seen in younger women. They are typically hormone secreting and usually affect one ovary.

- Dysgerminoma – this is the most common type of germ cell tumour which is derived from the primordial germ cells and secretes LDH.
- Yolk sac tumour (endodermal sinus tumour) – this is histologically similar to the primitive yolk sac and secretes AFP.
- Non-gestational choriocarcinoma – this demonstrates trophoblastic differentiation with the absence of any paternal genes and secretes hCG; it is very rare.

○ **Sex-cord stromal tumour**

This develops from the stromal content of the ovary.

- Granulosa cell tumour – this is the most common sex-cord stromal tumour. It is a malignant proliferation of granulosa cells which is oestrogen secreting.
- Sertoli-Leydig cell tumour – this secretes androgens which leads to masculinisation (can be benign or malignant).

○ **Metastases to the ovary**

Colorectal adenocarcinoma is the most common primary cancer that metastasises to the ovary. Others include the breast, GI tract and lung.

- Kruckenberg tumours specifically refers to signet cell metastases to the ovary that originate in the GI tract, most commonly the stomach.

- **Ovarian cancer**

This refers to a malignant proliferation of cells originating from one of the cell types of the ovary, which is usually seen in postmenopausal women.

Risk factors

- Increased age (postmenopausal)
- Higher number of ovulations (damages ovary) – associated with nulliparity, early menarche, late menopause
- HRT
- Genetics – BRCA1/2, Lynch syndrome

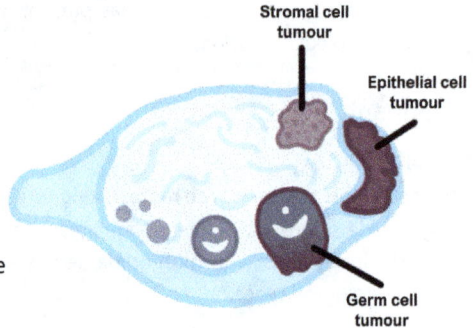

Stromal cell tumour

Epithelial cell tumour

Germ cell tumour

Symptoms

- Any of these persistent symptoms should prompt suspicion of ovarian cancer, especially in women ≥ 50 years of age:
- Abdominal distension (bloating)
- Pelvic or abdominal pain
- Early satiety or loss of appetite
- Urinary urgency and/or frequency
- Women > 50 yrs with IBS symptoms

Key tests

- Initially is a blood test to measure tumour marker CA-125
- If this is raised (e.g. > 35 IU/ml), refer for transvaginal ultrasound scan
- If USS appearance is suggestive of cancer, urgent 2-week referral to gynaecology
- Women who have ascites or pelvic/abdominal mass on examination should get 2-a-week referral immediately (without waiting for a scan)

Once a patient has been referred to gynaecology, they have additional test.
- In women < 40 yrs, measure AFP, LDH and beta-hCG (check for germ cell tumours).
- Calculate the risk of malignancy index (RMI) which gives you indication of the malignancy risk.

RMI = Ultrasound score × menopausal status × CA-125 level
- Menopausal status is scored out of 3 (pre-menopause = 1, post-menopause = 3)
- Ultrasound scored out of 3 depending on the number of suspicious features
- 0 feature = score 0   1 feature = score 1   ≥ 2 features = 3
- Worrying features include multilocular, bilateral, solid areas, ascites or metastases

Management

- If RMI of ≥ 250 refer to specialist MDT team (some units may use a lower cut off)
- Perform a CT chest-abdo-pelvis AP for staging of the disease and an MRI pelvis
- Management involves a combination of surgery and chemotherapy depending on the stage and functional status of the patient

Surgery (debulking) is offered if it is felt all the disease can be removed (complete cytoreduction). Surgery entails total hysterectomy, bilateral salpingo-oophorectomy, omentectomy and removal of any other sites of disease +/- lymphadenectomy.
- Women with suspected or confirmed early-stage disease will undergo surgery.

Where complete or optimal cytoreduction is not possible, neo-adjuvant chemotherapy (before surgery) is given which comprises of carboplatin and paclitaxel (first-line).
- If surgery is after 3 cycles of chemotherapy (interval debulking), a further 3 cycles of chemotherapy are usually given.
- If surgery is after 6 cycles of chemotherapy (delayed debulking), no further chemotherapy is usually given.

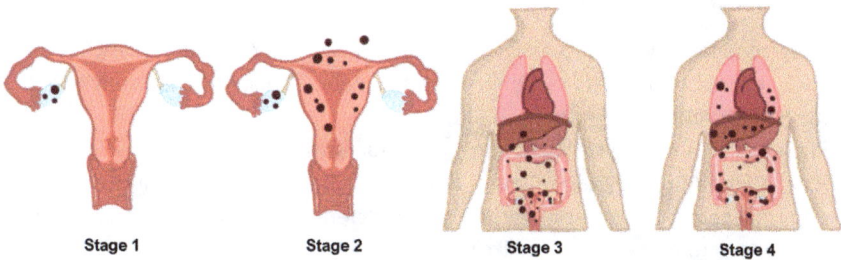

Stage 1   Stage 2   Stage 3   Stage 4

After surgery, patients can be started on additional drugs to prevent recurrence:
- Anti-angiogenic agents e.g. bevacizumab – this is a monoclonal antibody that targets vascular endothelial growth factor (VEGF), stopping tumour angiogenesis.
- PARP inhibitors (e.g. olaparib) have revolutionised ovarian cancer management.
- They inhibit DNA repair mechanisms and so are especially effective in ovarian cancer patients who have cancers which have errors in DNA repair genes, known as homologous recombination deficiency. As the cancer cells cannot repair DNA damage, they die (allowing targeted treatments to the cancer cell).

- **Ovarian cysts (benign)**

This refers to the presence of cysts which do not metastasise to other organs.

- Most of these are asymptomatic but can give similar symptoms to ovarian cancer.
- They can also cause acute complications e.g. rupture, torsion, infection.

Key tests

- This uses the same pathway as for ovarian cancer
- The CA-125 and ultrasound scan are used to calculate the RMI
- If a premenopausal woman has simple cyst on US, a CA-125 is not needed
- CA-125 can give false positives as the level will be raised by conditions such as fibroids, pelvic infection, endometriosis and adenomyosis
- In postmenopausal women, there is a greater risk of malignancy so both CA-125 and USS are performed

Management

- If RMI indicates high risk of malignancy, management is as ovarian cancer (above)
- The management of benign cysts depends on the size and the menopausal status of the women (according RCOG guidelines)

In pre-menopausal women, the management depends on the size of the cyst:
- Physiological/simple cysts < 50 mm – no follow-up (usually self-resolve within 2–3 menstrual cycles)
- Physiological/simple cysts 50–70 mm – yearly follow-up
- Physiological/simple cysts > 70 mm – further imaging (MRI) +/- surgical intervention
- Cysts that persist or increase in size are usually offered surgical intervention (cystectomy or oophorectomy) as they are unlikely to be simple

In post-menopausal women:
- If asymptomatic, simple and < 5 cm, reassess cyst in 4–6 months (CA-125, TVUS)
- Can discharge after 1 year if cyst is stable/reduces in size and CA-125 is normal
- If symptomatic, non-simple or > 5 cm, offer surgical removal with open/laparoscopic bilateral salpingo-oophorectomy

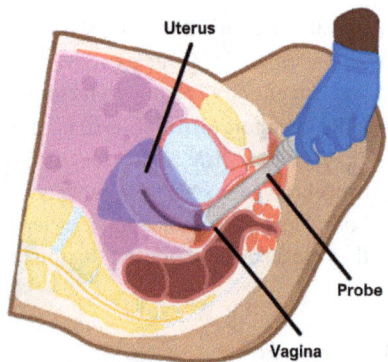

Uterus

Probe

Vagina

- **Ovarian torsion**

This is a condition when the ovary twists on its supporting ligaments (infundibulopelvic and utero-ovarian).

- It is a gynaecological emergency which reduces the blood supply to the ovary resulting in ischaemia.

Risk factors

- Ovarian mass > 5 cm (more likely to be benign)
- Ovulation induction (e.g. IVF)

Symptoms

- Sudden onset of sharp, intermittent, unilateral lower quadrant abdominal pain
- Nausea and vomiting
- There may also be a low-grade pyrexia (if the ovary is necrotic)

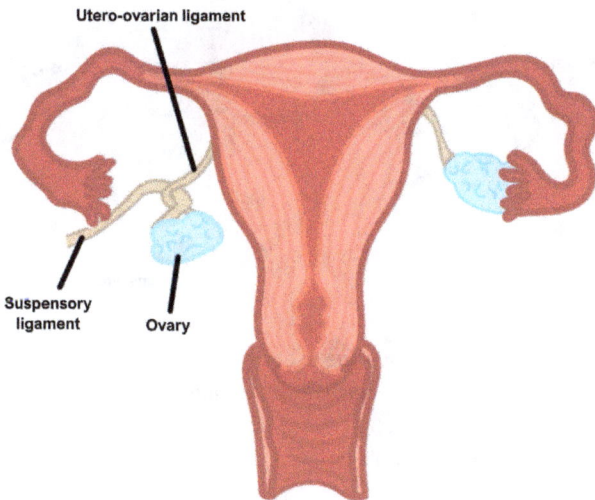

Utero-ovarian ligament

Suspensory ligament

Ovary

Key tests

- Transvaginal ultrasound – shows unilateral ovarian enlargement, oedema, "whirlpool" sign (twisted ovarian pedicle). However, the ovary may not be torted at the time of ultrasound so ultrasound cannot be used to rule out ovarian torsion
- Laparoscopy is diagnostic

Management

- Emergency laparoscopy to untwist the torted ovary +/- cystectomy if cyst is present

- **Polycystic ovary syndrome (PCOS)**

This is a condition of unknown cause which is associated with hormonal abnormalities and ovarian dysfunction.
- In this syndrome, increased insulin resistance results in hyperinsulinemia.
- The hyperinsulinemia, coupled with increased LH production by the anterior pituitary gland, leads to excessive androgen production by theca cells of the ovaries.
- In addition, hyperinsulinemia causes reduced production of sex-hormone binding globulin in the liver, which results in higher levels of free testosterone.
- High androgens lead to disordered follicle development and prevent ovulation.
- Instead, follicles remain in the ovaries leading to the development of multiple cysts.

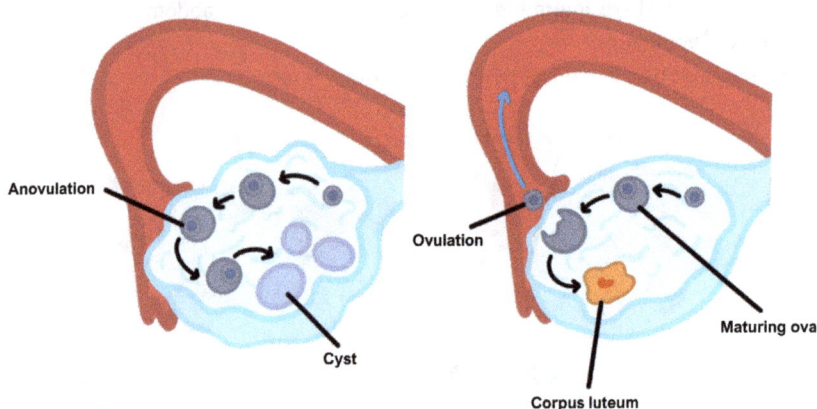

Anovulation
Cyst
Ovulation
Corpus luteum
Maturing ova

Symptoms

- Oligomenorrhoea and subfertility – due to anovulation
- Hirsutism, acne – due to excessive circulating androgens
- Weight gain, difficulty losing weight – due to insulin resistance
- May also cause psychological problems like depression

Complications

- Increased risk of T2DM, hypertension, and cardiovascular disease
- Increased risk of endometrial hyperplasia and carcinoma – as ovulation does not occur, ovarian oestrogen production remains high, causing endometrial hyperplasia

Key tests

- Blood tests show high total and free testosterone, low sex hormone binding globulin, high LH, normal FSH (LH:FSH ratio often > 3), high lipids and cholesterol
- Impaired glucose tolerance test
- Ultrasound – polycystic ovaries have 12+ follicles or an increased volume > 10 cm^3

Diagnosis
- PCOS should be diagnosed according to the Rotterdam criteria
- It is diagnosed if the patient has at least 2 out of:
i) Polycystic ovaries on USS
ii) Oligo or anovulation
iii) Clinical or biochemical signs of hyperandrogenism

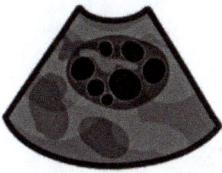

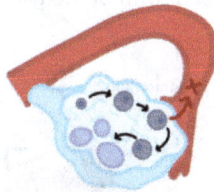

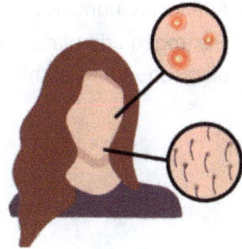

Management
- Weight loss helps to reduce hyperinsulinism, hyperandrogenism and restores menstrual regularity to improve fertility
- Metformin can also be used to reduce insulin resistance

For oligo/amenorrhoea
- If < 1 period every 3 months, can give medroxyprogesterone to induce a bleed
- Refer for TVUS to assess endometrial thickness (to check for hyperplasia/cancer)
- If the endometrium is normal, give treatment to prevent endometrial hyperplasia
- Options include cyclical progesterone (e.g. medroxyprogesterone), COCP, IUS

For hirsutism
- 1st line is the COCP (also helps to stop acne and regulated the menstrual cycle)
- Advice on hair removal methods
- Topical eflornithine is an option for facial hirsutism

For subfertility
- Ovulation induction agents such as clomiphene citrate or letrozole

Uterine Conditions

● **Endometrial cancer**

This refers to a cancer of the cells lining of the uterus.

- The most common type is an adenocarcinoma which is a malignant proliferation of the endometrial glands, which is associated with higher oestrogen levels.
- It usually occurs in post-menopausal women who present with uterine bleeding.
- Adenocarcinoma is preceded by hyperplasia of the glands, stimulated by oestrogen.
- Oestrogen stimulates endometrial growth of the glands whereas progesterone stimulates shedding of this tissue.

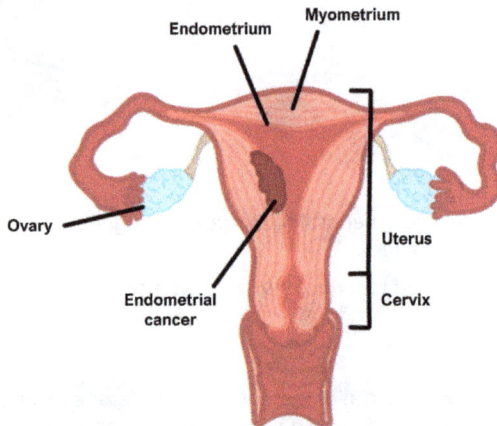

The hyperplasia of the glands is subdivided into two types:

- Endometrial hyperplasia without atypia – this carries a low risk of progression to cancer (< 5% over 20 years)
- Endometrial hyperplasia with atypia – this is characterised by disorganisation of glands, a high gland: stroma ratio. This carries a much higher risk of progression to cancer (27.5% after 19 years)

Endometrial carcinomas have been divided into two types:
- Type I – this includes the majority of endometrial cancers.
- It is composed mostly of endometrioid adenocarcinomas.

- Type II – these are mainly serous carcinomas, oestrogen independent.
- When compared to type I tumours, they are less well differentiated and carry a poorer prognosis.

Risk factors

- Early menarche/late menopause
- Obesity
- Infertility with anovulatory cycles
- Nulliparity
- Oestrogen only HRT
- Tamoxifen
- Polycystic ovarian syndrome
- Lynch syndrome

Protective factors

- COCP, parity, breastfeeding, smoking

Symptoms

- Abnormal uterine bleeding – usually present with post-menopausal bleeding (bleeding 1 year after the last menstrual period)
- In premenopausal women it can present as a change in menstrual bleeding or inter-menstrual bleeding
- Pyometra (pus in endometrial cavity)
- Advanced or metastatic disease may present with fatigue, weight loss, rectal bleeding, haemoptysis

Key tests

- Vaginal examination to assess the cervix, uterus and ovaries
- 1st line imaging is transvaginal ultrasound – used to measure endometrial thickness
- It also looks for free fluid, heterogeneity and invasion of the endo/myometrium
- A Pipelle biopsy is also used to obtain a sample from the endometrium
- If thickness < 4 mm, no further investigations required in the absence of any irregularity of the endometrial profile (such as presence of fluid, difference in endometrial thickness measurements) unless there is recurrent bleeding
- If thickness > 4 mm (post-menopause) or > 7 mm (premenopause), go to 2nd step
- 2nd step is hysteroscopy for direct visualisation of the uterine cavity and biopsy

Management

If hyperplasia without atypia there is a low risk of cancerous progression

- 1st line is manage risk factors e.g. obesity, HRT use
- If it is possible to reverse risk factors, can observe and follow up with repeat endometrial biopsies

If a failure to regress or symptomatic abnormal uterine bleeding
- 1st line is progesterone treatment with Mirena coil (LNG-IUS)
- 2nd line is oral progestogens (medroxyprogesterone or norethisterone)
- Repeat endometrial biopsy is recommended at a minimum of 6 monthly intervals and two 6 monthly negative biopsies are required prior to considering discharge

If hyperplasia with atypia, there is a high risk of cancerous progression
- If post-menopausal, hysterectomy and bilateral salpingo-oophorectomy
- If pre-menopausal, hysterectomy and salpingectomy with ovarian conservation
- If pre-menopausal and wanting to maintain fertility, can use the progesterone coil to induce regression (review every 3 months until ×2 negative biopsies)
- Once fertility is no longer required, offer hysterectomy and bilateral salpingectomy

If adenocarcinoma confirmed, the FIGO staging system is used to guide treatment
- Stage I – disease confined to uterus
- Stage II – disease extends to the cervix
- Stage III – disease with local or regional spread (adnexa, vagina, parametria, pelvic or para-aortic lymph nodes)
- Stage IV – spread to the bladder, bowel or distant metastasis e.g. lung, liver

Surgical options include a total hysterectomy with bilateral salpingo-oophorectomy and sentinel lymph node sampling.
- For later stages, debulking palliative surgery can play a role in symptom relief.

Additional treatment options include radiotherapy, vaginal brachytherapy as well as chemotherapy.
- This is dependent on the stage and grade of the endometrial cancer, the fitness of the patient and should be discussed in an MDT setting.

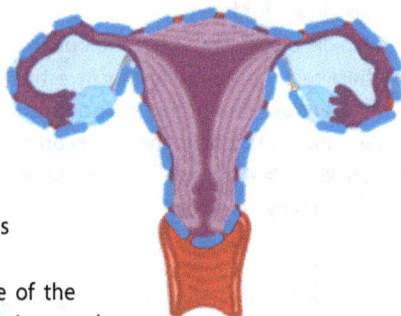

NICE referral guidelines
Urgent (2 weeks): if age > 55 with post-menopausal bleeding

- **Adenomyosis**

This is a condition in which the endometrium (lining of the uterus) is present within the myometrium (muscle layer) of the uterus.
- Although misplaced, it is functional (thickens, sheds, bleeds during menstrual cycle).
- The cause is unknown, but it may be related to a break between the myometrial and endometrial barrier. It is typically seen in multiparous women aged 40–50 years old.

Risk factors

- Uterine trauma – multiparity, surgery
- Increased age

Symptoms

- Dysmenorrhoea
- Menorrhagia
- Enlarged, boggy uterus

Key tests

- Transvaginal ultrasound or MRI

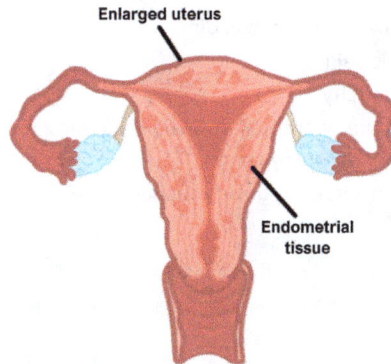

Management

- Non-hormonal – tranexamic acid to relieve menorrhagia, NSAIDs (mefenamic acid)
- Hormonal – COCP, oral progestogens, Mirena, GnRH agonists (Zoladex) to induce temporary menopause
- Medical – uterus-conserving (e.g. endometrial ablation, uterine artery embolisation)
- Surgical options include a hysterectomy

- **Fibroids (leiomyomas)**

These are benign tumours of the uterine wall which are composed of smooth muscle.

Fibroids are classified according to their wall position.
- Intramural – these develop completely within the myometrium and do not extend into the uterine or peritoneal cavity.
- Submucosal – these develop in the inner aspect of myometrium (under the inner mucosa) and extend into the uterine cavity; may impact fertility.
- Subserosal – these develop in the outer aspect of the myometrium (under the serosa) and extend into the peritoneal cavity.
- Pedunculated – these grow on a stalk either in to or outside of the uterine cavity.

Risk factors

- Advancing age, early menarche, obesity
- Ethnicity (more common in black and Asian women)

Symptoms

- Can by asymptomatic
- Heavy menstrual bleeding
- Pelvic pain
- Subfertility
- Pressure symptoms – urinary frequency, bloating, constipation
- A firm, large, irregularly shaped uterus on bimanual exam

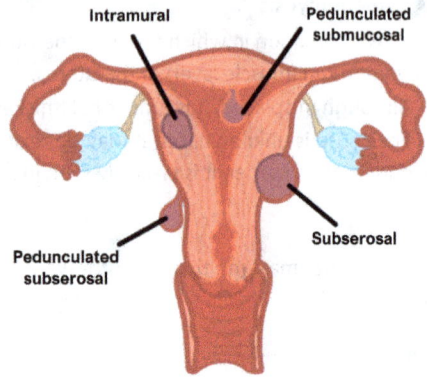

They can cause red degeneration
- This refers to ischaemia, infarction and necrosis that usually occurs during pregnancy (2nd and 3rd trimester)
- It leads to heavy bleeding and acute pelvic pain

Key tests

- Transvaginal ultrasound is the diagnostic test

Management

- To reduce bleeding, 1st line is insertion of a Mirena (progesterone coil)
- If the coil is not suitable – COCP, oral progestogen
- Mefenamic acid for analgesia and bleeding
- Tranexamic acid can also be used to reduce bleeding

To reduce the fibroid size, GnRH analogues (Zoladex), can only be used for 6 months due to osteoporosis risk. Therefore, they are often used pre-operatively.
- Uterine artery embolisation reduces blood flow causing fibroids to reduce in size.
- However, this is not suitable for women wanting future pregnancies.

If symptoms are not controlled with medical management, surgical options include:
- Hysteroscopic resection of fibroids – can be used for submucosal fibroids.
- Myomectomy – if the woman wishes to preserve her fertility.
- Hysterectomy is the most effective way of preventing recurrence.

- **Asherman's syndrome**

This refers to the development of intrauterine adhesions.

- It is mostly caused by procedures performed on the uterus, such as surgical management of miscarriage, termination of pregnancy, surgical treatment of retained placenta but also by polypectomy, fibroid surgery.
- It is caused by damage to the basal layer of the endometrium in opposing areas leading to formation of adhesions.

Symptoms

- Amenorrhoea/lighter periods as adhesion tissue does not respond to oestrogen
- Dysmenorrhoea occurs due to menstrual flow being obstructed by the adhesions
- Can lead to infertility

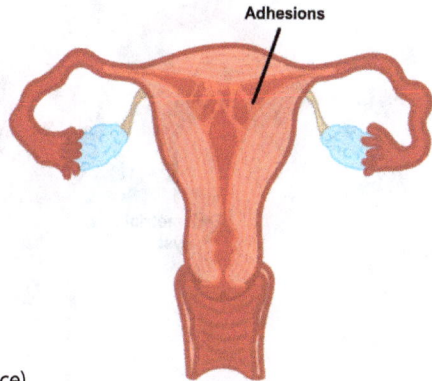

Key tests

- Hysteroscopy is the gold standard (ultrasound is not as useful in this instance)

Management

- Surgical excision of the adhesions

- **Endometriosis**

A condition characterised by growth of endometrial tissue outside the uterine cavity.

- The deposits are mostly found within the pelvis (e.g. ovaries, pouch of Douglas, bladder, rectum) but in rare cases may be seen in extra-pelvic locations like the diaphragm and pleural cavity.
- As endometrial tissue responds to oestrogen, symptoms vary with the menstrual cycle (as with the endometrial lining of the uterus).
- At the time of menstruation there may be bleeding at the location of the ectopic tissue which can lead to pain and inflammation at these sites in a cyclical fashion.
- It results in subfertility, potentially due to the altered pelvic anatomy.

Symptoms

- Pain – chronic pelvic pain (> 6 months), dysmenorrhea
- Deep dyspareunia (pain during intercourse)
- GI symptoms – dyschezia (difficulty passing stool)

- Urinary symptoms – dysuria, haematuria
- Subfertility
- On examination there may be reduced organ mobility, enlargement and tender nodules in posterior vaginal fornix

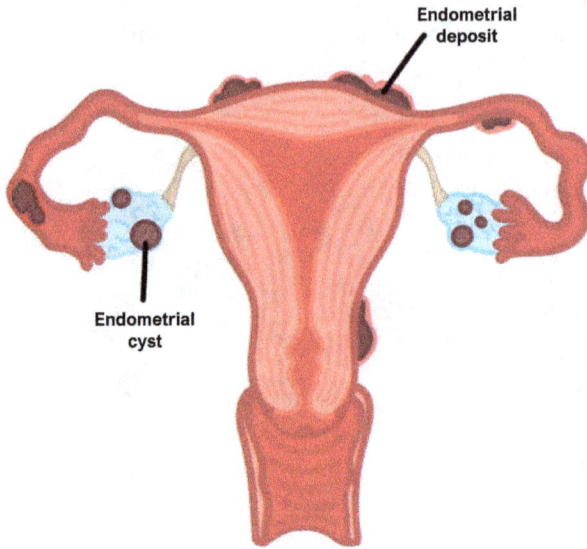

Endometrial deposit

Endometrial cyst

Key tests
- Transvaginal ultrasound can show endometriomas, though a negative scan does not rule out endometriosis
- Pelvic MRI for deep, infiltrating endometriosis
- Laparoscopy is gold standard for diagnosis

Management
- Pain management with the following which can be trialled in primary care
- NSAIDs and/or paracetamol
- Hormonal treatment such as COCP, progestogens (pill, implant, injection), LNG-IUS

If these are ineffective, not tolerated or contraindicated, refer to gynaecology
- GnRH agonists may be given in the short-term to induce temporary menopause (also given pre-operatively)
- Surgical treatment involves laparoscopic excision +/- ablation of endometriosis
- Surgical interventions can improve the chance of spontaneous pregnancy

Cervical Conditions

- **Cervical ectropion**

This is a condition in which simple columnar epithelium (lining the endocervix) is present on the ectocervix. It is a normal variant in women of reproductive age.

- Columnar epithelium is more fragile than the stratified squamous epithelium that usually lines the ectocervix and so may bleed after sexual intercourse.
- Ectropion can also lead to increased vaginal discharge as the simple columnar cells are mucus-producing.
- It is diagnosed after ruling out other more sinister pathologies like cervical cancer.

Causes

- Raised oestrogen levels (e.g. pregnancy, COCP)

Symptoms

- Mostly asymptomatic
- Post-coital bleeding
- An increase in vaginal discharge
- Pain/bleeding during cervical screening

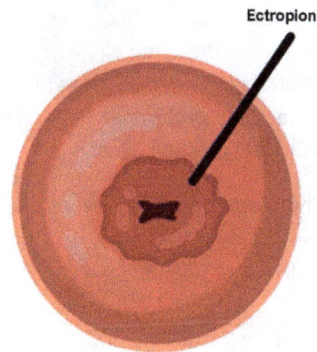

Ectropion

Key tests

- Speculum examination – red, velvety area on the ectocervix
- Triple swabs to rule out infection
- Smear +/- colposcopy to rule out CIN/cervical cancer

Management

- It usually does not require treatment unless it is symptomatic
- Stop underlying causes e.g. oestrogen containing contraception e.g. COCP
- Can offer silver nitrate cauterisation or electrocautery of the columnar epithelium

- **Cervical polyps**

These are benign growths on the cervix which result from epithelial hyperplasia.
- Most cases are benign (malignant in up to 1.5% of cases).

Symptoms

- Normally asymptomatic and discovered incidentally
- Abnormal vaginal bleeding (menorrhagia, IMB, PCB, PMB) and discharge

Key tests
- Swabs and smear to rule out infection and dysplasia

Management
- Remove polyp and send for histological evaluation to exclude malignancy

- **Cervical cancer**

This refers to an invasive carcinoma of cells in the lining of the cervix.
- It is usually seen in sexually active women aged between 30–45 years of age, although prevalence is increasing in the 25–29 years of age category.

Cervical cancer is typically preceded by cervical intraepithelial neoplasia (CIN).
- CIN describes premalignant dysplasia of the cervical epithelium.
- This is primarily due to the human papilloma virus (HPV) and most frequently occurs at the squamocolumnar junction of the cervix.
- CIN is characterised by nuclear changes and increased mitosis.

The proportion of the cervical epithelium consisting of the dysplastic cells determines the CIN grade:
- CIN 1 is < 1/3rd
- CIN 2 is 1/3rd – 2/3rd
- CIN 3 is > 2/3rd

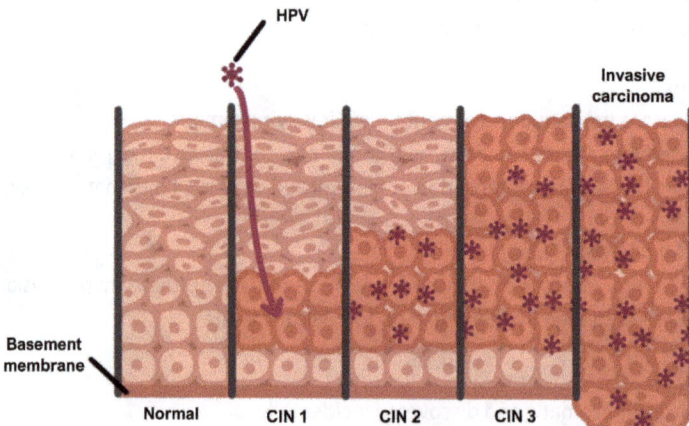

CIN classically progresses in stepwise fashion. CIN 1 can regress spontaneously whilst CIN 3 tends to require treatment to avoid progression to cancer.

Risk factors

- The main risk factor is infection with human papilloma virus (HPV) types 16 and 18
- These viruses make the proteins E6 (interferes with tumour protein p53) and E7 (interferes with retinoblastoma protein) which increases the risk of cancer
- Factors which increase the risk of HPV infection – multiple sexual partners, young age of first sexual intercourse, coinfection with other genital infections
- Factors which directly increase the risk of cancer – immunosuppressed patients (AIDS), smoking, inadequate cervical screening, COCP use

Symptoms

- Most cases of CIN asymptomatic and detected on screening
- If symptomatic, cervical screening (commonly called "smears") can be done out of the standard 3–5 yearly programme
- Can cause intermenstrual bleeding, postcoital bleeding, postmenopausal bleeding
- Blood-stained, mucoid or purulent vaginal discharge
- Dyspareunia

Vaccination

- Vaccination against HPV has been offered to all girls in school year 8 since September 2008 and all boys in school year 8 since September 2019 in the UK
- The vaccine currently used (since July 2022) is Gardasil 9 which protects against HPV types 6, 11, 16, 18, 31, 33, 45, 52 and 58

Screening

- There is currently a cervical screening programme for women aged 25–64
- A brush is inserted into the cervical os to obtain a sample of cells
- The best time to take a smear test is mid-cycle (bleeding may invalidate the smear)
- Women aged 25–49 years are offered 3-yearly screening and those aged 50–64 years are screened 5-yearly in England and Northern Ireland

Cancerous tissue

- The sample is screened for the presence of high-risk variants of HPV (hrHPV)
- If this is positive, cytological examination of the cells is automatically carried out on the same sample

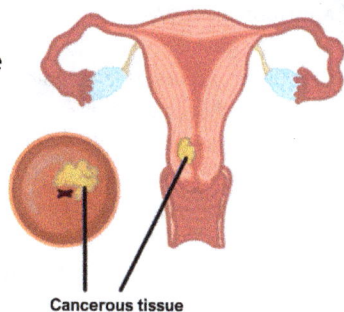

The results of the smear test can be:

i) Inadequate – due to problems and so should repeat the smear test within 3 months
- If you have 2 consecutive inadequate samples, refer for colposcopy

ii) Patient is hrHPV negative – return to routine 3-year screening or 5-year screening

iii) Patient is hrHPV positive with negative cytology – repeat cervical screening in 12 months

iv) Patient is hrHPV positive and positive cytology – refer for colposcopy

Cytological results include borderline changes, low-grade dyskaryosis, high-grade dyskaryosis, invasive squamous cell carcinoma and glandular neoplasia.

Key tests
- Colposcopy and biopsy are used to definitively measure the degree of CIN
- If there is a high suspicion of high-grade disease from cytology and colposcopy, the patient may be offered treatment at the time of colposcopy appointment

Management
- CIN 1 – surveillance with review in colposcopy clinic
- CIN 2 – may offer large loop excision of transformation zone (LLETZ) or surveillance depending on individual circumstances
- CIN 3 – LLETZ

Large loop excision of the transformation zone (LLETZ)
This is a procedure that removes abnormal cells from the cervix.
- Short term risks include bleeding, infection and pain.
- Long term risks include pre-term labour/cervical incompetence (depends on number of LLETZ procedures and amount of cervix removed), cervical stenosis.

For invasive carcinoma, treatment depends on the stage and whether the patient wants to preserve their fertility.
- For early-stage cancers, they can be managed surgically, e.g. radical hysterectomy, bilateral salpingectomy +/- oophorectomy and pelvic lymphadenectomy.
- Later stage cancers will require surgery and chemo-radiotherapy.

Vaginal Conditions

- **Bartholin's abscess**

This is an abscess which forms on the Bartholin's glands.

- These are located slightly posterior to the left and right of the opening of the vagina.
- A cyst can arise when one of the ducts carrying fluid from the gland becomes blocked, forming a fluid filled lump.
- The cyst can then become infected by bacteria, leading to the formation of a Bartholin's abscess.
- They generally occur in women of reproductive age.

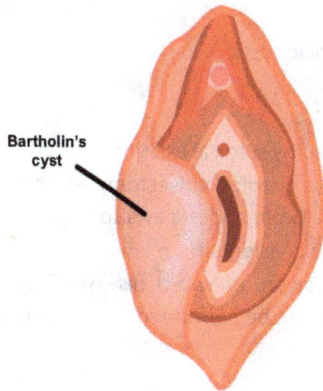

Bartholin's cyst

Symptoms

- Vaginal pain and redness
- Unilateral swelling near the vaginal introitus

Key tests

- Usually diagnosed clinically by physical examination

Management

- 1st line is antibiotics
- If abscess does not respond or is very painful, cyst drainage can be performed (using word catheter or marsupialisation)

- **Vulval carcinoma**

This describes a rare type of carcinoma which affects part or all of the vulva, usually the outer labia. Approximately 90% of these are squamous cell carcinomas.

- It is mostly seen in elderly women with incidence highest in those > 90 years of age.

Risk factors

- HPV infection
- Inflammation, secondary to lichen sclerosus and lichen planus

Symptoms

- Vulval lump, ulceration or bleeding
- An irregular fungating mass
- Might have palpable groin nodes

Key tests

- Physical examination
- Incisional tissue biopsy is diagnostic

Carcinoma

Management

- Small tumours are managed by surgical excision
- Larger tumours may require a radical vulvectomy +/- excision of other structures e.g. urethra +/- reconstruction. Groin nodes may also require removal
- Chemoradiotherapy can be considered
- Surgery is rarely considered in advanced disease (Stage IV – distant metastases) although palliative surgery can be performed for symptomatic relief

- **Atrophic vaginitis**

This refers to thinning of the vaginal epithelium due to low oestrogen levels.

- It typically occurs in 50% post-menopausal women, where low oestrogen is a natural physiological result of menopause.
- It is almost always secondary to menopause due to declining oestrogen levels, but can also be caused by breastfeeding and anti-oestrogen medication.

Symptoms

- Vaginal dryness, burning or itching
- Superficial dyspareunia
- Spotting or postcoital bleeding (any postmenopausal bleeding needs checking for endometrial cancer)
- Urgency, urethral pain, recurrent UTIs

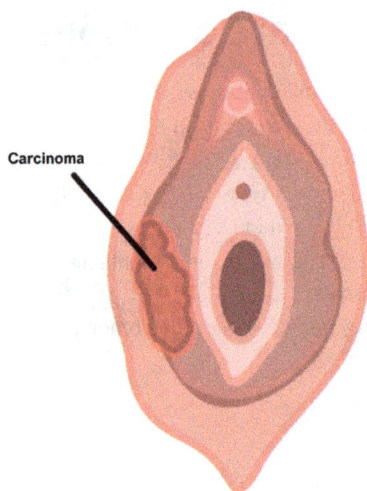

Key tests

- Clinical examination is diagnostic – the vagina shows fissuring and signs of friction
- These include reduced subcutaneous fat with lower volume of mons pubis, labia majora, labia minora and inflammation with erythematous patches +/- petechiae

Management

- Vaginal lubricants and moisturisers for symptomatic relief
- Intravaginal oestrogen (cream, tablets, ring) with a tapering down dose

- **Female genital mutilation (FGM)**

The world health organisation defines FGM as "the partial or total removal of external female genitalia or other injury to the female genital organs for non-medical reasons".
- It is practiced in multiple African countries (Somalia, Guinea and Djibouti having the highest prevalence) as well as in some Middle Eastern and Asian countries.
- FGM can be classified into 4 types.

Type	Description
1	Partial or total removal of the clitoral glans and/or the prepuce/hood (clitoridectomy)
2	Partial or total removal of the clitoris and labia minora +/- removal of the labia majora
3	Infibulation: the narrowing of the vaginal opening through the creation of a covering seal by cutting and appositioning the labia minor +/- with or without excision of the clitoris
4	All other harmful procedures to the female genitalia for non-medical purposes (e.g. pricking, piercing, incising)

Short term complications

- Pain and bleeding
- Infection
- Urinary retention
- Genital swelling

Long term complications

- Scar tissue formation
- Genital infection – increased risk of bacterial vaginosis, HSV

- Menstrual – haematocolpos, dysmenorrhoea
- Sexual – dyspareunia, reduced satisfaction
- Urinary – dysuria, UTIs
- Obstetric – perineal trauma, prolonged labour, postpartum haemorrhage
- Psychological – depression, anxiety, PTSD

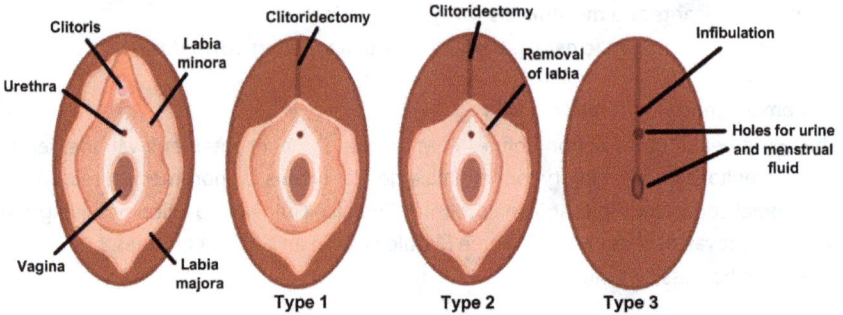

The Female Genital Mutilation Act 2003 in England, Wales & Northern Ireland states the following:

1. It is illegal unless it is a surgical operation on a girl/woman irrespective of her age:
(a) which is necessary for her physical or mental health.
(b) she is in any stage of labour, or has just given birth, for purposes connected with the labour or birth.

2. It is illegal to arrange, or assist in arranging, for a UK national or UK resident to be taken overseas for the purpose of FGM.

3. It is an offence for those with parental responsibility to fail to protect a girl from the risk of FGM.

4. If FGM is confirmed in a girl under 18 years of age (either on examination or because the patient or parent says it has been done), reporting to the police is mandatory and this must be within 1 month of confirmation.

Management
- As a resident doctor, if you suspect a case of FGM, you should escalate to your senior and raise a safeguarding referral

Menstrual Conditions

- **Premenstrual syndrome (PMS)**

This describes the distressing physical, psychological and behavioural symptoms that occur during the luteal phase of the menstrual cycle and affect daily functioning.

- PMS encompasses a whole spectrum of severity from mild to debilitating.
- The aetiology is unknown, but it may be related to progesterone sensitivity or the neurotransmitters serotonin and γ-aminobutyric acid (GABA).

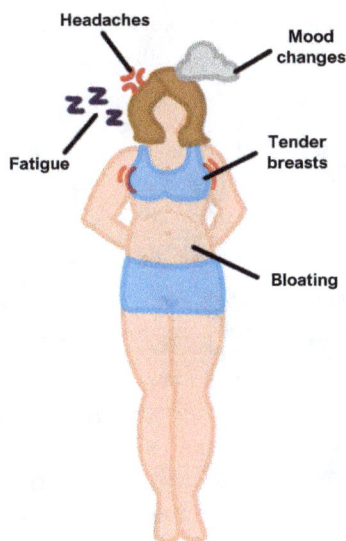

Headaches

Mood changes

Fatigue

Tender breasts

Bloating

Symptoms

- Psychological – depression, anxiety, irritability
- Physical – fatigue, bloating, mastalgia

Key tests

- It is a clinical diagnosis. It can help to use a symptom diary over two cycles (daily Record of Severity of Problems is widely used)

Management

- Conservative – exercise, smoking cessation, regular sleep and sleep reduction
- Complementary treatments include multivitamins and CBT
- Medical management includes the COCP (usually 1st line), as well as SSRIs (taken continuously or during the luteal phase)
- If symptoms unresolving, options include the oestrogen patch, GnRH analogues and surgery (bilateral salpingo-oophorectomy with or without hysterectomy)

- **Menorrhagia**

This refers to excessive menstrual blood loss that occurs regularly and interferes with a woman's quality of life. In up to 50% of women no underlying cause is found – this is known as dysfunctional uterine bleeding.

- Menorrhagia can also occur secondary to other underlying causes.

Causes

- Uterine – endometriosis, adenomyosis, fibroids, PID, endometrial cancer
- Iatrogenic – copper IUD
- Endocrine – PCOS, hypothyroidism, hyperprolactinaemia
- Haematological – anticoagulants, coagulopathy

Key tests

- Physical examination to assess for any obvious abnormalities
- Bloods with FBC to check for iron-deficiency anaemia due to excessive bleeding

NICE advises that the investigation for the cause depends on the presentation:

i) If menorrhagia with low risk of fibroids, uterine cavity abnormality, endometriosis or adenomyosis, you can start treatment without further investigation

ii) If menorrhagia and intermenstrual bleeding, pelvic pain or pressure symptoms, this suggest an underlying pathology so additional investigations are recommended:

- If hypothyroidism suspected – thyroid function tests
- If coagulation disorder suspected (suspect if menorrhagia since menarche and family/ personal history suggesting coagulation disorder) – do a coagulation screen
- If infection suspected – vaginal or cervical swab
- If structural uterine cause suspected (e.g. fibroids) – refer for USS +/- hysteroscopy

Management

- If an underlying cause is found, correct the underlying cause
- If no cause found, 1st line is the LNG-IUS (progesterone coil)
- 2nd line hormonal options include the COCP or cyclical oral progestogen
- Non-hormonal options include tranexamic acid or NSAID (mefenamic acid)
- If persistent, can consider uterine artery embolisation
- Surgical interventions include endometrial ablation or a hysterectomy

- **Dysmenorrhoea**

This term refers to excessive amount of pain experienced during the menstrual cycle.
- It is sub-classified into 2 types:

○ **Primary dysmenorrhoea**

This refers to excessive pain without an underlying organic pathology.
- The onset is usually in adolescence, about 6–24 months after menarche.
- It is thought to be related to excessive endometrial prostaglandin synthesis during the menstrual cycle.

Symptoms

- Cramping lower abdominal pain which can radiate to the back or down the thigh
- Pain starts just before/within a few hours of the period starting
- The pain usually improves later in the period
- The pain may be accompanied by other symptoms including nausea, vomiting, fatigue, headache and emotional symptoms

Management

- 1st line NSAIDs (these inhibit prostaglandin synthesis) +/- paracetamol
- 2nd line is hormonal contraceptives e.g. COCP, LNG-IUS

○ **Secondary dysmenorrhoea**

This refers to excessive pain due to an underlying anatomical or pelvic pathology.
- It occurs any time after menarche, normally after years of normal, painless periods.

Causes

- Endometriosis, adenomyosis
- Pelvic inflammatory disease, fibroids, IUD

Symptoms

- Painful periods during the menstrual cycle
- There will also be accompanying symptoms of the underlying pathology

Management

- Identify underlying cause and treat accordingly

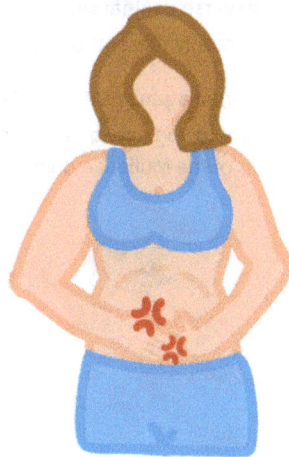

- **Amenorrhoea**

This is defined as the absence of a normal period. It is typically divided into two types.

○ **Primary amenorrhea**

This is defined by the absence of menarche (first period) by the age of 15 in the presence of secondary sexual characteristics (such as pubic hair growth) or the age of 13 in the absence of secondary sexual characteristics.

Constitutional delay refers to a delay in pubertal development, but it is not pathological, and normal maturation usually occurs by 18 years of age.
- In constitutional delay, there is often a family history of late puberty/menarche.
- It occurs more commonly in boys and is a diagnosis of exclusion.

There are many pathological causes of primary amenorrhea:

Outflow tract anomalies

These conditions are associated with a structural anomaly which results in the lack of a normal period. They are characterised by normal hormonal levels (normal FSH, normal oestrogen levels) and pubertal development.

▪ **Imperforate hymen**

This may cause amenorrhoea with cyclical pelvic pain (as the endometrium builds up but cannot shed via the vagina).

▪ **Transverse vaginal septum**

This commonly presents as cyclical pelvic pain due to haematocolpos.

▪ **Mullerian agenesis (Mayer-Rokitansky-Küster-Hauser, MRKH syndrome)**

This refers to vaginal agenesis (to varying degrees) and the absence of a uterus due to agenesis of the Mullerian duct.

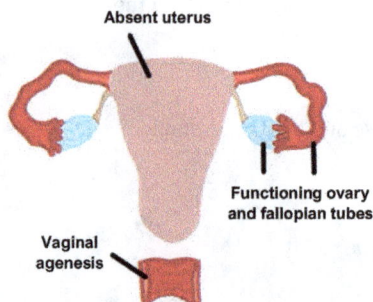

Absent uterus

Functioning ovary
and fallopian tubes

Vaginal
agenesis

Primary ovarian insufficiency

This refers to a primary problem with the ovaries, which results in low oestrogen levels and as a consequence absent secondary sexual characteristics.
- The FSH levels will be high due to lack of negative feedback.

- **Genetic abnormalities**
- Turner syndrome (45XO) – a syndrome characterised by having only one X chromosome, which causes ovarian dysgenesis
- Swyer syndrome (46XY) – a condition where there is a mutation in the SRY gene, the sex-determining region of the Y chromosome. It produces phenotypic females with female external genitalia but non-functional "streak gonads"
- Pure gonadal dysgenesis (46XX) – females with non-functional streak ovaries
- Congenital adrenal hyperplasia – an autosomal recessive disease resulting from deficiency in an enzyme required for cortisol synthesis in the adrenal cortex
- In most cases, it is caused by partial deficiency of 21-hydroxylase which leads to precursor build up and androgen excess causing ambiguous genitalia in girls

- **Injury**
- Damage to the ovaries – secondary to chemotherapy, infection (mumps oophoritis)

Endocrine conditions

These conditions interfere with the hypothalamic-pituitary-adrenal axis, resulting in low FSH and oestrogen levels, which causes a lack of normal periods.

- **Hypothalamic causes**
- Functional – eating disorders, stress, malnutrition, excessive exercise
- Idiopathic hypogonadotrophic hypogonadism – about 60% present with anosmia, which is known as Kallman syndrome
- Tumours e.g. craniopharyngioma

- **Pituitary causes**
- Medications – antipsychotics such as phenothiazines, antidepressants such as mono-amine oxidase inhibitors, opiates
- Stalk compression or damage e.g. tumours

- **Other causes**
- Hormonal imbalance – hyperprolactinaemia, Cushing's, thyroid disease, PCOS

○ **Secondary amenorrhea**

This refers to the cessation of established regular menstruation for ≥ 6 months.
- Many conditions that cause secondary amenorrhoea also give primary amenorrhoea if they occur before menarche.
- Natural causes include pregnancy, breastfeeding and menopause.
- However, it can also occur due to pathological causes, which affect the hypothalamic-pituitary-adrenal axis and the reproductive organs including the ovaries and uterus.

Gynaecological causes

- Cervical stenosis
- Asherman's syndrome
- Hysterectomy, oophorectomy
- Premature ovarian failure
- Polycystic ovary syndrome

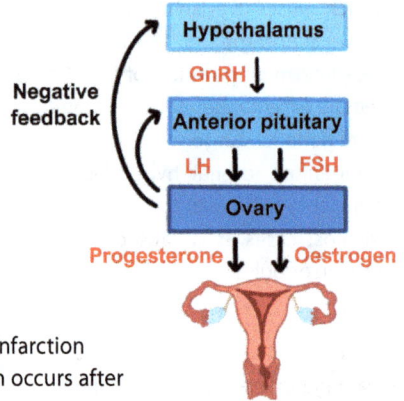

Endocrine causes

- Prolactinomas – prolactin suppresses GnRH secretion
- Sheehan syndrome – this refers to pituitary infarction due to massive obstetric haemorrhage which occurs after a complicated delivery
- Contraception – COCP taken continuously, progestogen implants/injections
- Endocrine conditions – hyper/hypothyroidism, Cushing's syndrome
- Hypothalamic amenorrhoea – dysfunction of the hypothalamus caused by factors such as excessive stress or excessive exercise which affects GnRH secretion
- Eating disorders – reduced calorie intake affects the HPA axis
- Chronic diseases – heart, kidney, liver disease, IBD all inhibit the hypothalamus

Key tests

- Primary amenorrhoea is usually referred to a specialist for investigations
- Pregnancy test
- Blood tests – sex hormones (FSH/LH, total testosterone levels), TFTs, prolactin
- Imaging includes transvaginal ultrasound to assess for structural causes
- Genetic tests and karyotyping are used to assess for genetic/chromosomal causes

Management

- Treat the underlying cause

Menopause

Menopause refers to the natural halting of the menstrual cycle due to depletion of ovarian follicles. It is defined as the cessation of menstruation for $\geq$ 12 months.
- The average age of menopause in the UK is 51.
- Perimenopause refers to the period of the final years of a woman's reproductive life.
- It begins with the onset of menstrual irregularity and ends after one year of amenorrhoea has occurred.

Each woman is born with a finite number of oocytes (ovarian reserve) and as women grow older, this reserve diminishes.
- In the perimenopausal period, declining follicle numbers result in reduced inhibin B which leads to increased FSH levels.
- Sustained high FSH causes an increase in cycle length variability due to normal length ovulatory cycles and superimposed ovulatory cycles (ovulations follow each other quickly with minimal follicular phase length).
- Declining levels of oestrogen result in more anovulatory cycles, giving irregular periods and menopausal symptoms.
- Eventually follicular development stops altogether and amenorrhoea occurs.
- Menopause is characterised by low oestrogen and high FSH and LH levels.

Symptoms
- Vasomotor – hot flushes, night sweats
- Psychogenic – mood changes, sleep disturbance, loss of concentration
- Urogenital – vaginal atrophy, decline in libido, pruritus, dyspareunia (pain during sexual intercourse), urinary frequency, urinary urgency
- Joint and muscle pain

Complications
- Osteoporosis – as oestrogen protects bone mass by reducing osteoclast activity
- Increased risk of ischaemic heart disease (IHD)
- Increased risk of dementia

Key tests
- Can be diagnosed clinically by the presence of symptoms and amenorrhoea
- Blood tests – high FSH and LH, low oestrogen levels

Management
- Lifestyle modifications include exercise, weight loss, sleep and stress reduction

Hormone replacement therapy (HRT)
- If vaginal symptoms only, can prescribe oestrogen topical gel
- If no uterus or IUS (coil), can prescribe oestrogen only HRT
- If they have a uterus, prescribe combined oestrogen and progesterone HRT
- If perimenopausal (last period < 1 year ago), use a cyclical regime
- If postmenopausal (last period > 1 year ago) use a continuous regime

HRT tablets are associated with a higher risk of VTE. This is often why in clinical practice, patches, gels and coils are offered.

If HRT is rejected or contraindicated, there are other options available.
- For vasomotor symptoms – options include SSRIs (paroxetine, citalopram), venlafaxine, gabapentin, pregabalin and clonidine
- Vaginal dryness – lubricant or moisturizer
- Mood disturbances – self-help groups, CBT, antidepressants

HRT (except the progesterone coil) does not work as a contraceptive.
- Therefore, to avoid pregnancy, contraception is still required until a woman is no longer considered fertile
- Women < 50 are considered potentially fertile for 2 years after their last period
- Women > 50 are considered potentially fertile for 1 year after their last period

- **Premature ovarian failure/premature ovarian insufficiency**
This is when menopause occurs before the age of 40 years.
- Causes include idiopathic, autoimmune (e.g. Hashimoto's thyroiditis), iatrogenic (e.g. chemotherapy, radiotherapy), genetic (e.g. Turner Syndrome).
- It causes similar symptoms to menopause.
- To be diagnosed, women should have menopausal symptoms and high FSH (on 2 blood samples taken 4–6 weeks apart).
- If there is diagnostic doubt, anti-Mullerian hormone (AMH) levels may be used, which is a more direct measure of ovarian reserve.
- Symptoms can also be managed with hormone replacement therapy.

Urogynaecology

- **Urinary incontinence**

This is defined as a "complaint of an involuntary loss of urine". Urinary incontinence is experienced by 10% of all women and more than 20% of women aged over 70 years.

There are different types of urinary incontinence:
- Stress urinary incontinence (SUI) – this is the involuntary leakage of urine due to increased intra-abdominal pressure e.g. sneezing, coughing.
- It is also associated with pregnancy and childbirth.

- Urge urinary incontinence (UUI) – this is the involuntary leakage of urine associated with a sense of urinary urgency due to detrusor overactivity.

- Mixed urinary incontinence – a mixture if SUI and UUI.

- Overflow urinary incontinence – the involuntary leakage of urine from an over-distended bladder due to bladder outlet obstruction or impaired detrusor contractility.

Risk factors

- Ageing
- Diet (caffeinated beverages)
- Constipation
- Exercise – lower levels are associated with a higher rates of SUI
- Obesity
- Surgery – hysterectomies increase the risk of SUI
- Parity – childbirth is associated with increasing incontinence symptoms

Key tests

- Abdominal examination to look for a palpable, enlarged bladder suggesting retention
- Vaginal/rectal examination – assess for pelvic organ prolapse and faecal impaction
- Urine dipstick and culture – this is to rule out a urinary tract infection
- Post-void residual bladder scan – assess for incomplete bladder emptying
- Bladder diaries – ask the patient to complete a bladder diary for a minimum of 3 days, allowing you to identify any triggers and how much fluid the patient drinks
- Cystoscopy – used to identify a structural cause of incontinence

Urodynamic studies are used to assess concerns regarding bladder filling/emptying.
- They consist of different tests which are typically performed together in one study.
- Cystometry – this is a measure of detrusor pressure during bladder filling and the capacity and compliance of the bladder.
- Electromyography – this measures the electrical activity of the pelvic floor muscles.
- Urethral pressure profile – this measures the competence of the urethra.
- Uroflowmetry – this measures the quantity and speed of the urine during voiding.
- Voiding pressure study – this measures the detrusor muscle pressure and resulting flow during urination.

The test involves catheters in the bladder and the rectum or vagina. Two common diagnoses on urodynamic studies are detrusor overactivity and SUI.

Detrusor overactivity (DO)
This is characterised by involuntary detrusor contractions during the filling stage.
- These contractions can be spontaneous or provoked.
- There will be a rise in the detrusor pressure due to increased intravesical pressure.
- The abdominal pressure remains stable.
- DO is associated with urgency but may or may not result in incontinence.

Stress incontinence
This is observed during filling or provocation.
- The leakage of urine accompanies an increase in abdominal pressure.
- The detrusor pressure remains stable.
- Provocations include cough or Valsalva causing a rise in abdominal pressure.

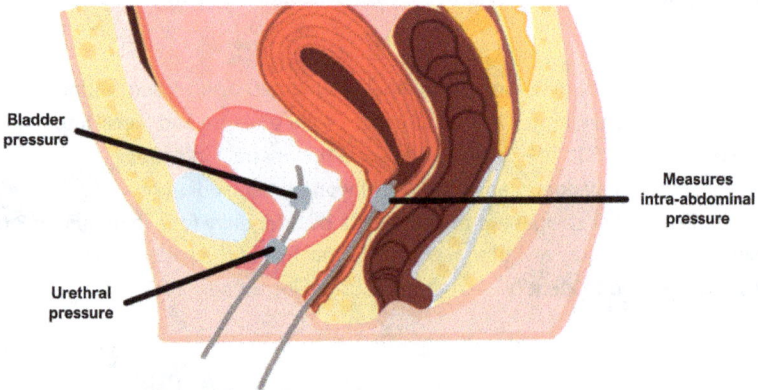

Management
- Common to all types of urinary incontinence – reduce caffeine, regulate fluid intake
- Weight loss (if BMI 30+), stop smoking and avoidance of constipation

For urge incontinence
- Conservative measures – bladder retraining (at least 6 weeks)
- Medical management – 1st line is anticholinergic medications e.g. oxybutynin (avoid in older women), tolterodine or solifenacin
- 2nd line is mirabegron (B$_3$ agonist) if antimuscarinics are contraindicated
- Desmopressin can be used specifically to reduce nocturnal polyuria
- Intravaginal oestrogens in postmenopausal women with UUI and vaginal atrophy

If the following are unsuccessful, consider surgical options.
- Intra-detrusor injection with botulinum toxin type A – side effects include urinary retention so patients must be aware of the potential need to self-catheterise
- Sacral nerve stimulation and percutaneous tibial nerve stimulation
- Augmentation cystoplasty to increase the bladder size

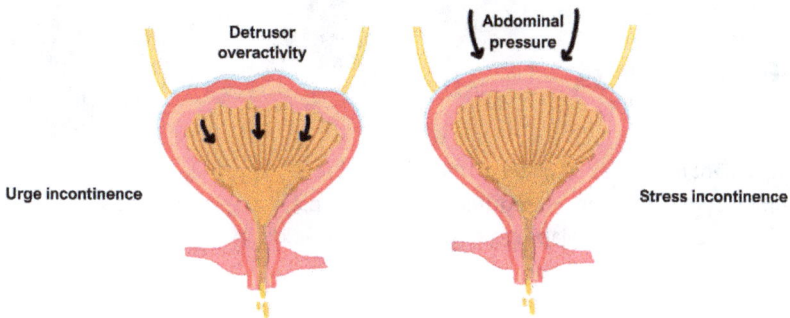

For stress incontinence
- Pelvic floor muscle exercises (3-month trial of 8 contractions, 3 times/day)
- Medical – duloxetine is offered if surgical management is unsuitable/declined

Surgical options include:
- Colposuspension (laparoscopic or open) – sutures to support the bladder neck
- Autologous rectus fascial sling – abdominal wall fascia is used to form a sling to support the bladder neck and urethra
- Urethral bulking agents – to narrow the walls of the urethra and prevent leakage
- Synthetic mesh or tape procedures – placement of synthetic material to support the urethra. Its use is currently restricted in the UK due to complications

- **Pelvic organ prolapse (POP)**

This refers to descent of the pelvic structures due to ligament or muscular weakness.

- The type of prolapse is described by the organ which prolapses through the vagina.
- Anterior vaginal prolapse (cystocele) is when the bladder pushes into the vagina.
- A rectocele is a prolapse of the rectum into the posterior vaginal wall.
- An apical prolapse is of the uterus or post hysterectomy vaginal vault.
- Procidentia is a severe form of organ prolapse (POP) that occurs when the anterior, posterior, and apical vaginal compartments herniate through the vaginal introitus.

Risk factors

- Higher parity
- Vaginal childbirth
- Advancing age
- Previous hysterectomy
- Obesity

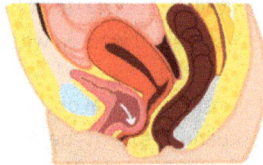

Anterior prolapse

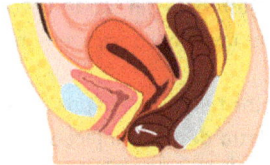

Posterior prolapse

Symptoms

Uterine prolapse

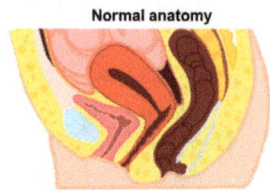

Normal anatomy

- Dragging sensation of heaviness in the vagina
- Feeling that something is coming out of the vagina
- The patient may be able to feel a protruding bulge
- Urinary symptoms – increased frequency, incomplete emptying, weakened stream, manual reduction of prolapse to start or complete voiding

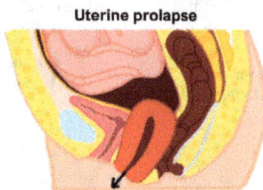

Staging

- It is staged according to the distance of prolapse from the hymenal ring
- Stage 0 – no prolapse
- Stage 1 – most distal part of the prolapse is > 1 cm proximal to the level of the hymen
- Stage 2 – most distal part of the prolapse is < 1 cm proximal or distal to the level of the hymen
- Stage 3 – the most distal part of the prolapse is < 1 cm beyond the hymen but protrudes no further than 2 cm less than the total vaginal length
- Stage 4 – complete vaginal inversion

Key tests
- Pelvic examination resting and straining both supine and standing

Management
- Conservative measures – pelvic floor exercises
- Medical management involves a pessary – these are available in different shapes and sizes with the ring pessary being the most common
- They are changed every 3–6 months

- Surgical management aims to restore pelvic anatomy, eliminate POP symptoms and improve bowel, bladder and sexual function. The operations can be combined depending on the individual's presenting complaints.

Type of prolapse	Surgical repair (reconstructive)
Anterior segment	Anterior colporrhaphy
Posterior segment	Posterior colporrhaphy +/- perineorrhaphy
Apical	Sacrospinous fixation, sacrocolpopexy or sacrohysteropexy

For apical prolapses, surgical options include:
- Sacrospinous fixation – the cervix or vaginal vault is attached to the sacrospinous ligaments with a suture. This is performed vaginally. There is a risk of pudendal nerve (leading to buttock pain) and pudendal vessel injury.
- Sacrocolpopexy – attach the vagina to the sacrum or coccyx using a synthetic mesh.
- Sacrohysteropexy – attach the cervix to the sacrum or coccyx using a synthetic mesh. This can be performed with an open or minimally invasive approach.

In women with apical (uterine) prolapse, vaginal hysterectomy can be offered along with an apical suspension procedure should the patient not wish to preserve the uterus.

- **Pelvic inflammatory disease (PID)**

This is inflammation of the upper genital tract involving the uterus, fallopian tubes +/- ovaries, typically due to an ascending infection arising from the lower genital tract.
- Chronic inflammation gives scarring and fibrosis casuing symptoms such as pain.
- Inflammation can cause adhesions and obstruction of the fallopian tubes.
- This increases the risk of infertility, chronic pelvic pain and ectopic pregnancy.

Causes

- Sexually transmitted infections – Chlamydia trachomatis (most common), Neisseria gonorrhoeae
- Cervical microbes – Mycoplasma genitalium
- Pathogens responsible for bacterial vaginosis – Bacteroides species
- Enteric pathogens – Escherichia coli, Group B Streptococcus

Symptoms

- Fever
- Pelvic and lower abdominal pain
- Dyspareunia
- Vaginal discharge
- Abnormal vaginal bleeding

Key tests

- Pelvic examination – adnexal tenderness, cervical excitation (pain elicited when two fingers used to move cervix), abnormal discharge
- Pregnancy test to exclude ectopic pregnancy
- High vaginal swab and chlamydia and gonorrhoea swabs ("triple" swabs)
- Blood tests may show raised inflammatory markers (raised WBC and high CRP/ESR)
- Consider pelvic ultrasound, especially if concern regarding a tubo-ovarian abscess

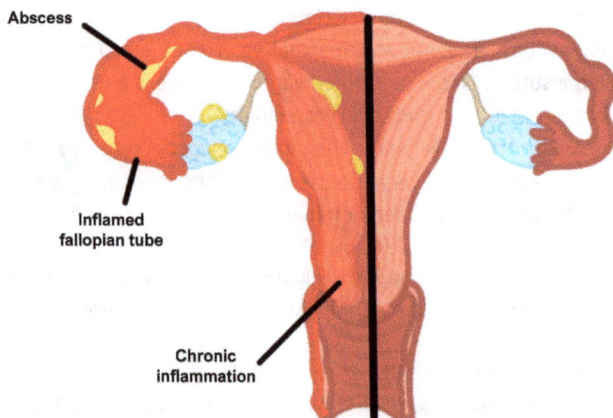

Abscess

Inflamed
fallopian tube

Chronic
inflammation

Management

- PID is a clinical diagnosis and if suspected, start empirical antibiotic treatment
- The BNF recommends a 14-day course of doxycycline and metronidazole and single-dose IM ceftriaxone or 14 days of ofloxacin and metronidazole
- If severe, can give doxycycline and IV metronidazole and ceftriaxone

Breast Anatomy

Although the breast is not typically covered under gynaecology, conditions which affect the breast are an important part of womens' health.

The breast is a sexual organ which is made of fat, connective tissue and glands.
- Glands are arranged in 15–20 lobules which secrete milk into lactiferous ducts.
- Milk drains from smaller ducts to the major ducts and to the lactiferous sinus (a reservoir behind the nipple) and ultimately onto the nipple.
- The pectoralis major muscle is the base of the breast.
- Bands of connective tissue called Coopers' ligaments run from the pectoralis major fascia to the dermis of the breast to maintain its shape.
- The breast can produce bilateral nipple discharge naturally.

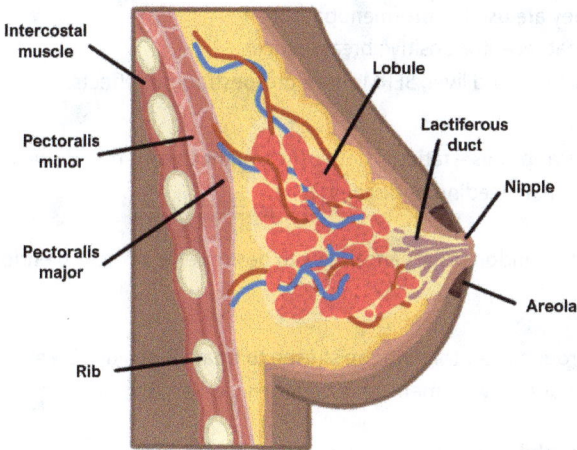

Blood supply: Axillary, posterior intercostal arteries (lateral aspect), internal thoracic arteries (medial aspect)

Lymph drainage: Axillary nodes (which drain to apical nodes in the apex of axilla) and internal mammary (parasternal) nodes

The breast is hormone sensitive, and development is mainly driven by the sex hormones oestrogen and progesterone.
- Oestrogen increases cell proliferation and hypertrophy of the milk duct system.
- Progesterone increases cell differentiation and proliferation of the lobules.

Endocrine Therapies

These drugs are used to treat breast cancer which is positive for oestrogen and progesterone receptors.

- **Selective oestrogen receptor modulators (SERMs) – Tamoxifen, toremifene**

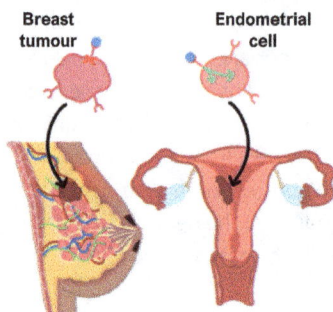

Breast tumour

Endometrial cell

These modulate activity of the oestrogen receptor.
- They have oestrogenic and anti-oestrogen effects depending on the tissue on which they are acting.
- In the breast, SERMs inhibit oestrogen receptors, so inhibit proliferation of oestrogen-dependent cancers.
- Therefore, they are used in pre-menopausal women to treat receptor positive breast cancer.
- In the uterus, bone and liver, SERMs have pro-oestrogenic effects.

Side effects
- Menopausal symptoms – fatigue, hot flushes, night sweats, mood swings
- Abnormal vaginal bleeding or discharge
- Increased risk of VTE
- Increased risk of endometrial cancer, due to oestrogenic effects on endometrium

- **Fulvestrant**

This is an oestrogen receptor antagonist used to treat ER-positive breast cancer.
- It is given to patients with metastatic breast cancer (e.g. spread to the lymph nodes).

- **Aromatase inhibitors – Anastrozole, letrozole**

These drugs inhibit the aromatase enzyme which converts testosterone to oestrogen.
- They are used in postmenopausal women with ER-positive breast cancer.

Side effects: Hot flushes, increased risk of osteoporosis

- **GnRH agonists – Leuprolide (Prostap), goserelin (Zoladex)**

These are analogues that bind and stimulate the GnRH receptor.
- Over time, this results in inhibition of LH and FSH secretion.
- This has downstream effects to decrease levels of testosterone and oestrogen.
- They are used in pre-menopausal women who have ER+ breast cancer.
- These drugs are also used to treat prostate cancer in men.

Side effects: Menopausal symptoms

Breast Conditions

Many breast conditions present with a lump. When this happens, the standard procedure is to conduct a triple assessment, which includes the following:
- Clinical examination – should offer patient a chaperone (not a family member).
- Radiology – ultrasound for < 35 years; mammography and ultrasound if > 35 years.
- Histology – core biopsy for new lumps.

- **Mastitis**

This is a condition which refers to inflammation of the breast.
- It is associated with breastfeeding: milk stasis can cause an inflammatory response which can lead to a secondary infection, usually due to S. aureus.
- It can also be caused by damage to the nipple.

Symptoms

- Erythematous, tender, swollen area of breast
- Systemic upset with fevers, chills and fatigue

Management

- 1st line is to continue breastfeeding, ensuring that the breast is fully emptied
- If symptoms do not improve, treat with antibiotics (e.g. flucloxacillin)

Inflamed lobules

Erythema

If mastitis is left untreated, it may develop into a breast abscess.
- It gives a tender, red fluctuant mass, often associated with history of mastitis.
- This will require antibiotics and may require surgical aspiration and drainage.

- **Mammary duct ectasia**

This is a benign condition which involves the dilation and shortening of the subareolar ducts. It causes ducts to become blocked and the secretions to stagnate.
- It classically arises in peri-menopausal women.

Symptoms

- Green or brown nipple discharge
- A lump behind the nipple (near the clogged duct) or an inverted nipple
- Tenderness of the nipple or areola

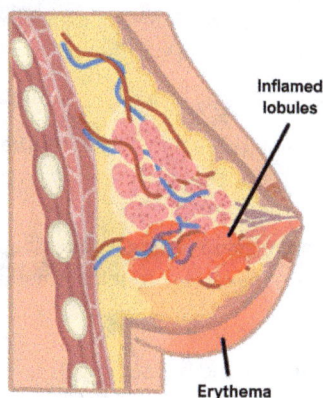

Management

- It is usually self-limiting
- Conservative measures – warm compress, breast pads to absorb discharge
- Consistent or recurrent symptoms may warrant excision of the duct and the surrounding areolar tissue

• Periductal mastitis

This refers to an inflammatory condition of the subareolar ducts.
- Unlike mammary duct ectasia, it tends to occur in younger women.
- The cause of this inflammatory condition is unknown, but smoking is a risk factor.

Symptoms

- Can lead to nipple discharge/inversion, breast lump, mastitis, abscess formation
- Can lead to the development of mammary fistulae (communication between subareolar ducts and the skin)

Management

- Empirical antibiotics and surgical excision

• Fat necrosis

This refers to necrosis of breast adipose tissue, usually occurring following injury to the breast tissue (e.g. by minor trauma, breast biopsy, radiotherapy or surgery).

Symptoms

- Firm, round breast lump
- May be accompanied by changes of the overlying skin (e.g. red, bruised)

Key tests

- Triple assessment to rule out breast cancer

Management

- No treatment is needed once the diagnosis is confirmed as it self-resolves

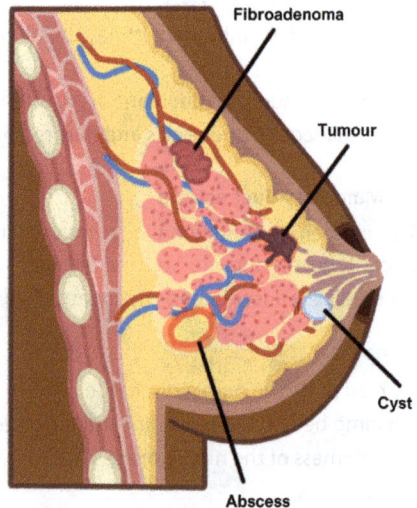

- **Fibrocystic change (fibroadenosis)**

This refers to the development of fibrosis and cystic changes in the breast.
- It most commonly occurs in women aged 30–50.

Symptoms

- Lumpy, nodular breasts – fibrosis is firm/rubbery, cysts are soft and fluctuant
- May be accompanied by breast pain
- Symptoms may fluctuate throughout the menstrual cycle, getting worse just before the time of menstruation

Management: Analgesia

- **Fibroadenoma**

This is a benign tumour that forms from a breast lobule and is composed of both stroma and glandular tissue. It occurs most commonly in women aged 14–35.
- There is no increased risk of malignancy.

Symptoms

- Well circumscribed, non-tender highly mobile marble-like mass
- 1/3 get larger, 1/3 reduce, 1/3 stay the same

Management

- Usually none needed
- Surgical excision is considered if large or painful

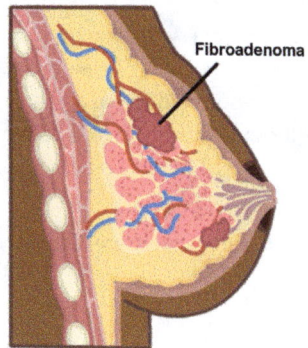

Fibroadenoma

- **Intraductal papilloma**

This is the growth of a benign wart-like lump that develops in large mammary ducts.
- It can occur in all ages but is most common in women 35–55 years old.

Symptoms

- Clear or blood-stained nipple discharge, but they are too small to be palpated

Key tests

- Can be detected on ultrasound. Galactogram (ductogram) is the definitive test

Management: Surgical excision

- **Breast cancer**

This is the most common cancer in women in the UK.
- The main risk factors for breast cancer are related to oestrogen exposure.

Risk factors

- Age (most breast cancers occur in women > 50 years)
- Early menarche, late menopause
- Obesity
- Not breastfeeding
- Combined oral contraceptive pill (risk returns to normal 10 years after stopping)
- Combined HRT
- Genetics – 1st degree relative with breast cancer, BRCA1 and 2 gene mutations
- Alcohol intake

Screening: In the UK, women aged 50–70 are offered a mammogram every 3 years

Key tests: Breast lumps should undergo a triple assessment

Li-Fraumeni syndrome

A syndrome due to an autosomal dominant mutation in p53 tumour suppressor gene.
- It is associated with a high incidence of sarcomas and leukhaemias.
- It can be diagnosed if a patient develops a sarcoma < 45 years and has a first-degree relative and family member who develops cancer < 45 years old.

There are many different terms which are used to describe breast cancer:

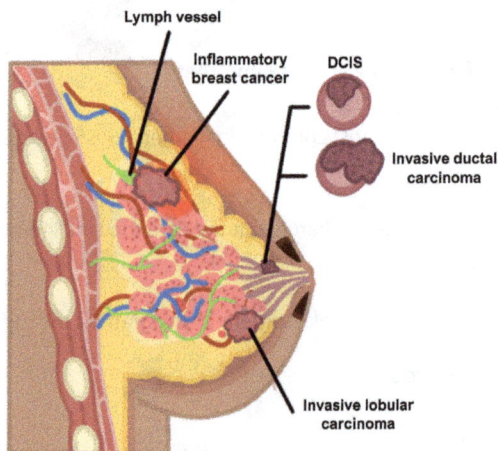

○ **Ductal carcinoma in situ (DCIS)**

This is a proliferation of ductal cells with no invasion of the basement membrane.

○ **Invasive ductal carcinoma**

This is a malignant proliferation of ductal cells, which tends to occur in older women.
- This is the most common invasive carcinoma in the breast.

○ **Lobular carcinoma in situ (LCIS)**

This is a proliferation of cells in lobules with no invasion of the basement membrane.
- This does not produce a mass or calcification and is discovered incidentally.
- It may develop into a malignant cancer.

○ **Invasive lobular carcinoma**

This is a malignant proliferation of lobule cells associated with e-cadherin mutations.
- It is the second most common type of breast cancer.

○ **Inflammatory breast cancer**

This is a type of breast cancer where cancerous cells block lymph drainage giving the inflamed "orange-peel" (peau d'orange) appearance of the breast.

○ **Paget's disease of the breast**

This term refers to a rare skin change at the nipple which is associated with an underlying breast cancer.
- It presents as nipple ulceration and erythema (looking like eczema) that can give bloody discharge.

○ **Hereditary breast cancer**

These are associated with BRCA1 and BRCA2 mutations (autosomal dominant).
- This gives 50% lifetime risk of breast cancer so women can opt to undergo bilateral mastectomy to reduce the risk of developing cancer.

NICE referral guidelines. Urgent 2WW referral if:
- Age > 30 with unexplained breast lump with or without pain
- Age > 50 with any of following symptoms in one nipple only: discharge, retraction or other changes that are concerning

Non-urgent referral if age < 30 and unexplained breast lump with or without pain

Management

- This is dependent on the type and stage of cancer
- Local treatment involves surgery and radiotherapy whilst systemic treatment involves chemotherapy, hormone therapy, targeted therapy and immunotherapy

Most women will have surgery as part of their treatment.
- Wide local excision (also known as lumpectomy) – this refers to removal of the cancer and a margin of normal breast tissue (breast conserving surgery). This is normally followed by radiotherapy to reduce the risk of recurrence.
- Mastectomy refers to removal of the entire breast.

Drug treatments include chemotherapy, hormone therapy, as well as targeted and immunotherapy drugs.
- They can be used before surgery to reduce the size of the cancer, known as neoadjuvant therapy.
- They can also be used after surgery to reduce the risk of recurrence, known as adjuvant therapy.

To determine which drug treatment will be most effective, breast cancers are tested for the presence of oestrogen receptors (ER), progesterone receptors (PR) and human epidermal growth receptors (HER2).

○ **ER positive cancer**
These can be treated with hormone therapy used, usually used as adjuvant therapy.
- In pre-menopausal women, consider tamoxifen or GnRH analogues.
- In post-menopausal women, aromatase inhibitors (anastrozole) are used.

○ **HER-2 positive cancers**
Targeted drugs such as trastuzumab are used on a neoadjuvant or adjuvant basis.
- Trastuzumab should be avoided in cardiac patients due to cardiac toxicity
- An ECG and echocardiogram should be perfromed before treatment is started

○ **Triple negative cancers**
These carry the worst prognosis as there are no targeted treatments available.
- In addition to surgery, they are treated with chemotherapy, as well as an increasing role for immunotherapy (such as pembrolizumab).

Haematology

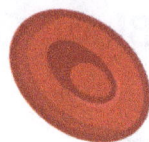

Blood Cells

Blood cells are produced from haematopoietic stem cells in the bone marrow.
- These cells can differentiate into either common myeloid or lymphoid progenitors.

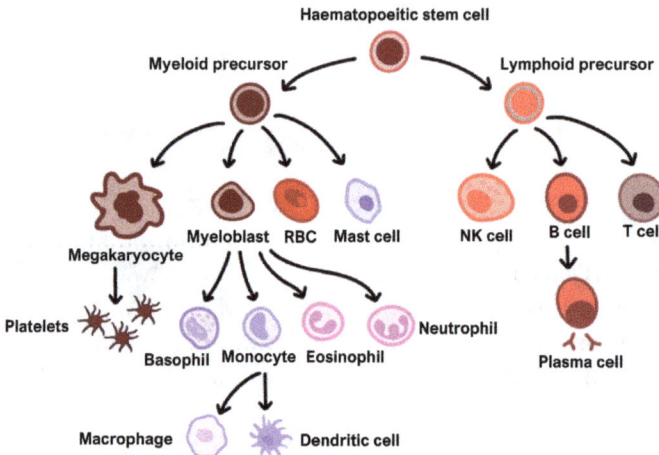

The cells which transport oxygen around the body are known as erythrocytes (red blood cells). These are formed from an erythroid progenitor called a reticulocyte.

To produce red blood cells, the body needs to synthesise both the cellular precursors and haemoglobin, the main oxygen carrying component.

Haemoglobin
Haemoglobin is the functional molecule of red blood cells.
- It is composed of four polypeptide chains – two alphas and two betas.
- Each chain contains a prosthetic haem group, responsible for binding oxygen.
- The haem group consists of an iron (Fe^{2+}) ion held in porphyrin rings, where the nitrogen atoms of the rings bind to the central Fe^{2+} ion.
- In adults, the most common form of haemoglobin is haemoglobin A, a tetramer consisting of two alpha and two beta subunits. These subunits are non-covalently bound and each chain consists of 141 and 146 amino acid residues respectively.

Iron is a key element in haemoglobin, which is acquired in animal and vegetable foods.
- The iron content in the body is regulated by controlling its absorption in the gut.
- Fe^{2+} ions are absorbed across the brush border of the small intestine.
- The protein ferroportin transports iron across the intestinal wall into the blood.

The clotting pathway is activated simultaneously with the fibrinolytic system, which works in the opposite fashion.

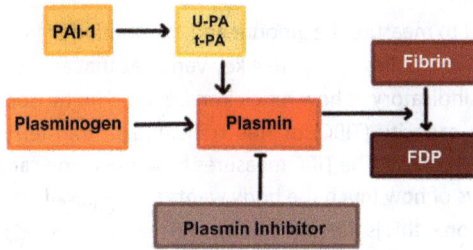

Most thrombolytic medicines work by producing the serine protease plasmin.
- Plasmin cuts the fibrin mesh at various places producing fragments that can be cleared by the kidney and liver.
- It also assists in the breakdown of other clotting factors.

Thrombus formation

The chances of a thrombus occurring depend on three types of factors, which is known as Virchow's triad:

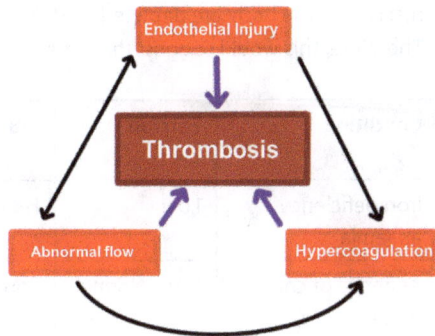

- **Changes in blood constituents**

These are changes to the blood components which increase the tendency for blood to coagulate.
- Genetic – deficiency of antithrombin III or protein C resistance (factor V Leiden).
- Acquired – malignancy, smoking, hyperlipidaemia, oral contraceptive pill.

- **Changes in vessel wall**

These factors induce endothelial cell injury or activation of the clotting cascade.
- Examples include ischaemia, hypoxia, infection and immunological damage (due to immune complexes).

- **Changes in blood flow**

Turbulent flow puts platelets in contact with the endothelium.
- This leads to poor delivery of anticoagulants and activation of the endothelium.
- Arterial changes include narrowing, heart valve disease, aneurysm and arrhythmias.
- Venous changes include right-sided heart failure and varicose veins.

Tests and Investigations

- **Iron studies**

Iron studies are used to measure the amount and distribution of iron in the body.
- When requesting iron studies, there are 4 key variables that are usually measured.
- Ferritin – this is an indicatory of how much iron is stored in the body.
- Total iron binding capacity (TIBC) or free transferrin – transferrin is a protein that transports iron in the blood. The TIBC measures how much iron can bind to transferrin. These are indicators of how much the body wants to use iron.
- Transferrin saturation – this is the percentage of transferrin bound to iron.
- Serum iron – measures the amount of iron circulating in the blood. It can vary throughout the day, so it is used in combination with other tests.

By putting the results of these investigations together, it can help determine whether the body is depleted of iron and the underlying cause.
- For example, if the ferritin is low and the TIBC is high, this shows that the natural reserves in the body are depleted, and the body wants iron.
- Therefore, this would suggest the patient has an iron-deficiency anaemia.

Condition	Ferritin	TIBC	Transferrin saturation	Serum iron
Iron deficiency anaemia	Low	High	Low	Low
Anaemia of chronic disease	High/Normal	Low	Low	Low
Sideroblastic anaemia	High	Normal/Low	Normal/High	High
Iron overload	High	Low	High	High

- **Group and save**

A group and save is the processing of a patient's blood.
- It consists of a blood test with an antibody screen to determine the patient's blood group and whether or not they have atypical red cell antibodies in their blood.
- If atypical antibodies are present the laboratory will do additional work to identify them, which helps to reduce the risk of a hypersensitivity reaction during transfusion.

- **Crossmatch**

A crossmatch involves physically mixing the patient's plasma or serum with the donor's red blood cells (or vice versa) to check for any incompatibility.
- If no reaction is observed, the donor blood is compatible and can be issued for a blood transfusion.

- **Coagulation studies**

The coagulation cascade converts fibrinogen to fibrin.
- Coagulation factors are produced in the liver in an inactive state.
- The extrinsic pathway requires tissue factor (activates factor VII).
- The intrinsic pathway is activated by subendothelial collagen.

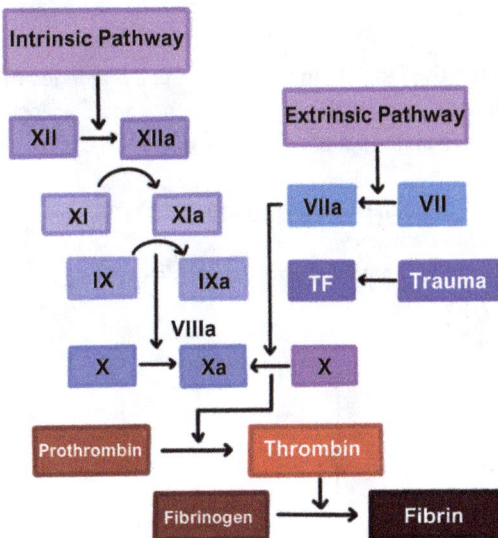

○ **Prothrombin time (PT)**

Prothrombin time (PT) is a blood test that measures the time it takes for the liquid portion (plasma) of your blood to clot. It is an assay for evaluating the extrinsic pathway and common pathway of the coagulation cascade.
- It is prolonged by vitamin K deficiency, liver disease as well as drugs like warfarin.

○ **Internalized normalized ratio (INR)**

This is the PT expressed as a ratio to a control.
- This makes it easier to compare against a frame of reference.

The INR is the most commonly used test to monitor the effect of warfarin.
- The target for many patients with atrial fibrillation is 2.5 (with a range 2–3) to balance the thrombosis versus bleeding risk.
- If the INR gets too high or the patient experiences bleeding, there are guidelines on how to reverse the effect of warfarin, which may differ between hospital trusts.
- Specialist advice should usually be sought from a haematologist, as it may require their approval to obtain certain blood products such as prothrombin complex.

○ **Activated partial thromboplastin time (APTT)**
This is another test which measures the blood's time to clot.
- In contrast to the PT, this measures the intrinsic pathway of the coagulation cascade.
- It is prolonged in haemophilia, von Willebrand disease and heparins.

○ **APTT mixing study**
This is a laboratory test used to determine the cause of a prolonged APTT result.
- It differentiates between coagulation factor deficiency and presence of an inhibitor.
- The APTT is performed on the patient's plasma, the normal control plasma and a 50:50 mix.
- If the APTT fully corrects to the normal range, then the prolongation of the APTT is due to a coagulation factor deficiency.
- If it does not correct to the normal range, then it is most likely due to the presence of an inhibitor.

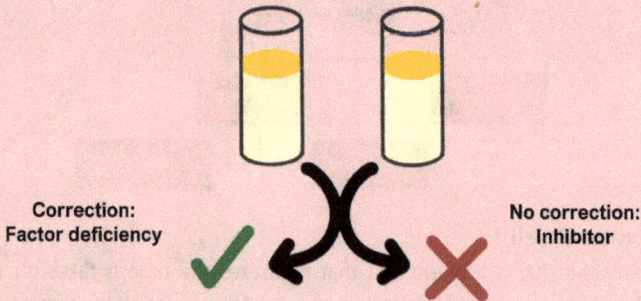

Correction:
Factor deficiency

No correction:
Inhibitor

○ **Thrombin time**
This is a test that measures how quickly a blood clot forms when thrombin is added to a sample of plasma. It assesses the functionality of the fibrinogen molecule, a key protein in the coagulation process.
- It is prolonged in by substances that inhibit thrombin such as heparin.

- **Bone marrow aspiration and biopsy**

This involves the analysis of bone marrow samples obtained through a trephine biopsy and a bone marrow aspiration.

- These procedures are typically performed on the posterior iliac crest.
- The aspirate provides semi-liquid bone marrow, which can be examined under a microscope and analysed using flow cytometry or polymerase chain reaction.
- The trephine biopsy provides a solid piece of marrow for histological examination.

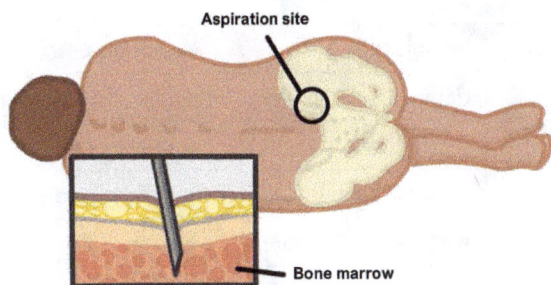

- **Immunophenotyping with flow cytometry**

This is a technique which allows the analysis of cell types in a bone marrow aspirate using a flow cytometer.

- Immunophenotyping is a flow cytometry test that uses fluorophore-conjugated antibodies to detect surface marker antigens expressed by cells.
- Cells are labelled with the conjugated antibodies, and thousands of cells per second can be processed in a flow cytometer using laser-based detection.
- This technique is commonly used to detect cell types in leukemia and lymphoma and to quantify CD4+ T cells in patients with HIV.

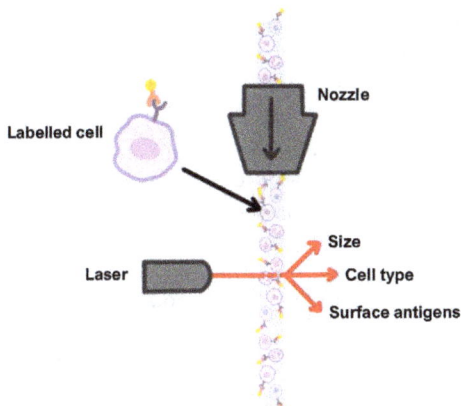

Blood Transfusions

This is where you can transfuse donor blood into a patient.
- RBCs have a H antigen on their surface which can be modified in 2 ways (A and B).
- Patients produce an antibody against the antigen which they do not possess.
- Therefore, if the wrong blood group is given, this results in an antibody-mediated hypersensitivity reaction.

Blood group	Modification	Antibodies
O	Unmodified H antigen	Anti-A and anti-B antibodies
A	A modification	Anti-B antibodies
B	B modification	Anti-A antibodies
AB	A and B modifications	No antibodies

Whilst the majority of blood transfusions are safe, complications can occur, which can be life threatening.

- **Anaphylactic reaction**

This is a type I hypersensitivity reaction which leads to the release of histamine.
- This causes symptoms within seconds to minutes and can be life threatening.

Symptoms: Urticaria to anaphylaxis with hypotension, dyspnea, wheezing and stridor

Management
- If mild urticaria, pause the transfusion and give an antihistamine
- Trial restarting the transfusion at a slower rate
- If severe, stop the transfusion permanently and follow anaphylaxis protocol
  (IM adrenaline, oxygen, hydrocortisone, chlorphenamine)

- **Acute haemolytic transfusion reaction**

This is an immediate reaction due to an ABO blood group mismatch.
- This results in massive intravascular haemolysis due to pre-formed antibodies in donor blood. If left untreated, it can lead to DIC and renal failure.

Symptoms: Fever, abdominal and chest pain, hypotension

Management: Immediate transfusion termination and fluid resuscitation

- **Transfusion associated circulatory overload (TACO)**

A single pack of red blood cells contains about 350 mls of fluid.

- Therefore, a common complication of blood transfusion is fluid overload causing fluid to third space and accumulate in the lungs causing cardiogenic pulmonary oedema.
- This can lead to hypertension (increased afterload) and shortness of breath.

Symptoms

- Pulmonary oedema – shortness of breath, cough, chest pain

Management

- Diuretics (e.g. furosemide) to reduce fluid in lungs
- Ideally, TACO should be prevented by giving the transfusion slowly or with diuretics, particularly in at-risk individuals

- **Transfusion-related acute lung injury (TRALI)**

Blood transfusions can cause immune-mediated damage to the lungs leading to non-cardiogenic pulmonary oedema.

- This leads to hypoxia and acute respiratory distress syndrome, usually within about 6 hours of the transfusion.

Symptoms

- Fever, dyspnoea, severe hypoxaemia and hypotension

Management

- Discontinue transfusion immediately
- Supportive treatment with oxygen therapy and monitoring for complications
- Corticosteroids usually not recommended, but can be considered in severe cases

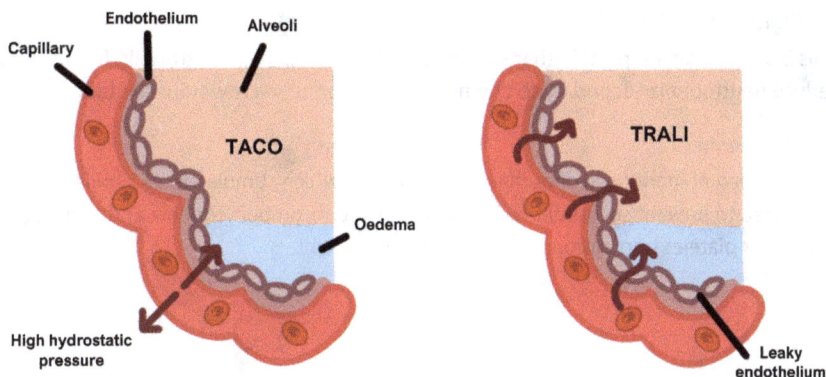

Blood Products

These drugs include those which stimulate the production of types of blood cells as well as direct replacements of blood constituents.

- **Erythropoiesis-stimulating agents – Erythropoietin (EPO)**

Erythropoietin is a glycoprotein released by the kidneys that stimulates the production of reticulocytes, which are precursors of red blood cells.
- EPO synthesis is triggered by hypoxia, which increases the proliferation of red blood cell precursors and their release into the bloodstream.
- It is used to treat anaemia in AIDS patients, chemotherapy-induced anaemia, and anaemia in chronic kidney disease (CKD).

Side effects

- Hypertension, seizures, headaches, secondary to rapid expansion of blood volume

- **Myeloid growth factors**

These are glycoproteins which are produced by various cells, including fibroblasts, macrophages, and immune cells.
- They stimulate the proliferation and differentiation of cells in the myeloid lineage.

○ **Sagramostim (GM-CSF)**

This is a recombinant protein that stimulates the macrophage pathway.
- It helps reduce neutropenia and infection for patients receiving chemotherapy or bone marrow transplantation.

Side effects

- Granulocytosis (increased white blood cells) and bone pain

○ **Filgrastim (G-CSF)**

This is a recombinant protein that stimulates the production of neutrophils. It is used to reduce neutropenia secondary to chemotherapy or bone marrow transplantation.

○ **Oprelvekin**

This is a recombinant form of human interleukin-11, which stimulates cell proliferation.
- It is used to prevent severe chemotherapy-induced thrombocytopenia and reduce the need for platelet transfusions following chemotherapy.

- **Packed red blood cells**

This refers to isolated red blood cells which are obtained through the centrifugation of whole blood. The universal donor blood type is O, and the universal recipient is AB.
- RBCs should be stored at 4°C prior to transfusion.
- They are typically transfused over 90–180 minutes (though can be slower).
- They are used in patients to treat both acute and chronic anaemia. The transfusion threshold is usually 70 g/L, or 80 g/L for those with ischaemic heart disease.

- **Fresh frozen plasma (FFP)**

This is a product obtained by centrifuging blood to collect the plasma. It is made from a single unit of blood, containing immunoglobulins, clotting factors and albumin.
- Unlike red blood cells, the universal donor for fresh frozen plasma is AB blood, as the plasma lacks anti-A or anti-B antibodies, while the universal recipient is O.
- It is commonly used as bleeding prophylaxis before surgery or invasive procedures to correct clotting in patients with liver failure.
- It is most suited for patients with a prothrombin time (PT) or activated partial thromboplastin time (APTT) > 1.5 and is typically given in volumes of 150–220 mL.

- **Cryoprecipitate**

A blood product made from plasma, typically transferred as a 6-unit pool. It contains factor VIII (100 IU), fibrinogen (250 mg), von Willebrand factor and fibronectin.
- The volume is approximately 1/10th of fresh frozen plasma (FFP), around 15–20 mL.
- It is commonly used to replace fibrinogen, such as after large transfusions, in disseminated intravascular coagulation (DIC), liver failure, or before surgery.
- It is also used to replace factor VIII in conditions like von Willebrand disease and haemophilia A.

- **Prothrombin complex concentrate**

Prothrombin complex concentrate is composed of factor II, IX, and X.
- It is used for the emergency reversal of warfarin in patients with major haemorrhage.

- **Irradiated blood**

This is where the blood is treated with radiation (X-rays) to inactivate the donor's lymphocytes, preventing them from proliferating and attacking the recipient's cells.
- It is used to avoid transfusion graft versus host disease (TA-GVHD) caused by the transplant of viable donor T lymphocytes, associated with haematological cancers like lymphomas.

Coagulation Drugs

Thrombolytics

These drugs work to break down a clot once it has already formed, e.g. in stroke.
- Fibrinolysis is achieved by producing the serine protease plasmin.
- Tissue plasminogen activators (t-PA) convert inactive plasminogen to plasmin.
- Fibrinolytics mimic activators to increase plasmin production to break down clots.

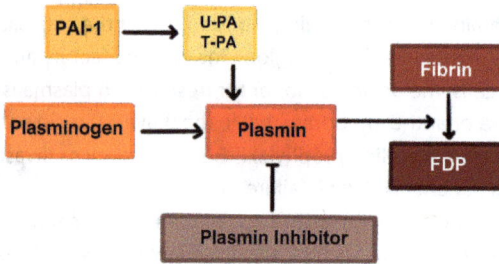

- **Streptokinase**

This is made by Streptococcus bacteria and binds to plasminogen to form plasmin.

- **Alteplase, duteplase**

These are recombinant tissue plasminogen activators. They are genetically engineered forms of human t-PA which have localised action on fibrin in clots.

- **Anistreplase**

This is a combination of streptokinase and plasminogen. It has a longer half-life than streptokinase and does not require circulating plasminogen.

- **Urokinase**

This is a protease found in the urine which activates plasminogen.
- It is used as an alternative in patients who are sensitive to streptokinase.

Side effects

- Allergic reactions and anaphylaxis
- Bleeding
- Hypotension
- Problems due to reperfusion

Contraindications

- These include conditions which predispose to bleeding

Anticoagulants

These drugs work by inhibiting specific aspects of the clotting cascade.

- **Heparin**

Heparin is a natural anticoagulant produced by basophils and mast cells.
- Heparins work by binding to and activating antithrombin-III (AT-III).
- AT-III inactivates several clotting factors.
- Different types of heparins are used therapeutically.

o **Unfractionated heparin** (aka "standard" heparin)

This is a type of heparin which has a shorter duration of action.
- It binds AT-III leading to the inactivation of several clotting factors including II and X.
- It is preferred for patients who are at high risk of bleeding because of its shorter duration of action and those with severe renal impairment.
- UFH is generally given as an IV infusion and monitored using the APTT.

o **Low molecular weight heparins – Dalteparin, enoxaparin, tinzaparin**

These have a longer duration of action then unfractionated heparin.
- They bind AT-III leading to more specific inactivation of factor X.
- They are usually preferred because they carry a lower risk of heparin-induced thrombocytopaenia, and they are given by subcutaneous injection.

o **Fondaparinux**

This is a drug which is chemically related to LMWH.

Side effects

- Haemorrhage – protamine sulphate is used to reverse the effects
- Heparin-induced thrombocytopaenia
- Skin reactions
- Osteoporosis
- Priapism
- Hyperkalaemia
- Alopecia

Contraindications

- Should not be given in people who are bleeding (peptic ulcer)
- Caution should be taken if patient is taking aspirin/antithrombotic agents

- **Warfarin**

This is a drug which blocks the enzyme vitamin K epoxide reductase.

- The enzyme is needed to produce the active form of vitamin K.
- Less active vitamin K leads to reduced production of vitamin-K-dependent proteins.
- This include clotting factors II, VII, IX, X and factors C, S, Z.
- It is given orally and has 100% bioavailability, and a slower course of action.

Side effects

- Bleeding – it is monitored by measuring the prothrombin time/INR
- Skin necrosis and skin reactions
- Blue toe syndrome
- Metabolised by CYP450 enzyme, so affected by many other drugs and liver disease

Contraindications

- Highly teratogenic so not used in pregnancy
- Can be used while breastfeeding as significant levels are not found in breast milk

- **Novel oral anticoagulants – Dabigatran, apixaban, rivaroxaban**

These are newer anticoagulants which directly inhibit certain clotting factors.

- They are used in treatment and prevention of venous thromboembolism.
- They are also used in the prevention of embolism in individuals with atrial fibrillation (in the absence of severe mitral stenosis).

- **Dabigatran** – this is a direct inhibitor of thrombin (factor IIa), and is reversed by the antidote idarucizumab.

- **Apixaban/rivaroxaban** – these are direct inhibitors of factor Xa.

Anti-platelet

These drugs work to reduce the chances of thrombus formation by inhibiting the normal action of platelets interacting with the endothelium.

- **Aspirin**

This is an acetylsalicylate which irreversibly acetylates and inhibits COX-1.

- It decreases thromboxane A_2 production in platelets which is a vasoconstrictor.
- It also inhibits prostaglandin I_2 production in the endothelium which is a vasodilator.

However, the endothelium can make new COX-1 whereas platelets cannot, which shifts the balance towards net vasodilation.
- This inhibits platelet aggregation reducing the chance of clot formation.
- It is 1st line for patients with ischaemic heart disease and thrombotic stroke.

Side effects
- Peptic ulcer formation
- Reye's syndrome, seen in children under the age of 16
- Salicylism if taken in overdose

● **Dipyridamole**

This inhibits uptake of adenosine and a PDE3 inhibitor which allows for vasodilation.

● **Ticlopidine, clopidogrel, prasugrel**

They inhibit platelet aggregation by stopping ADP binding to the platelet P2Y receptor.
- This interaction is usually responsible for platelet aggregation and stabilisation.
- They are used in high-risk thromboembolism patients and coronary disease.

● **GPIIb/IIIa inhibitors – Eptifibatide, tirofiban, abciximab**

The GPIIb/IIIa is an integrin which allows fibrinogen-mediated platelet aggregation.

Pro-thrombotic agents

These drugs are used to stop bleeding and can be used if the INR becomes too high.
- They are also indicated in hypocoagulable states such as vitamin K deficiency.

● **Vitamin K**

This is required for the maturation of clotting factors II, VII, IX and X.
- It is given to newborns to reduce hypothrombinaemia of the new-born in premature infants and also given to reverse the effects of warfarin in patients.

● **Aminocaproic acid, tranexamic acid**

These bind to plasminogen and prevent conversion to the active form plasmin.
- They are used to stop bleeding (menorrhagia/epistaxis) and used to prevent/treat significant haemorrhage following trauma.

● **Desmopressin acetate**

This works by increasing synthesis of factor VIII, and so is used in haemophilia A.

Anti-cancer Drugs

Chemotherapy drugs were traditionally designed to kill rapidly dividing cells, which is a characteristic hallmark of malignant cells. Chemotherapy is administered in cycles, allowing normal tissue to recover between treatments.
- Combination chemotherapy involves using a combination of drugs with different mechanisms to reduce resistance and minimise toxicity.

There are several classes of chemotherapy drugs:
- Adjuvant – given after the initial treatment (surgery) to reduce the risk of relapse.
- Neoadjuvant – used to shrink tumours before surgical or radiological treatment.
- Palliative – this prolongs survival and relieves symptoms rather than aim to cure.

Inhibitors of DNA replication

One of the hallmarks of cancer is uncontrolled cell proliferation, which relies on high rates of DNA synthesis. As a result, many chemotherapy drugs are designed to target this process, effectively halting cancer progression.

Covalent DNA binders

These compounds have an electrophilic centre, allowing them to form covalent bonds with nucleophilic bases in DNA.

- **Nitrogen mustards**

These are very reactive and form a positive ion which allows them to bind the oxygen/ nitrogen in bases and cause crosslinking of the DNA.
- They usually lead to bone marrow suppression and can cause a secondary cancer.

○ Cyclophosphamide

This is one of the most commonly used nitrogen mustards with broad applications.
- It can be used to treat both cancers as well as autoimmune conditions like vasculitis.

Side effects

- Myelosuppression (neutropenia)
- SIADH
- Haemorrhagic cystitis (as broken down to irritant acrolein) – this is prevented with MESNA, which binds to acrolein and inactivates it
- Increased rise of transitional cell carcinoma (usually in the bladder)

○ **Melphalan, chlorambucil**

These drugs can be used for chronic lymphocytic leukaemia (and lymphomas).

● **Nitrosoureas – Lomustine, carmustine**

These drugs are also alkylating agents which work similarly to the nitrogen mustards to cause crosslinking of the DNA strands.
- They can cross the blood-brain-barrier and so are useful in treating brain tumours and Hodgkin's disease.

● **Busulfan**

This is an alkylating agent which is used to treat chronic myelogenous leukaemia.

Side effects: Pulmonary fibrosis of the lower lobes

● **Platinum compounds – Cisplatin**

This drug contains platinum which forms crosslinks with the DNA between neighbouring bases.
- This causes bending of the DNA helix which inhibits DNA replication and transcription.
- It is typically used in the treatment of testicular, ovarian and bladder cancers.

Side effects

- Nephrotoxicity, ototoxicity
- Peripheral neuropathy
- Hypomagnesiumaemia

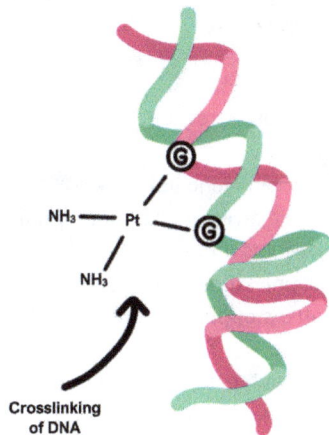

NH_3 — Pt

NH_3

Crosslinking
of DNA

Anti-tumour drugs

These compounds also cause DNA damage in a different way to drugs above.

● **Anthracyclines – Daunomycin, doxorubicin, actinomycin, mitoxantrone**

These drugs non-covalently intercalate in the DNA to block DNA and RNA synthesis.
- They also generate free radicals which result in strand breakage.

Side effects: Doxorubicin can cause dilated cardiomyopathy leading to heart failure

● **Mitomycin**

This is an alkylating agent which is activated intracellularly.
- It causes free radical formation which causes DNA strand breaks.

Side effects: Myelosuppression (condition where bone marrow activity is decreased)

- **Bleomycin**

This intercalates in the DNA grooves and generates radicals to cause strand breaks.

Side effects: Pulmonary fibrosis

Anti-metabolites

These inhibit the production of key metabolites which are required for DNA synthesis.

- **Methotrexate**

This is an inhibitor of dihydrofolate reductase which stops the synthesis of folic acid.
- It is important to check FBC, U&Es and LFTs before starting and then monitoring weekly until stable, then every 2–3 months.
- It is given alongside folic acid once weekly, usually more than 24 hours after methotrexate dose.

Side effects

- Myelosuppression
- Mucositis
- Liver and lung fibrosis
- Avoid giving with trimethoprim or co-trimoxazole due to bone marrow aplasia
- Women should avoid pregnancy for 3–6 months after stopping treatment

To counter the side effects of this, patients are given leucovorin/folinic acid, a folic acid precursor which can be converted to tetrahydrofolate without the DHFR enzyme.
- This helps direct the toxicity to cancerous cells and it also used to "rescue" from methotrexate toxicity.

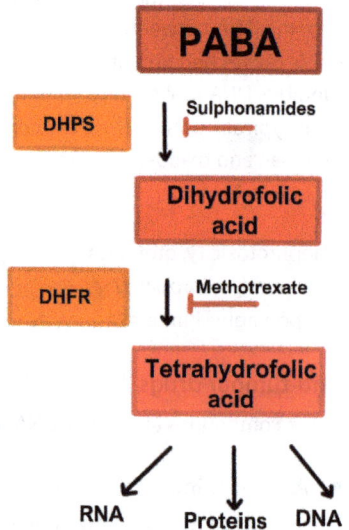

- **5-Fluorouracil**

This is a pyrimidine analogue which inhibits the thymidylate synthetase enzyme.
- It inhibits the production of thymine, which is needed to synthesise DNA.
- Inhibition causes the cell to undergo apoptosis during mitosis.
- It is classically used in treatment of colorectal cancer.

Side effects: Myelosuppression, mucositis and dermatitis

- **6-Mercaptopurine**

This is a purine analogue that is activated by the enzyme HGPRTase.
- It decreases purine synthesis stopping proliferation of the cancerous cells.

Side effects: Myelosuppression

- **Cytarabine**

This is a pyrimidine antagonist which interferes with DNA polymerase.
- This inhibits DNA synthesis at the S-phase of the cell cycle.

Side effects: Myelosuppression, ataxia

DNA topoisomerase inhibitors

These drugs inhibit the topoisomerase enzymes which organize the DNA.

- **Etoposide**

An inhibitor of DNA topoisomerase type II, used commonly in testicular tumours.

- **Topotecan, irinotecan**

These are inhibitors of DNA topoisomerase type I. Irinotecan is classically used for treating metastatic colon cancer in combination with 5-fluorourcal and leucovorin.

Side effects: Myelosuppression

Inhibitors of mitosis

These drugs inhibit formation of the spindle assembly made of microtubules.
- Microtubules are made of tubulin dimers which are arranged in filaments.
- The free dimers are added to the growing filament in a reversible reaction.

- **Taxanes –** Paclitaxel, docetaxel

These drugs shift the equilibrium towards building more microtubules.
- This results in abnormal microtubule formation causing cell arrest in mitosis.

Side effects: Neutropenia, peripheral neuropathies

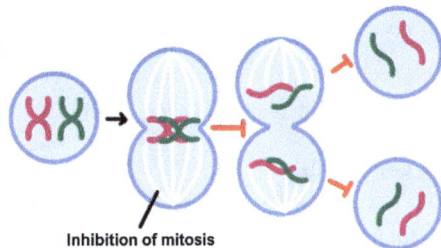

Inhibition of mitosis

- **Vinca alkaloids –** Vinblastine, vincristine

These bind free tubulin dimers to prevent microtubule assembly.
- They are classically used in the treatment of lymphomas.

Side effects: Vincristine causes peripheral neuropathy and paralytic ileus

Small molecule inhibitors

This refers to small molecules which are designed to target particular proteins, receptors or other molecules that may be unregulated in specific cancer.
- This allows for targeted treatment and reduced toxicity to other tissues.

- **Imatinib**

This is a tyrosine kinase inhibitor specific for the Bcr-Abl oncoprotein.
- It is specific for chronic myeloid leukaemia, due to the Bcr-Abl chromosome translocation which codes the Philadelphia chromosome.
- It is also used to treat GI tumours displaying the tyrosine kinase c-kit.

Monoclonal antibodies (mAb)

These are antibodies directed against particular antigens. They slow the tumour either by enhancing host immunity and can also be conjugated with chemotherapy.

- **Rituximab**

This is mAb against CD20 on B cells. It can be used to treat lymphoma as well as many autoimmune conditions due to its depletion of B cells.

- **Trastuzumab (Herceptin)**

This is a mAb against epidermal growth factor 2 (HER2) found in breast cancer cells.
- It is used to treat HER2+ breast cancers.

Side effects

- Cardiovascular toxicity – usually avoided in patients with ischaemic heart disease

- **Bevacizumab (Avastin)**

This is a mAb which inhibits VEGF, a factor which stimulates angiogenesis.

Side effects

- Interferes with wound healing

- **Cetuximab**

This is a mAb that binds epidermal growth factor receptor (EGFR). It prevents growth factor from binding and is often used in colorectal cancers with 5-flourouracil.

- **Alemtuzumab**

This binds CD52 on lymphocytes, targeting T cells for destruction.
- It is used to treat various leukhaemias and lymphomas due to widespread attack on lymphocytes, as well as being used in kidney transplants to prevent rejection.

Anaemia

Anaemia is defined as a low concentration of haemoglobin (Hb), due to a reduction in the amount of haemoglobin or increased plasma volume (e.g. during pregnancy).
- The thresholds are < 135 g/L for men and < 115 g/L for women.
- We can categorise anaemia by the mean corpuscular volume (MCV) into microcytic (MCV < 80 μm^3), normocytic (80–100 μm^3), and macrocytic (MCV > 100 μm^3).

General symptoms

- Weakness, fatigue and dyspnoea
- Pale conjunctiva and skin
- Headaches and light headedness
- Angina, especially if there is pre-existing coronary artery disease
- Can be signs of a hyperdynamic circulation due to compensation (tachycardia, heart enlargement)
- If left untreated for too long, can lead to heart failure

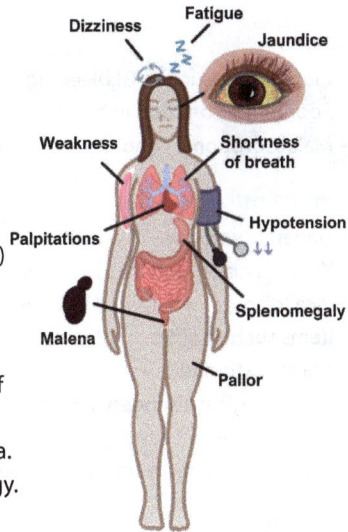

To diagnose the underlying cause, follow a series of diagnostic steps:
- FBC to check if the Hb is low, confirming an anaemia.
- Assess the MCV to help narrow down the aetiology.
- If microcytic anaemia, proceed with iron studies.
- If macrocytic, folate and B_{12} levels and send a blood film to distinguish between megaloblastic and normoblastic anaemia.
- If normocytic, assess the reticulocyte count.
- An increased reticulocyte count suggests a destructive problem.
- A decreased reticulocyte count points to a production issue or early blood loss (since the bone marrow has not had enough time to compensate).

General management

- Address the underlying cause, supplement any deficiencies
- Blood transfusion if Hb below thresholds (usually < 70, or 80 with IHD)

Microcytic Anaemia

This refers to an anaemia with a mean corpuscular volume of $< 80 \ \mu m^3$. Errors in haemoglobin structure result in improper folding in RBCs causing reduced cell mass.
- Causes include problems in synthesis of the haem group or the polypeptide chains.

- **Iron deficiency anaemia (IDA)**

Iron deficiency anaemia is a microcytic anaemia caused by decreased iron levels.

Causes

- Blood loss – such as GI bleeding or menstruation (often seen in young women)
- Poor diet – common in babies or children
- Malabsorption – conditions like coeliac disease, due to inflammation of the bowel

Symptoms

- General symptoms of anaemia
- Koilonychia (spoon-shaped nails)
- Pica (disorder where patients eat non-food items such as dirt)
- Angular stomatitis
- Atrophic glossitis (beefy red tongue)
- Plummer-Vinson syndrome – iron deficiency anaemia plus oesophageal web and atrophic glossitis

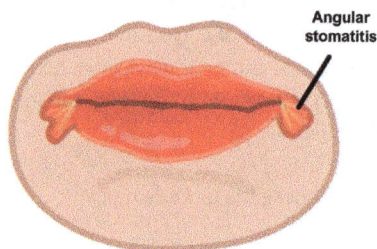

Angular stomatitis

Key tests

- Iron studies – low ferritin, high TIBC, low serum iron, low % saturation
- Blood film – shows microcytic, hypochromic RBCs. There may also be pencil poikilocytosis (abnormal shape) and target cells
- Raised free erythrocyte protoporphyrin (FEP) – this makes up the other component of haem with iron, so more is unbound in low Fe^{2+}

Management

- Investigate for underlying causes e.g. menorrhagia, check coeliac serology
- Consider referral for gastroscopy and colonoscopy to rule out malignancy
- 1st line is treating with oral iron supplements (e.g. ferrous sulphate), or intravenous if patient does not tolerate oral therapy. Blood transfusion if Hb level very low

- **Anaemia of chronic disease**

This refers to an anaemia associated with chronic inflammatory states, for example auto-immune conditions or cancer.
- It is the second most common anaemia worldwide.
- Chronic disease results in production of acute phase reactants from the liver such as hepcidin, limiting iron transfer to RBC precursors and stopping renal EPO release.
- The aim is to prevent bacteria from accessing iron, which is necessary for their survival. However, this causes a fall in haemoglobin resulting in anaemia.

Key tests

- Iron studies – raised ferritin, low TIBC, low serum iron, low transferrin saturation
- Bloods show raised free erythrocyte protoporphyrin (FEP)

Management: The mainstay of Management is correcting the underlying cause

- **Sideroblastic anaemia**

This is a microcytic anaemia which occurs due to defective protoporphyrin synthesis.
- Usually, protoporphyrin is made in a series of enzyme-controlled reactions.
- One of the key enzymes in this pathway is ALAS.
- Fe^{2+} ions are transferred to RBC precursors and enter mitochondria to form haem.
- If protoporphyrin is deficient, Fe^{2+} remains trapped in the mitochondria.
- Iron then accumulates to form a ring around the nucleus of RBC precursors, hence they are called ringed sideroblasts.
- This anaemia is characterised by ineffective RBC production, with increased Fe^{2+} deposition in the liver and heart.

Causes

- Congenital defect in ALAS enzyme (involved in protoporphyrin synthesis)
- Acquired causes – lead poisoning or vitamin B_6 deficiency (cofactor for ALAS)

Key tests

- Iron studies – raised ferritin, low TIBC, high serum iron, transferrin high saturation
- Bone marrow biopsy shows disease defining sideroblasts

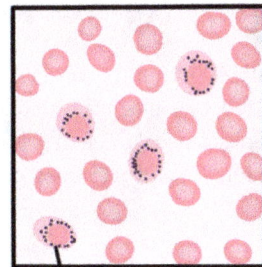
Sideroblasts

Management

- In lead poisoning, give dimercaprol and pyridoxine (vitamin B_6)

- **Thalassemia**

This is an anaemia due to decreased synthesis of the globin chains of haemoglobin.

- Thalassemias are common in the Mediterranean and Africa and divided into alpha and beta-thalassemia based on the chain affected.
- The normal form of haemoglobin is HBA (a_2B_2) and normal variants include HbA_2 ($a_2\delta_2$) and foetal HbF in infancy ($a_2\gamma_2$).
- Thalassemia results in reduced synthesis of one of the haemoglobin chains, producing RBCs which are microcytic and hypochromic.
- It also results in excess of the unaffected chain which precipitates as inclusions damaging cell membranes.

Key tests

- Iron studies to exclude iron deficiency anaemia
- Blood film shows hypochromic cells and target cells (Mexican hat cells)
- Hb electrophoresis is the definitive diagnostic test

- **Alpha-thalassemia**

The α-chain are encoded by two duplicated genes on chromosome 16, each which contribute 25%.

- If 1 gene copy is deleted ($-\alpha/\alpha\alpha$) – asymptomatic.
- If 2 genes are deleted ($-\alpha/-\alpha$) – known as α-thalassemia trait. The RBCs will be hypochromic and microcytic, but the Hb level is usually normal.
- 3 genes deleted ($--/-\alpha$) – this leads to HbH disease. The lack of α chains means there is formation of β_4 tetramers. However, this is less serious than β-thalassemia as they are more soluble than α-chains.
- 4 genes deleted ($--/--$) – known as Bart's disease and leads to death in utero.

Symptoms

- Moderate anaemia – tiredness, lethargy, dyspnea etc.
- Splenomegaly, due to extramedullary haematopoiesis
- Jaundice and gallstones, due to haemolysis

Key tests

- Hb electrophoresis is diagnostic

Management

- Supportive care with blood transfusions, splenectomy can be considered
- Curative treatment is a complete bone marrow transplant

○ **Beta-thalassemia**

This is a condition which occurs due to a mutation in the genes which encode the beta-polypeptide chain. Two β-genes are present on Chr 11.
- A mutation can result in the loss of the chain (β^0) or diminished synthesis (β^+).

■ **β-thalassemia trait (β/β^+)**
This is autosomal recessive disease which is asymptomatic.
- It causes a mild microcytic hypochromic anaemia – the microcytosis is characteristically disproportionately lower than the anaemia.
- Hb electrophoresis shows reduced levels of HbA ($\alpha_2\beta_2$) with a compensatory increase in HbA$_2$ ($\alpha_2\delta_2$) and increased HbF ($\alpha_2\gamma_2$).

■ **β-thalassemia major (β^0/β^0)**
This is a severe form due to mutations giving complete absence of β-globin genes.
- It often presents in first year of life with failure to thrive and a microcytic anaemia.
- α-tetramers aggregate damaging RBCs leading to haemolysis.
- The significant anaemia results in compensatory extra-medullary hematopoiesis causing skull enlargement (crewcut appearance) and facial bones (chipmunk facies) as well as hepatosplenomegaly.

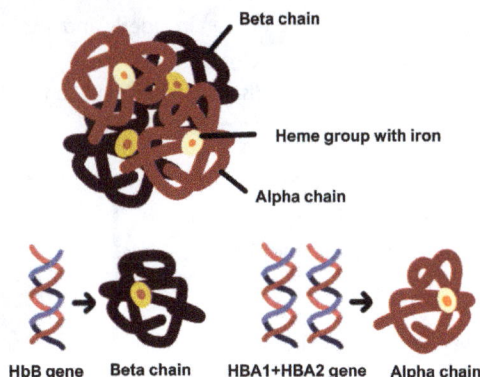

Beta chain

Heme group with iron

Alpha chain

HbB gene   Beta chain   HBA1+HBA2 gene   Alpha chain

Key tests
- Hb electrophoresis shows absent HbA with raised HbA$_2$ (> 3.5%) and HbF

Management
- Lifelong transfusions required, often leads to iron overload (haemochromatosis)
- Iron overload is managed with subcutaneous infusions of desferrioxamine
- Splenectomy if the hypersplenism remains
- Cure is complete bone marrow transplant

Macrocytic Anaemia

This refers to an anaemia with a mean corpuscular volume > 100 um^3, which is often due to folate or vitamin B_{12} deficiency, which are required for DNA synthesis.

Causes of macrocytic anaemia can be remembered by the acronym **FAT RBC MC**.
Foetus
Alcohol excess
Thyroid (hypothyroid)
Reticulocytosis (due to haemolytic anaemia as RBC precursors are bigger)
B$_{12}$/folate deficiency
Cirrhosis (liver)
Myeloproliferative disorders (precursors larger than RBC increasing average volume
Cytotoxic drugs (e.g. 5-fluorouracil)

- **Folate deficiency**

Folate is found in leafy vegetables, nuts and liver and is absorbed in the jejunum.
- Deficiency leads to an inability to synthesise enough DNA for RBC production.

Causes

- Reduced supply – secondary to poor diet seen in elderly and alcoholics
- Increased demand – pregnancy, cancer
- Malabsorption – conditions like coeliac disease giving small bowel inflammation
- Antifolate drugs – methotrexate, sulphonamide antibiotics

Symptoms

- Anaemia – fatigue, weakness, syncope
- Glossitis, angular cheilosis (not koilonychia)

Key tests

- Blood film – hypersegmented neutrophils (> 5 lobes)
- Blood tests – low folate, high homocysteine (as it is not converted to methionine), low methylmalonic acid
- It is very important to also check serum B_{12}

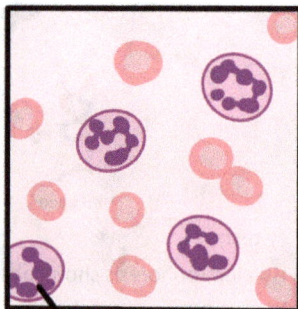

Hypersegmented neutrophils

Management: Folic acid supplements, manage the underlying cause

- **Vitamin B$_{12}$ deficiency**

This is a deficiency of vitamin B$_{12}$, which Is usually seen in elderly people and vegans.

- It is less common than folate deficiency. It often takes longer to develop B$_{12}$ deficiency unlike folate deficiency due to large hepatic stores of vitamin B$_{12}$.

Causes

- Reduced supply – seen in vegans as vitamin B$_{12}$ as it is only found in animal products
- Malabsorption – Crohn's disease, tapeworms affect absorption in terminal ileum
- Pernicious anaemia – autoimmune destruction of parietal cells in stomach which produce intrinsic factor, which is required for B$_{12}$ absorption
- Nitrous oxide usage

Symptoms

- Anaemia symptoms – fatigue, weakness, syncope, glossitis, angular cheilosis
- Lemon tinge to skin due to pallor and mild jaundice (haemolysis)
- Can lead to subacute degeneration of spinal cord

Key tests

- Same as folate deficiency, except there is raised methylmalonic acid

Management

- B$_{12}$ replacement (e.g. 3 times/week for 2 weeks, then once/3 months by IM injection)
- Treat the underlying cause. If also folic acid deficient, the B$_{12}$ deficiency should be treated first to avoid precipitating spinal cord degeneration

---

Subacute degeneration of spinal cord

Vitamin B$_{12}$ acts as a cofactor in the conversion of methylmalonic acid to succinyl CoA.

- In B$_{12}$ deficiency, methylmalonic acid builds causing demyelination of the spinal cord giving neurological symptoms.
- It affects the dorsal columns affecting proprioception and sensory fibres.
- It also gives a mix of upper and lower motor neuron signs, such as absent knee jerks and ankle jerks but hyperreflexia of the extensors.
- Can also give neuropsychiatric symptoms (mood changes) and ataxia.

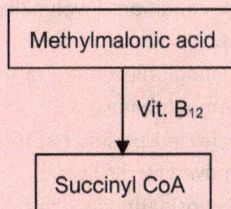

Methylmalonic acid

Vit. B$_{12}$

Succinyl CoA

Normocytic Anaemia

Normocytic anaemia refers to an anaemia with a normal mean corpuscular volume.
- It usually occurs due to underproduction of RBCs by the bone marrow (aplastic anaemia, chronic kidney disease) or increased peripheral destruction (haemolytic anaemias).

To distinguish between peripheral destruction and bone marrow underproduction, the reticulocyte count (RC) is assessed.
- This measures the number of young RBCs released from the bone marrow.
- A functioning marrow responds to anaemia by increasing the reticulocyte count (RC) to > 3% of total RBCs.
- The RC is corrected by multiplying the reticulocyte count by the haematocrit (Hct) divided by 45.
- A corrected count > 3% indicates a good marrow response, suggesting peripheral destruction of RBCs.
- A corrected count < 3% indicates a poor marrow response, suggesting bone marrow underproduction.

Within peripheral destruction, it is important to determine whether the destruction is occurring intravascular or extravascular.
- Once this distinction is made, specific tests can be performed to diagnose the underlying condition.

Intravascular haemolysis

These conditions involve destruction of RBCs within blood vessels and lead to following signs.
- Haemoglobinaemia – raised free plasma Hb in serum.
- Haemoglobinuria – this causes tea-coloured urine.
- Decreased plasma haptoglobin – haptoglobin mops up free plasm Hb, and is then removed by the liver.
- Haemosiderinuria – this occurs when the haptoglobin-binding capacity is exceeded causing Hb to be filtered and freely absorbed by tubule cells which store it as hemosiderin, which is then shed in the urine.
- Jaundice – released hemoglobin leads to an increase in bilirubin, a yellow pigment.

- **Paroxysmal nocturnal haemoglobinuria (PNH)**

This is an acquired disorder which is characterised by the destruction of red blood cells by the complement system, a part of the body's innate immune system.

- It occurs due to a deficiency in the glycosylphosphatidylinositol (GPI) anchor, a molecule that helps anchor proteins to the surface of blood cells.
- GPI anchors decay accelerating factor (DAF) to the cell which inhibits complement.
- The lack of DAF makes cells susceptible to complement lysis, which results in the release of bilirubin and LDH within blood vessels.

PNH leads to intravascular haemolysis occasionally, especially in night during sleep.

- This is because shallow breathing during sleep gives a mild respiratory acidosis which activates complement.
- The lack of CD59 on platelet membranes also causes platelet aggregation leading to thrombosis.

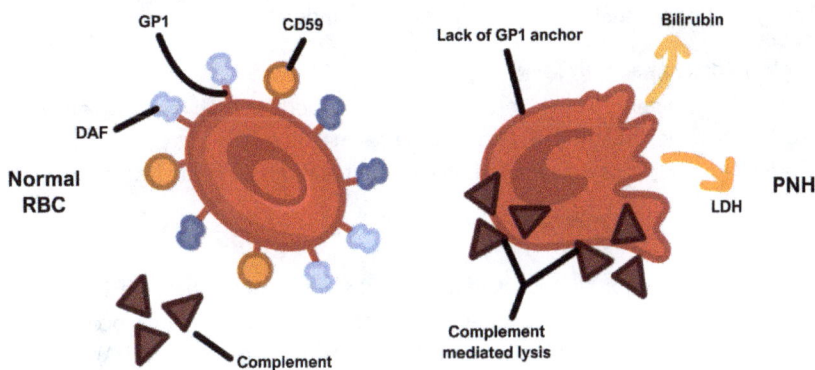

Normal RBC — GP1, CD59, DAF, Complement. PNH — Lack of GP1 anchor, Bilirubin, LDH, Complement mediated lysis.

Symptoms

- Anaemia symptoms
- Haemoglobinuria (tea-coloured urine in the morning)
- Thrombosis – hepatic veins (Budd-Chiari syndrome), cerebral veins
- May evolve to an aplastic anaemia and acute myeloid leukhaemia

Key tests

- Flow cytometry detects lack of CD55 and CD59 on blood cells

Management

- Supportive management for anaemia
- Anticoagulation to reduce chances of thrombosis
- Other drugs include eculizumab (mAb which inhibits the complement system)

- **Autoimmune haemolytic anaemia (AIHA)**

This refers to antibody-mediated destruction of RBCs, usually due to IgG or IgM antibodies. The disease may be primary, or secondary to another condition.

Causes

- Primary AIHA is idiopathic, accounting for more than half of cases
- Lymphoproliferative disorders – lymphoma, chronic lymphoid leukaemia
- Autoimmune conditions – SLE, Crohn's, rheumatoid arthritis
- Infections – HIV, EBV, mycoplasma
- Drugs – penicillins, methyldopa

○ **IgG mediated haemolysis**

This type is characterised by the presence of IgG antibodies which coat RBCs allowing them to be removed by the spleen (causing extravascular haemolysis).
- The IgG antibody usually binds RBCs in warmer temperatures.

○ **IgM mediated haemolysis**

This type is characterised by the presence of IgM antibodies which coat RBCs and result in complement dependent lysis (intravascular haemaolysis).
- The IgM antibody causes haemolysis in cold temperatures i.e. in the extremities.

Key tests

- The diagnostic test for AIHA is called the Coombs test, of which there are 2 types
- Direct Coombs test – anti-IgG is added to the patient RBCs; agglutination occurs if RBCs are already coated with antibody. (Most important diagnostic test for AIHA)
- Indirect Coombs test – anti-IgG and donor RBCs are mixed with the patient's serum. If there are anti-RBC antibodies in the patient's serum, it will cause agglutination

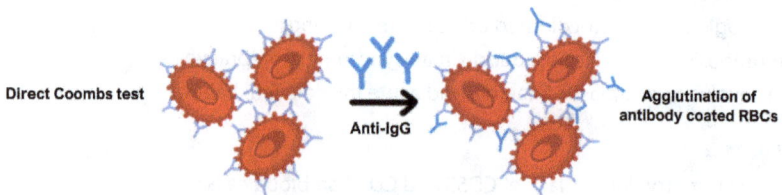

Direct Coombs test   Anti-IgG   Agglutination of antibody coated RBCs

Management

- Treat the underlying cause, and supportive management with transfusion
- In warm AIHA, first line is usually steroids for immunosuppression
- For cold AIHA, keep warm, rituximab can also be used
- Splenectomy can also be considered for AIHA

Extravascular haemolysis

These conditions are characterised by RBC destruction by the reticuloendothelial system (macrophages in the spleen and liver).

- The haemoglobin is broken down into amino acids and unconjugated bilirubin, which collects in the blood giving rise to jaundice.

General features

- Splenomegaly due to increased work by organs
- Jaundice (due to bilirubin release) increasing risk of bilirubin gallstones
- Bone marrow tries to compensate by increasing the reticulocyte count > 3%

• Glucose-6-phosphate dehydrogenase deficiency

This is an X-linked recessive disorder, which results in deficiency of the enzyme glucose-6-phosphate dehydrogenase (G6PD).

- This enzyme is involved in the synthesis of reduced glutathione. Without this, RBCs are susceptible to oxidative stress due to a variety of different causes such as drugs.
- The oxidative stress causes haemoglobin to precipitate as Heinz bodies which are removed by macrophages making bite cells.
- It has a higher incidence in Africans and Mediterranean, due to malaria protection.

Triggers

- Infections
- Drugs – primaquine, ciprofloxacin, sulphur-drugs (sulphasalazine)
- Fava beans

Symptoms

- Often presents with jaundice in newborn babies within the first 24 hours
- Gives acute attacks with symptoms of both intra- and extravascular haemolysis (e.g. anaemia, jaundice, gallstones, splenomegaly)

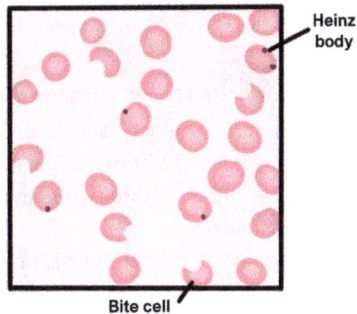

Heinz body

Bite cell

Key tests

- Blood film shows bite and blister cells, with Heinz bodies
- Definitive diagnosis by enzyme assay – this should be taken 8 weeks after attack

Management

- Prevention is key, Management is usually supportive

- **Hereditary spherocytosis**

This is an autosomal dominant condition which affects the red blood cell cytoskeleton, resulting in abnormally shaped, inflexible spherical RBCs.

- These RBCs are unable to move through the spleen sinusoids so get consumed by macrophages, resulting in extravascular haemolysis.

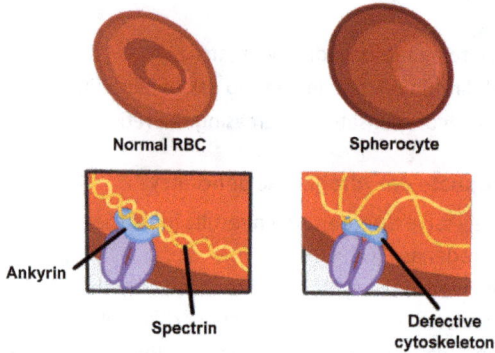

Normal RBC   Spherocyte

Ankyrin

Spectrin   Defective cytoskeleton

Symptoms

- In childhood, causes failure to thrive
- Anaemia with splenomegaly and jaundice
- Can lead to an aplastic crisis with a parvovirus infection

Key tests

- Bloods show raised MCHC (mean corpuscular hemoglobin concentration)
- Blood film shows characteristic spherocytes
- The osmotic fragility test was originally gold standard – spherocytes rupture in liquid solutions hypotonic solutions, due to increased permeability of the spherocyte membrane to salt and water
- Eosin-5-maleimide binding test is now diagnostic – test will demonstrate a reduced ability of the eosin-5-maleimide dye to bind to erythrocyte plasma membrane proteins

Management

- Supportive management if required
- Splenectomy is mainstay of treatment (stops the extravascular hemolysis)

- **Sickle cell anaemia**

This is an autosomal recessive condition caused by a mutation in the haemoglobin β-chain where a glutamate is replaced with valine, resulting in HbS rather than HbA.

- Homozygotes have HBSS (sickle cell anaemia) whereas heterozygotes have HbAS (sickle-cell trait). Patients still make foetal haemaoglobin HbF and HbA$_2$.

○ **Sickle-cell trait**

This is generally asymptomatic and does not usually cause an anaemia.
- It is protective against P. falciparum (malaria).
- RBCs do not sickle except in times of stress e.g. altitude or anaesthesia, which can lead to microscopic haematuria and acute kidney injury.
- It is important to screen high risk patients pre-surgery for this.

○ **Sickle cell anaemia**

HbS polymerizes in low oxygen, causing RBCs to sickle and get stuck.
- This results in both extravascular and intravascular haemolysis.

Symptoms

- It is characterised by periods of good health with intervening crises
- Sequestration crisis – blood becomes trapped in the spleen and liver (giving organomegaly). Can cause severe anaemia and shock, requiring urgent transfusion
- Aplastic crisis – sudden drop in Hb (often secondary to parvovirus infection)

Thrombotic (vaso-occlusive) crises occur when red blood cells occlude in blood vessels leading to infarction of organs and tissues.
- In infants, can cause hand-and-foot syndrome, swollen hands/feet due to occlusion.
- Splenic infarction leads to a shrunken, fibrotic spleen increasing infection risk.
- Ischaemia of bone marrow gives significant pain.

Acute chest syndrome refers to occlusion of the pulmonary microcirculation.
- This causes chest pain, dyspnea, haemoptysis and can result in death.

Key tests

- Blood film shows target and sickle cells
- Diagnostic test is Hb electrophoresis

Management

- Patients will often have a treatment plan in place – this involves strong analgesia, avoidance of triggers, supportive management with blood transfusions

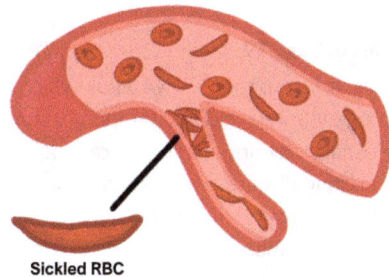

Sickled RBC

- Hydroxyurea is used to increase levels of HbF
- Regular vaccinations and prophylactic antibiotics in splenic infarction
- Other treatments include stem cell transplantation and gene therapy

Underproduction conditions

These conditions are marked by decreased red blood cell production, characterised by a low reticulocyte count. In the chronic setting, the 2 main conditions are renal failure (due to reduced production of EPO) and aplastic anaemia. It can also occur from infiltration of the bone marrow causing fibrosis secondary to malignancy.

- **Aplastic anaemia**

This is a stem cell disorder in which the bone marrow stops making cells, resulting in pancytopenia (reduction in cells of all lineages).

Causes

- Idiopathic
- Radiation
- Cytotoxic drugs
- Viruses (parvovirus)

- (Congenital) Fanconi anaemia – an autosomal recessive condition causing aplastic anaemia, short stature and microcephaly

Symptoms

- Bone marrow failure – anaemia, susceptibility to infections, bleeding

Key tests

- Full blood count shows pancytopenia
- Bone marrow biopsy reveals an empty, fatty marrow

Management

- Stop the offending drug if applicable, treat the underlying cause
- Supportive care – blood transfusions and marrow stimulating factors
- Other strategies include bone marrow transplant

Parvovirus B19

This is a respiratory DNA virus which usually affects children. This virus also infects progenitor red cells and temporary stops erythropoiesis for about a week.

- Usually asymptomatic but can cause an aplastic anaemia if the patient has a pre-existing disease (e.g. sickle cell anaemia or hereditary spherocytosis).
- If reticulocytes are very low (or not raised), suspect an aplastic crisis (this suggest that the bone marrow is not capable of mounting a compensatory reticulocytosis).
- Management is usually supportive as the infection is self-limiting.

Platelet Disorders

Platelet conditions are classified as quantitative (low platelet count due to reduced production or increased removal) and qualitative disorders (involving a defect in platelet structure or function).

- Clinical features typically involve mucosal and skin bleeding (petechiae, purpura > 3 mm, and easy bruising) as well as bleeding from mucosal membranes, e.g. epistaxis (most common symptom), gastrointestinal bleeding, and haematuria.

- **Immune thrombocytopaenic purpura (ITP)**

This is an autoimmune condition characterised by the production of antibodies against platelet antigens, such as glycoprotein IIb/IIIa or the Ib-V-IX complex.

- It can be associated with autoimmune haemolytic anaemia, called Evan's syndrome.
- ITP can occur acutely, which is often seen in children weeks after a viral infection
- This is usually self-limiting and resolves within weeks.
- A chronic form of the disease is more common in women of childbearing age and may be primary or secondary to other conditions (e.g. SLE).

Symptoms

- Bleeding – epistaxis, menorrhagia
- Purpura (especially on the extremities)

Key tests

- Bloods – low platelet count but normal PT/APTT, as the coagulation cascade is unaffected
- Bone marrow biopsy will show increased megakaryocytes

Management

- Mainstay of treatment is immunosuppression e.g. steroids
- IV immunoglobulin (IVIG) can be used
- Supportive treatment with blood products if required or patient is bleeding

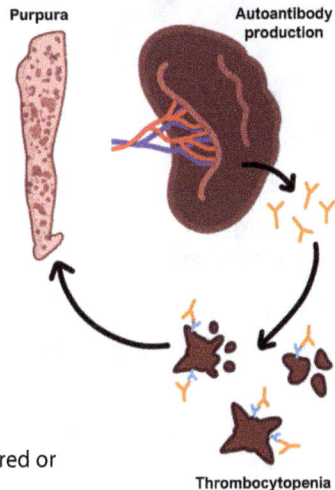

Purpura

Autoantibody production

Thrombocytopenia

- **Heparin-induced thrombocytopenia (HIT)**

This is one of the most severe side effects of heparin therapy, where antibodies form against the heparin platelet complex, which leads to platelet destruction.

- Paradoxically, the fragments of destroyed platelets can activate the remaining platelets, resulting in thrombosis.

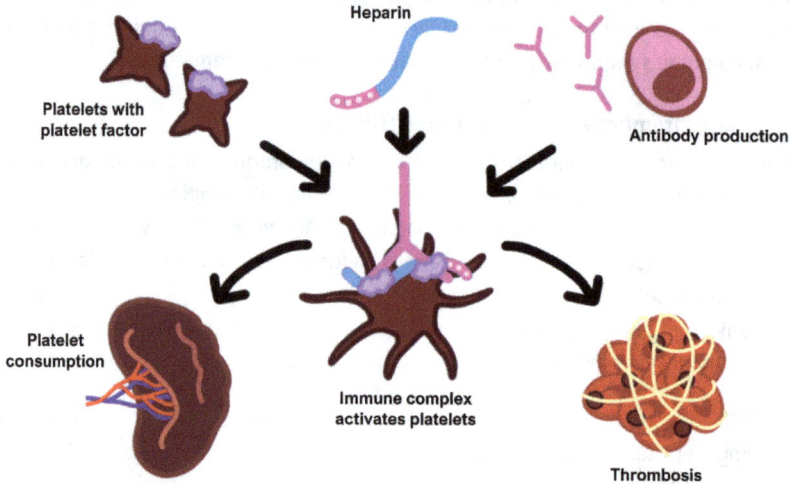

Heparin

Platelets with platelet factor

Antibody production

Platelet consumption

Immune complex activates platelets

Thrombosis

Symptoms

- May present as thrombotic events – stroke, myocardial infarction, DVT

Key tests

- FBC shows low platelet count
- HIT screen (looks for antibodies against the PF4/heparin complex)

Management

- Switch to alternative anticoagulants e.g. thrombin inhibitor lepirudin

- **Glanzmann thrombasthenia**

This is an example of a qualitative platelet disorder, where there is a problem in the structure or function of the platelet rather than the quantity.

- It is caused by a genetic deficiency platelet glycoprotein IIb/IIIa receptor, also known as αIIbβ3, which disrupts the process of platelet aggregation and clot formation.
- Glanzmann thrombasthenia can be inherited in an autosomal recessive manner or acquired as an autoimmune disorder.
- Understanding of the role of GpIIb/IIIa in Glanzmann thrombasthenia led to the development of GpIIb/IIIa inhibitors, a class of powerful antiplatelet agents.

The next 2 conditions are characterised by the pathological formation of platelet microthrombi within small blood vessels, leading to platelet consumption.
- As red blood cells pass through these microthrombi, they become sheared, resulting in haemolytic anaemia characterised by the presence of schistocytes.

- **Haemolytic uraemic syndrome (HUS)**

This is a condition which is usually seen in children, often after a bout of infective gastroenteritis (food poisoning), characterised by a triad of anaemia, thrombocytopaenia and acute kidney injury.
- Primary HUS (atypical) is due to one or several genetic mutations that cause chronic, uncontrolled and excessive activation of the complement system.
- Secondary HUS (typical) usually occurs due to the shiga-toxin from E. coli (STEC) 0157:H7, which releases inflammatory cytokines causing inflammation and vascular injury with microthrombi that are associated with HUS.

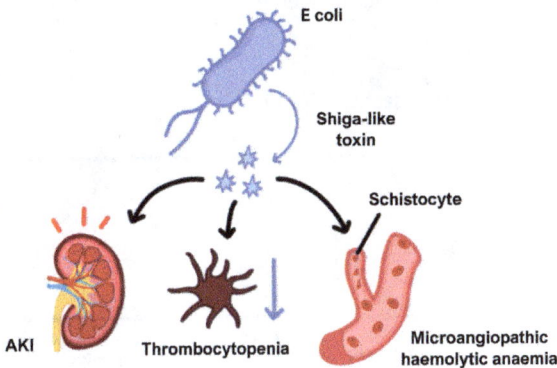

Symptoms
- History of diarrhoea
- Acute kidney injury (oliguria)
- Bleeding (purpura and epistaxis)
- Symptoms of anaemia

Key tests
- FBC shows anaemia and thrombocytopenia, U&Es shows AKI
- Stool culture should be sent if history of diarrhoea

Management
- Typically supportive with fluids and blood transfusion (no antibiotics required)
- Plasmapheresis (blood plasma exchange) can be used in severe cases

- **Thrombotic thrombocytopenic purpura (TTP)**

This is a haematological emergency, characterised by the formation of blood clots in small blood vessels throughout the body, leading to thrombocytopenia and anaemia.

- It usually occurs due to an antibody inhibits the enzyme ADAMTS13.
- This enzyme usually cleaves von Willebrand factor into monomers.
- Inhibition of this enzyme results in the presence of large, uncleaved vWF giving abnormal platelet adhesion, resulting in microthrombi formation. Red blood cells get sheared as they cross these microthrombi resulting in a haemolytic anaemia.
- It can be congenital or due to an acquired autoantibody (which is more commonly seen in adult females).

Symptoms

- There is a classic pentad of 5 symptoms
- Haemolytic anaemia
- Thrombocytopenia (which results in bleeding)
- Acute kidney injury
- Fever
- Neurological symptoms (headache, seizure)

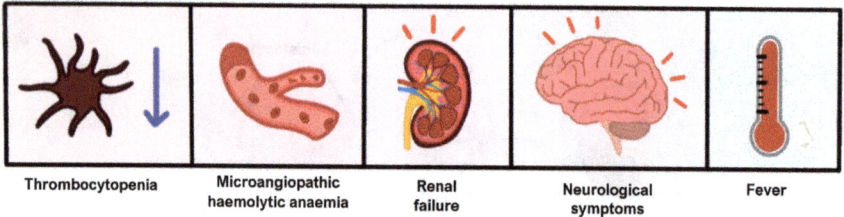

| Thrombocytopenia | Microangiopathic haemolytic anaemia | Renal failure | Neurological symptoms | Fever |

Key tests

- Clinical diagnosis. Aided by bloods which show low Hb, low platelets and AKI
- Enzyme assay of ADAMTS13 can be used in cases of diagnostic doubt

Management

- Plasma exchange – an exchange transfusion involving removal of the patient's plasma through apheresis and replacement with donor plasma
- Immunosuppression e.g. steroids

Coagulation Disorders

These disorders are due by a problem affecting to one or more coagulation factors.
- Typically, they lead to bleeding from joints and muscle as well as after surgery.

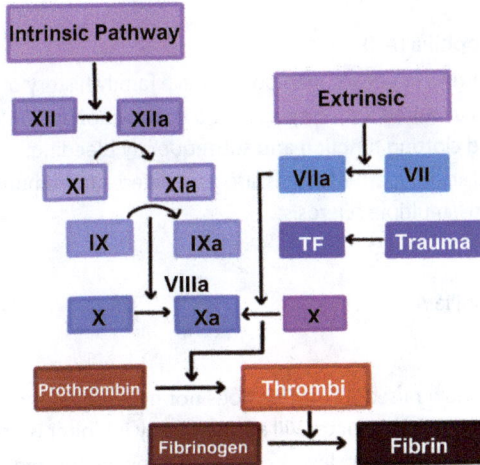

- **Haemophilia A**

Haemophilia A is a genetic deficiency of factor VIII.
- It is inherited in an X-linked recessive pattern, primarily affecting males.
- It can also result from spontaneous mutations.

Symptoms

- Deep tissue, joint (haemarthroses), and prolonged post-surgical or trauma bleeding
- Recurrent haemarthroses can lead to haemophiliac arthropathy (which resembles osteoarthritis but is caused by repeated joint bleeds)

Key tests

- Coagulation screen – raised APTT, normal PT, thrombin time and platelet count/ bleeding time
- The APTT corrects by mixing normal plasma with patient's plasma
- Low factor VIII assay

Management

- For minor bleeds, desmopressin helps to raise factor VIII levels
- For major bleeds recombinant factor VIII can be given (but 10% develop antibodies against factor VIII treatment)

- **Haemophilia B (Christmas disease)**

This is the same as Haemophilia A in all regards, except mutation is in Factor IX.

Management

- Recombinant factor IX

- **Acquired haemophilia (AH)**

A rare disorder occurring in people who do not have family history of bleeding.
- It occurs due to an acquired antibody against a coagulation factor (usually VIII) which results in deranged clotting function and subsequently bleeding.
- About half of cases are idiopathic but it is also associated autoimmune diseases e.g. SLE, rheumatoid arthritis, multiple sclerosis.

Symptoms

- Similar to Haemophilia A

Key tests

- Coagulation tests show raised APTT. This does not normalis by mixing normal plasma with the patient's plasma as a factor VIII autoantibody inhibitor is present
- Factor assay will show reduced levels of the affected factor and the presence of a factor VIII autoantibody

Management

- Immunosuppression e.g. steroids, cyclophosphamide
- Supportive management with blood transfusions and products

- **Vitamin K deficiency**

This is a vitamin activated by epoxide reductase, which is required for the carboxylation of factors II, VII, IX and X. Deficiency results in immaturation of these factors leading to a higher risk of bleeding.

Causes

- In newborns, lack of GI bacteria that make vitamin K
- Long term antibiotic therapy – this kills vitamin K producing GI bacteria
- Malabsorption of fat-soluble vitamins e.g. in liver failure

Management

- Newborns – IM vitamin K injection given prophylactically to prevent haemorrhage
- Adults – IV vitamin K; if significant bleeding, give human prothrombin complex

- ● **Von Willebrand disease**

This is a condition due to a genetic deficiency of von Willebrand factor (vWF).

- vWF is needed to activate the intrinsic pathway and cause platelet aggregation.
- It is the most common inherited coagulation disorder with an autosomal dominant-pattern of inheritance.
- In addition to poor platelet aggregation, vWF is needed to stabilise factor VIII.

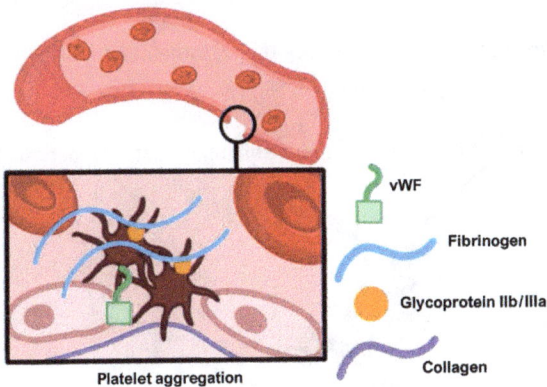

vWF

Fibrinogen

Glycoprotein IIb/IIIa

Collagen

Platelet aggregation

Symptoms

- These resemble a platelet disorder causing mucosal and superficial bleeding

Key tests

- Coagulation tests – high APTT (due to decreased factor VIII), normal PT
- Abnormal ristocetin test – ristocetin induces platelet agglutination by causing vWF to bind to platelets

Management

- Desmopressin increases vWF release from endothelium and stimulates factor VIII
- If bleeding, can give tranexamic acid
- If factor VIII deficient, give factor VIII concentrate

	Haemophilia	Von Willebrand's	Vitamin K deficiency
APTT	↑	↑	↑
PT	-	-	↑
Bleeding time	-	↑	-

- **Disseminated intravascular coagulation (DIC)**

This refers to the pathological activation of the coagulation cascade, due to leakage of tissue factor (TF) into the circulation.

- TF is released in response to cytokines (IL-1), TNF, endotoxins and trauma.
- It leads to the formation of multiple small clots resulting in depletion of the clotting factors in the coagulation cascade resulting in bleeding.

Causes

- Sepsis – endotoxins from bacteria induce the endothelium to make tissue factor
- Malignancy – mucin activates coagulation
- Trauma
- Pregnancy – amniotic fluid leak can induce an inflammatory reaction

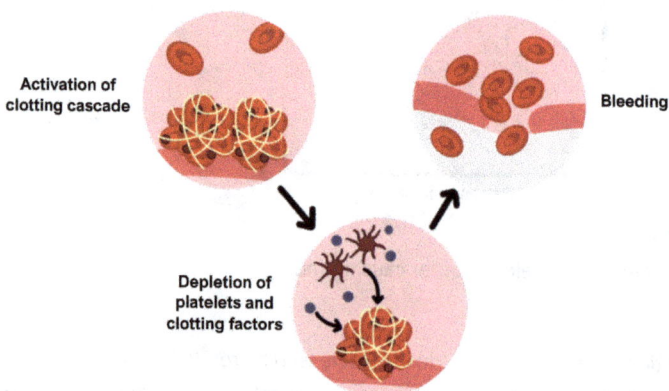

Symptoms

- Bleeding – due to the consumption of all clotting factors and platelets
- End-organ infarction – secondary to microthrombi formation
- Haemolytic anaemia – fibrin strands form haemolysing passing RBCs

Key tests

- Bloods show low platelets, low fibrinogen
- Coagulation tests show high PT, high APTT and high bleeding time
- Raised D-Dimer (good screening test for DIC)

Management

- Address the underlying cause
- Supportive management with blood products, e.g. platelets, RBCs, cryoprecipitate

Leukaemia

Leukaemia is a type of blood cancer that affects the blood and bone marrow due to a neoplastic proliferation of white blood cell lineages that do not function properly.

Leukaemia is usually diagnosed through the following pathway:
- Full blood count (FBC) reveals an elevated white blood cell count.
- Blood smear shows the presence of malignant cells in the circulation.
- Bone marrow biopsy with immunophenotyping – this is diagnostic, showing over 20% blasts along with specific cell surface markers.
- Staging scans – used to assess disease extent and identify organ involvement.

Acute leukaemia

This refers to the malignant proliferation of white blood cell (WBC) precursors, or "blasts", defined by > 20% blasts in the bone marrow.
- These excess blasts impair normal haematopoiesis, leading to bone marrow failure causing anaemia (fatigue), thrombocytopenia (bleeding), and neutropenia (infection).

- **Acute lymphoblastic leukaemia (ALL)**

This is a malignant proliferation of immature lymphoid precursors (lymphoblasts) within the bone marrow, causing bone marrow failure and infiltration of other tissues.
- It is the most common childhood cancer (less frequent in adults).
- The malignant cells express the enzyme terminal deoxynucleotidyl transferase (TdT) and are classified as either B or T lymphoblasts.
- B lymphoblasts are CD19+ but lack CD20+ and the B cell receptor.
- T lymphoblasts are CD3+ but have not yet developed CD4+ or CD8+ expression.
- Cure rates in children reach around 90%, depending on the cytogenetic features.

Symptoms
- Pancytopenia – anaemia (low Hb), infection (low WCC), and bleeding (low platelets)
- Fever may result from infection or cytokine release from leukaemia cells
- Tissue infiltration – hepatosplenomegaly, testicular enlargement, CNS involvement (headache, seizures)
- Bone pain, due to marrow expansion by malignant blasts

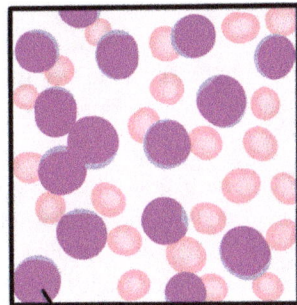

Lymphoblast

Key tests
- Bone marrow biopsy shows lymphoblasts

Management
- Chemotherapy induces and maintains remission
- Bone marrow transplantation may be curative in selected cases

- **Acute myeloid leukaemia (AML)**

This is a malignant proliferation of immature myeloid cells in the bone marrow. It is the most common form of acute leukaemia in adults, with incidence increasing with age.
- AML can develop secondary to other myeloproliferative disorders like CML, as well as following exposure to radiotherapy or alkylating chemotherapy agents.

AML is classified by the cytogenetic abnormalities, lineage and surface antigens.
- A common subtype is acute promyelocytic leukaemia, characterised by a translocation between chromosomes 15 and 17 which results in fusion of the PML and RAR-alpha genes and typically presents in younger adults.
- It can be treated with all-trans-retinoic acid, which targets the abnormal receptor to promote blast maturation.

Symptoms
- Bone marrow failure – anaemia, bleeding, and infection
- Tissue infiltration – hepatomegaly, splenomegaly, bone pain, gingival hypertrophy
- Leukaemia cutis – purple skin lesions from dermal infiltration by blasts

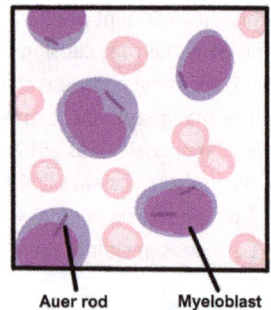

Auer rod   Myeloblast

Key tests: Bone marrow biopsy reveals myeloblasts containing Auer rods

Management
- Chemotherapy is the mainstay of treatment
- Bone marrow transplantation may be considered in high-risk or relapsed cases

NICE referral guidelines (refer to haematology if):
- Immediate referral if child with unexplained petechiae or hepatosplenomegaly
- Offer FBC to adults or child (within 48 hours) if pallor, persistent fatigue, unexplained bruising, lymphadenopathy, unexplained fever

Chronic leukaemia

This refers to the malignant proliferation of more mature white blood cells, which accumulate due to reduced apoptosis rather than rapid cell division.
- These cells may appear morphologically normal but are functionally impaired, leading to a slower onset with symptoms such as fatigue, lymphadenopathy, splenomegaly and increased susceptibility to infection.

• Chronic lymphocytic leukaemia (CLL)

This is a neoplastic proliferation of mature B cells that co-express CD5 and CD20, making it the most common leukaemia in adults.
- It is characterised by an accumulation of functionally ineffective B cells, leading to immune dysfunction and other complications.
- Unlike lymphoblasts in acute leukaemia, these are more differentiated cells with distinct surface markers.
- Mature B cells express CD19+, CD20+, and surface immunoglobulin (B cell receptor).
- Mature T cells express CD3+ along with either CD4+ or CD8+ markers.

Symptoms

- Often asymptomatic and detected incidentally on full blood count
- B cell-driven systemic features – anorexia, weight loss and night sweats
- Increased risk of recurrent infections
- Anaemia – light headedness, fatigue, pallor
- Lymph node involvement causes lymphadenopathy and splenomegaly

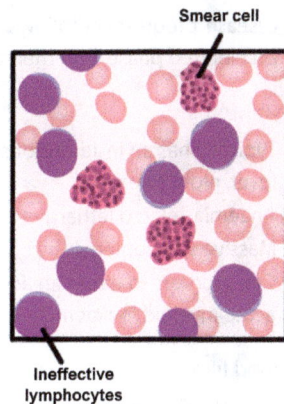

Smear cell

Ineffective lymphocytes

Blood film

- Characteristic finding of smear (smudge) cells due to fragile lymphocytes

Complications

- Autoimmune haemolytic anaemia
- Progressive marrow failure leads to anaemia and hepatosplenomegaly
- Hypogammaglobulinaemia (reduced IgG) increases susceptibility to infections, a leading cause of mortality in CLL

One of the most serious complications is **Richter's syndrome.**
- This is when CLL transforms into a high-grade non-Hodgkin's lymphoma.
- It can present with a rapid clinical deterioration with fever, weight loss, nausea, and marked lymphadenopathy.

Management

- In asymptomatic or early-stage cases, management is usually watchful waiting
- If symptomatic, rapidly increasing cell counts or complications, then chemotherapy is mainstay of treatment. An example regimen is FCR, fludarabine (a purine analogue inhibiting DNA synthesis), cyclophosphamide and rituximab

- **Chronic myeloid leukaemia (CML)**

This is a neoplastic proliferation of mature myeloid cells, including basophils and other granulocytes, which most commonly affects older adults, typically around age of 70
- It is caused by a translocation between chromosomes 9 and 22 (Philadelphia chromosome), resulting in a BCR-ABL fusion gene that encodes a constitutively active tyrosine kinase.
- Disease progression follows a triphasic course: initial chronic phase, followed by an accelerated phase, and then transformation into acute leukaemia (blast crisis).

Symptoms

- Typically has an insidious onset – weight loss, fatigue, fever, night sweats
- Anaemia-related lethargy
- Massive splenomegaly
- Can progress to either an acute lymphoblastic or acute myeloid leukaemia

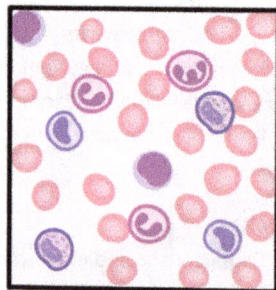

Abnormal proliferation of immature myeloid cell

Blood film

- Shows leukocytosis with myeloid cells at various stages of maturation
- Presence of band forms indicate circulating myeloid precursors

Management

- Due to the translocation, targeted therapy with a BCR-ABL tyrosine kinase inhibitor (e.g. imatinib) can be given
- Bone marrow transplantation is considered in younger or treatment-resistant patients

Lymphoma

Lymphoma refers to the neoplastic proliferation of lymphocytes, typically forming a mass in lymph nodes or extranodal tissue. It is divided into Hodgkin's lymphoma (characterised by Reed-Sternberg cells) and non-Hodgkin's lymphoma (NHL).

The **Ann-Arbor system** is one of the most popular methods used to stage lymphomas.
- It depends on the number of lymph nodes involves, their location in the body, as well as other features like B cell symptoms.
- Stage 1 – a single lymph node
- Stage 2 – >1 node on same side diaphragm
- Stage 3 – nodes on both sides of diaphragm
- Stage 4 – extra nodal site involvement

Some other variables can be included, depicted by a letter after the number.
- A: asymptomatic
- B: presence of B symptoms (including fever, night sweats and weight loss of $\geq$ 10% of body weight over 6 months)
- E: involvement of a single, extranodal site (only in stages I to III)
- S: splenic involvement
- X: bulky nodal disease

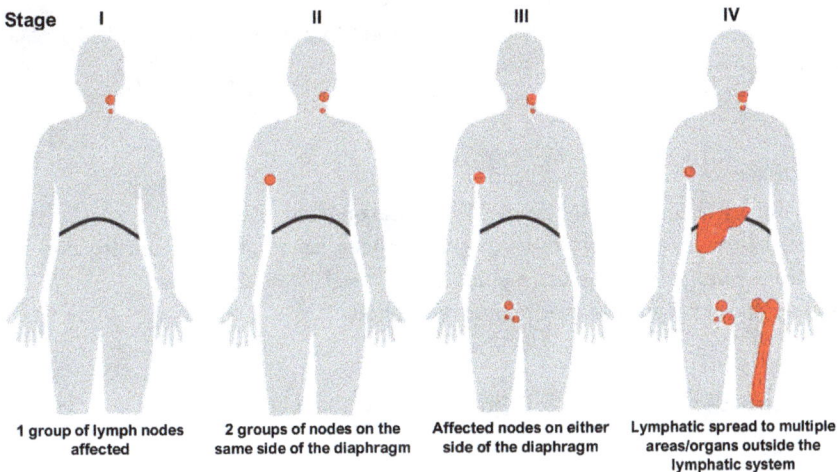

Stage I	II	III	IV
1 group of lymph nodes affected	2 groups of nodes on the same side of the diaphragm	Affected nodes on either side of the diaphragm	Lymphatic spread to multiple areas/organs outside the lymphatic system

- **Hodgkin's lymphoma (HL)**

This is a malignant proliferation of Reed-Sternberg (RS) cells – these are large B cells with multilobed nuclei and prominent nucleoli ("owl-eye" appearance).

- It has a bimodal age distribution, with a peak incidence in the 20s and again in patients aged 60–70 years old.
- RS cells express CD15 and CD30, and secrete cytokines which drive B symptoms to attract inflammatory cells (forming the tumour mass).
- Risk factors include Epstein-Barr virus infection.

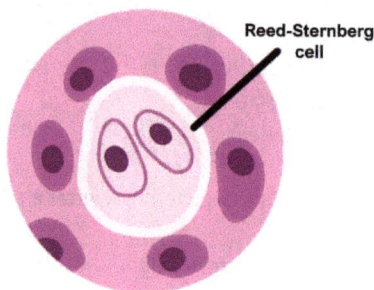

Reed-Sternberg cell

There are a few subtypes of HL, based on the cellular composition of the tumour:
- Nodular sclerosis – most common; shows fibrous bands within lymph nodes
- Lymphocyte-rich – this has the best prognosis
- Lymphocyte-poor – this carries the worst prognosis
- Nodular lymphocyte predominant – this features "popcorn cells" that are CD20+ and lack CD15/CD30
- Mixed cellularity

Symptoms

- Enlarged, painless lymph node (usually cervical or mediastinal)
- Can cause mass effect on lungs – cough, dyspnoea, haemoptysis, SVC obstruction
- B cell symptoms – weight loss, night sweats, cyclical (Pel-Ebstein) fever
- Lymph node pain can be precipitated by alcohol

Key tests

- Lymph node biopsy is diagnostic and shows Reed-Sternberg cells

Management

- Chemotherapy is the mainstay of treatment. An example regimen is ABVD
  ("**A**driamycin" – doxorubicin hydrochloride, **b**leomycin, **v**inblastine, **d**acarbazine)

- **Non-Hodgkin's lymphoma**

This is an umbrella term which describes lymphomas that lack Reed-Sternberg cells.

- These usually occur in older adults and are overall more common than HL.
- Risk factors include EBV, HIV, immunodeficiency, autoimmune conditions (e.g. Sjögren's syndrome).
- Low grade lymphomas are those which are less aggressive, though these are generally harder to cure.
- High-grade lymphomas are potentially curable but carry a worse prognosis.

○ **Follicular lymphoma**

This is a proliferation of small B cells forming follicle-like nodules. It is caused by Chr 14–18 translocation, overexpressing Bcl-2 (anti-apoptotic protein).

- It is a low-grade lymphoma, but can transform into diffuse a large B-cell lymphoma.

○ **Marginal zone lymphoma**

This is a proliferation of B cells expanding into the lymph node marginal zone.

- It is associated with chronic inflammatory states – Hashimoto disease, H. pylori.

○ **Diffuse large B-cell lymphoma**

This is a proliferation of large B cells growing in sheets.

- It is the most common form of non-Hodgkin's lymphoma and is very aggressive.

○ **Burkitt lymphoma**

This is a proliferation of medium-sized B cells, representing one of the most aggressive forms of lymphoma.

- It is caused by a translocation involving the c-Myc gene from chromosome 8 to 14.
- It is associated with the Epstein-Barr virus (EBV).
- Histology shows a "starry sky" appearance, due to interspersed macrophages among malignant B cells.
- The African (endemic) form typically affects the jaw and is linked to EBV and Plasmodium falciparum infection.
- The sporadic form more commonly involves the abdomen, often presenting with ileo-caecal tumours.

○ **T cell lymphoma**

This is a rare form of lymphoma affecting T-cells.

- Due to their rarity and high variability between the different subtypes, the prognosis of T-cell lymphoma is significantly worse than other non-Hodgkin's lymphoma.

Symptoms

- Superficial lymphadenopathy (without alcohol-induced pain)
- B symptoms may develop later than in HL – fever, night sweats, weight loss
- Extra-nodal involvement is more common, affecting the gastrointestinal tract, bone marrow and lungs

Key tests

- Lymph node biopsy confirms the diagnosis

Management

- Mainstay of treatment is chemotherapy +/- radiotherapy

- **Tumour lysis syndrome (TLS)**

This is a potentially fatal complication that can occur following chemotherapy for high-grade haematological malignancies. It results from the rapid breakdown of tumour cells, leading to the release of intracellular contents into the bloodstream.
- This causes significant electrolyte disturbances and associated clinical features.

Symptoms

- Acute kidney injury (AKI) – elevated uric acid can cause acute tubular necrosis
- Palpitations and arrhythmias, due to hyperkalaemia, often secondary to AKI

Key tests

- Bloods show high potassium, phosphate and uric acid levels with low calcium

Management

- Supportive treatment for AKI and hyperkalaemia
- Prevention is key. During chemotherapy, patients usually receive aggressive hydration, medications to lower uric acid levels (allopurinol or rasburicase) and close monitoring of electrolytes and kidney function

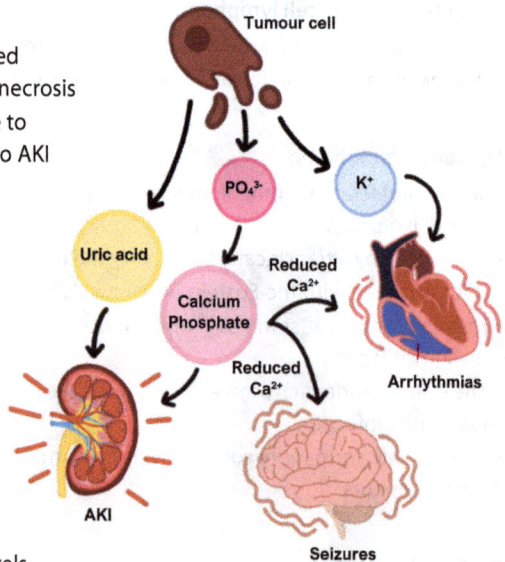

Plasma Cell Conditions

These conditions are characterised by abnormal plasma cell proliferation, which leads to excessive secretion of immunoglobin causing organ dysfunction.
- The urine of affected patients contains Bence Jones proteins (free Ig chains) which are filtered by the kidney.

● **Multiple myeloma**

This is a malignant proliferation of plasma cells within the bone marrow, which typically affects individuals around the age of 70.
- The abnormal plasma cells crowd out normal haematopoiesis, stimulate osteoclast activity and produce excessive quantities of immunoglobulins.

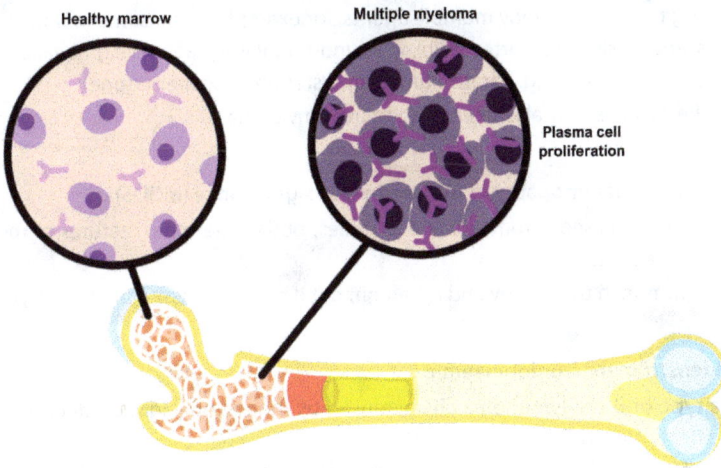

Healthy marrow   Multiple myeloma

Plasma cell proliferation

Symptoms
- Bone pain, usually in the hips and lower back, due to osteolytic lesions caused by increased bone resorption
- Hypercalcaemia (thirst, abdominal pain, constipation, confusion) resulting from the release of calcium during bone breakdown
- Renal damage – light chains (Bence Jones proteins) deposit in renal tubules, leading to real dysfunction
- Bone marrow failure – anaemia, increased bleeding tendency and susceptibility to infections (a common cause of death)

Key tests

- Bloods – anaemia, renal dysfunction
- Blood film shows rouleaux (linked RBCs)
- Serum or urine electrophoresis might show the presence of a paraprotein (monoclonal protein, or M protein) band. The paraprotein is a clonally restricted specific immunoglobulin and IgG is the most common
- Bone marrow biopsy shows > 10% plasma cells
- Whole body MRI – shows lytic bone lesions
- X-ray skull shows a "rain drop skull" appearance

Management

- It is a chronic relapse-remitting malignancy, so monitor and manage complications
- If aggressive disease, then use chemotherapy or bone marrow transplant
- Most drug therapies employ multiple agents, for example proteasome inhibitor which induces apoptosis (e.g. bortezomib), immunomodulatory agent (e.g. lenalidomide), monoclonal antibody (e.g. daratumumab) and steroid (dexamethasone)
- CAR-T therapy has now also been used to treat myeloma

- **Monoclonal gammopathy of undetermined significance (MGUS)**

This refers to increased serum clonal antibodies, but all the other features of multiple myeloma are absent.
- This is common in the elderly and is benign, but it can progress to multiple myeloma.

- **Waldenström macroglobinaemia**

This is a type of B-cell lymphoma characterised by monoclonal IgM production, which usually affects elderly males.
- The proliferation of B cells results in typical lymphoma features, alongside hyperviscosity symptoms caused by elevated IgM levels.

Symptoms

- B-cell symptoms – weight loss, fatigue, lymphadenopathy, hepatosplenomegaly
- IgM-related hyperviscosity – visual disturbances, neurological deficits
- Raynaud's phenomenon

Management

- Chemotherapy for lymphoma
- Plasmapheresis can be used for hyperviscosity (removes IgM from serum)

Amyloidosis

This is a condition caused by the deposition of amyloid, an insoluble fibrillar protein that is highly resistant to degradation.

- In addition to its fibrillar structure, amyloid also contains a non-fibrillar component known as the amyloid P-component.
- Amyloidosis is classified as either systemic or localised, and further characterised based on the precursor protein involved – for example, AL amyloidosis is associated with myeloma (A = amyloid, L = immunoglobulin light chain).
- The median survival is 1–2 years, with a poorer prognosis if associated with multiple myeloma.

○ **AL amyloid (primary amyloidosis)**

This is when a proliferation of plasma cells causes elevated levels of fibrillar immunoglobin light chains which get deposited in organs causing organ failure.

- It is associated with multiple myeloma and lymphoma.

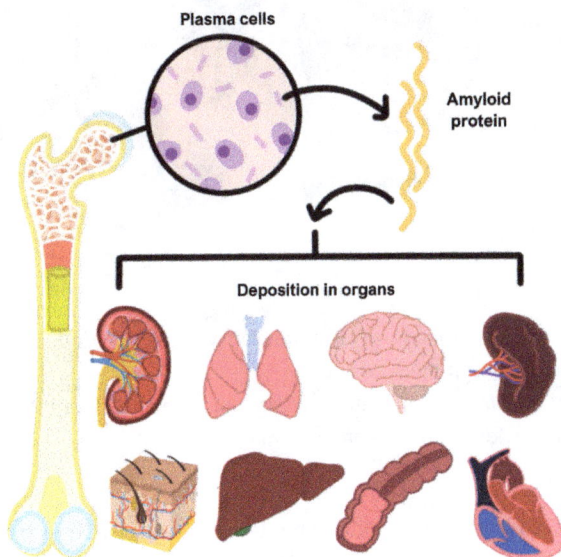

Symptoms

- Kidney – proteinuria and nephrotic syndrome
- Heart – restrictive cardiomyopathy, arrhythmias
- Nerves – peripheral and autonomic neuropathy
- Gut – macroglossia, weight loss, obstruction
- Periorbital purpura is characteristic

○ **AA amyloid (secondary amyloidosis)**

This is when amyloid is derived from serum amyloid A, an acute phase protein.

- It is seen in chronic inflammatory states, such as autoimmune conditions (rheumatoid arthritis, IBD) and chronic infections (TB).

Symptoms

- Similar to primary amyloidosis but usually no macroglossia or cardiac involvement

○ **Familial amyloidosis**

This is due to an autosomal dominant mutation in the liver which gives rise to elevated levels of amyloid in the blood.

Symptoms

- Sensory or autonomic neuropathy with possible cardio/renal involvement

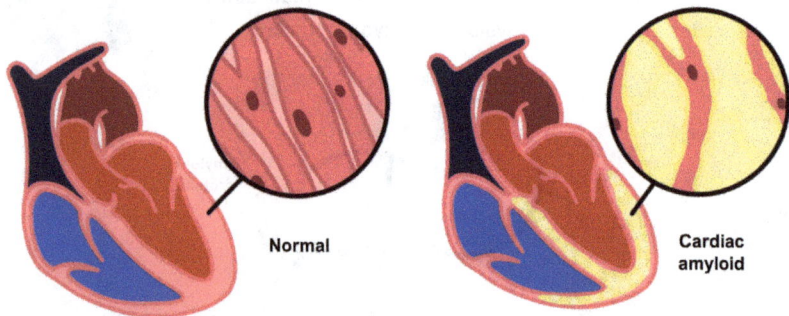

Normal

Cardiac amyloid

Key tests

- Biopsy of the affected tissue (usually a rectal biopsy is taken). A Congo Red stain is used which shows apple-green birefringence
- Serum amyloid precursor (SAP) scan shows amyloid precursor coating organs
- Blood tests show evidence of end organ damage

Management

- For AL amyloid, chemotherapy followed by stem cell transplant is recommended
- For AA amyloid, treat the underlying condition, usually with immunosuppression

Myeloproliferative Disorders

This is an umbrella term which describes a neoplastic proliferation of mature myeloid lineage cells, typically occurring in late adulthood.

- Although cells from all myeloid lineages can be elevated, the classification is based on the predominant cell type produced.
- These disorders are associated with mutations in the JAK2 kinase gene.
- Complications include elevated uric acid levels (leading to gout) due to increased cell turnover, bone marrow fibrosis and transformation into an acute leukaemia.

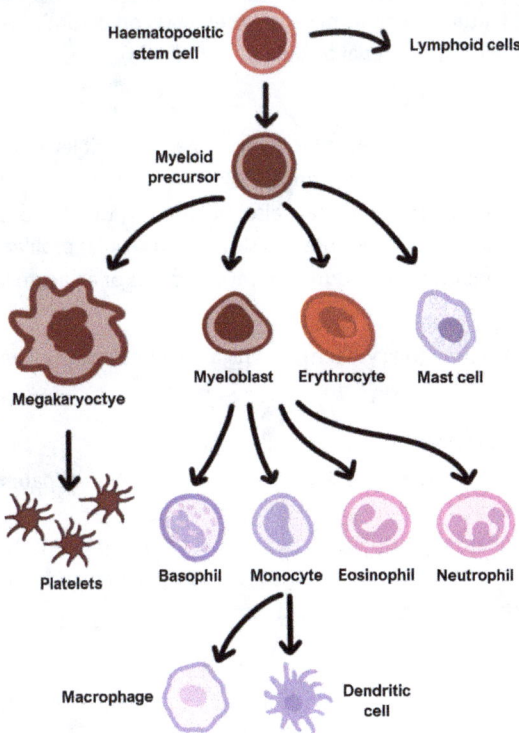

- ● **Polycythaemia vera (RBC)**

This is a clonal proliferation of red blood cells, notable by their independence from erythropoietin for survival.

- The majority of patients are over 60 years old and have a JAK2 kinase mutation.
- White blood cells and platelets are also elevated, contributing to blood hyperviscosity and an increased risk of thrombosis.

Symptoms

- Increased blood viscosity – headaches, blurred vision, dizziness, hypertension
- Itching after hot baths (triggered by histamine release from increased mast cells)
- Flushed face due to vascular congestion
- Splenomegaly
- Thrombotic events – deep vein thrombosis (DVT) and myocardial infarction (MI)

Key tests

- FBC shows high haematocrit
- Genetic testing for JAK2 mutation – however, a JAK2-negative diagnosis is still possible with supportive features, such as raised red cell mass on chromium-51 (^{51}Cr) studies, splenomegaly and normal arterial oxygen tension (PaO_2)

Management

- First-line treatment is phlebotomy to reduce the haematocrit levels
- Low dose aspirin to reduce the thrombosis risk
- Hydroxyurea (hydroxycarbamide) can also be used – this inhibits ribonucleotide reductase which inhibits DNA synthesis to slow down cellular proliferation
- If untreated, the condition can progress to myelofibrosis or an acute leukaemia

---

Patients can also develop polycythaemias, which are not associated with a JAK2 kinase mutation.

○ **Relative polycythaemia**

This is caused by a reduction in plasma volume, leading to an apparent increase in red blood cell concentration.
- Red cell mass studies help distinguish between relative and true polycythaemia.
- In true polycythaemia, total red cell mass > 35 ml/kg (males) and 32 ml/kg (females).
- Causes include dehydration, stress and burns.

○ **Secondary polycythaemia**

This refers to an actual increase in red blood cell production, driven by elevated erythropoietin (EPO) due to an underlying condition.
- Causes include chronic obstructive pulmonary disease (COPD), high altitude, obstructive sleep apnoea and hypernephroma.

- **Essential thrombocythaemia**

This is a clonal proliferation of platelets exceeding 600×10^9/L, with dysfunctional platelet activity that may lead to bleeding or thrombosis.

- Elevated platelets can also be a reactive response to bleeding, infection, malignancy, or iron deficiency anaemia – these causes must be excluded before confirming a diagnosis of essential thrombocythaemia.

Symptoms

- Increased risk of thrombosis – VTE, MI as well as abnormal bleeding
- Microvascular occlusion – headache, chest pain, and light-headedness
- A burning sensation in the hands (erythromelalgia) is characteristic

Key tests

- Full blood count – low Hb with raised WCC and platelets
- Testing for JAK2 mutation

Management

- Low dose aspirin to reduce thrombosis risk
- Hydroxyurea reduces platelet count, interferon-alpha can also be used

- **Myelofibrosis (megakaryocytes)**

This is a clonal proliferation of abnormal megakaryocytes that secrete platelet-derived growth factor (PDGF), which stimulate fibroblasts, resulting in bone marrow fibrosis.

- As a result, extramedullary haematopoiesis occurs in the spleen and liver.
- This condition is usually seen in elderly individuals.

Symptoms

- Anaemia (pale, tired, lethargic)
- Constitutional symptoms – fever, weight loss, night sweats, infections
- Massive splenomegaly due to extra-medullary haematopoiesis

Key tests

- Full blood count shows anaemia with high WBC count
- Blood film – teardrop poikilocytes
- Bone marrow biopsy shows a scarred, or fibrotic bone marrow

Management

- Bone marrow stem cell transplantation can be curative
- Otherwise, treatment is largely supportive with regular RBC and platelet transfusions
- Other options include dexamethasone, hydroxyurea and splenectomy

Porphyria

This refers to a group of rare diseases caused by various errors in porphyrin biosynthesis, which can be genetic or acquired.

- Porphyrins are synthesised through a series of enzyme-mediated reactions.
- Depending on the specific enzymatic defect, there may be an accumulation of porphyrinogens (unstable precursors of porphyrins) or early reactants such as δ-aminolaevulinic acid.
- Early reactants are neurotoxic, while porphyrins cause photosensitivity and promote free radical formation.

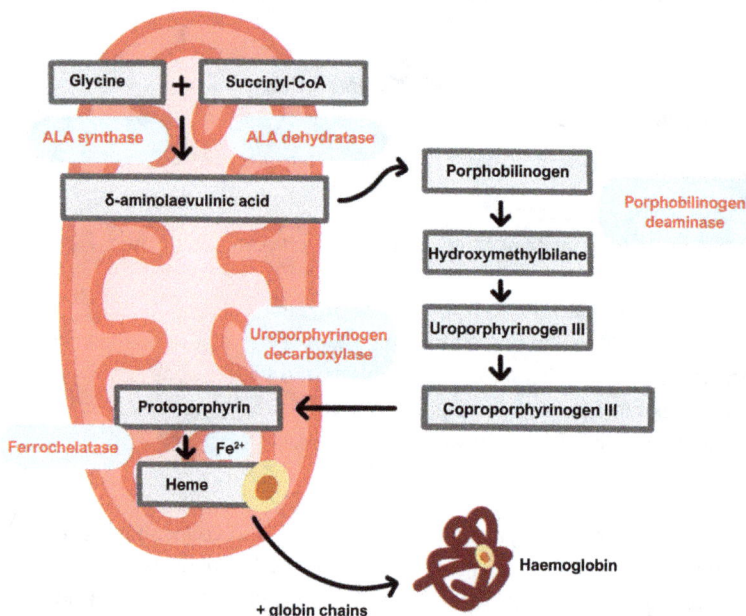

- **Acute intermittent porphyria (AIP)**

This is an autosomal dominant condition which occurs due to a defect in porphobilinogen deaminase, which is much more common in females.

- The results in the toxic accumulation of δ-aminolaevulinic acid and porphobilinogen.
- It characteristically presents in young women with intermittent attacks.

Triggers

- Infection
- Surgery

- Drugs
- Cytochrome P450 enzyme inducers

Symptoms

- GI – abdominal pain, vomiting (colic and fever)
- Neuro – seizures and motor problems
- Cardio – sympathetic overload gives hypertension and tachycardia
- Psychiatric – mood disturbances (depression and anxiety)

Key tests

- Elevated urinary porphobilinogen levels
- Urine turns deep red on standing
- Red blood cell enzyme essay – deficiency in the enzyme porphobilinogen deaminase
- Blood tests – raised levels of δ-aminolaevulinic acid and porphobilinogen

Management

- Involves treating the underlying cause and stopping causative substance
- Supportive management with fluids and electrolytes correction
- Medical management involves haematin (inhibits production of porphyrinogen precursors)

- **Porphyria cutanea tarda**

This is a liver-based porphyria which occurs due to a problem with the enzyme uroporphyrinogen decarboxylase.

- This is a chronic porphyria and does not present with acute intermittent attacks.
- It is usually due to a genetic defect in the enzyme or secondary to chronic liver damage (secondary to alcohol/viral hepatitis).

Symptoms

- Photosensitive rash on the face and hands with skin fragility and blisters
- Excess hair growth all over body with darkening of the skin

Key tests

- Urine test shows elevated levels of uroporphyrinogen
- Pink fluorescence of urine under UV light using a Wood's lamp

Management

- Phlebotomy (guided by serum iron levels). Chloroquine can be used

Obstetrics

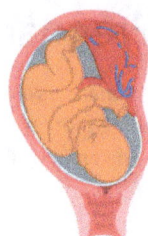

BACKGROUND

MEDICAL CONDITIONS

Pregnancy Basics

Pregnancies are dated by the number of weeks of gestation measured from the first day of the mother's last menstrual period (LMP), known as the gestational age.
- The embryonic or fertilisation age is equal to gestational age minus 2 weeks (because fertilisation occurs about 2 weeks after the LMP).

The gravida, parity, abortus system records the pregnancy count of a woman:
- Gravida = parity + abortus
- Gravida – this is the number of times a woman has been pregnant, regardless of the pregnancy outcome. The current pregnancy is included in this count.
- Parity – this is the number of pregnancies which have reached a viable (≥ 24 weeks) gestational age (including any live births and stillbirths).
- Abortus – this is the number of pregnancies that were lost prior to a viable (< 24 weeks) gestational age for any reason.

For example, a $G_3P_2A_1$ woman means that she has been pregnant a total of 3 times.
- In 2 of these times, it means that the foetus was carried > 24 weeks.
- In one of these times, she had a miscarriage (loss of pregnancy before 24th week).

The average duration of a pregnancy is 40 weeks (280 days).
- Preterm birth refers to a live birth before the completion of 37 weeks of pregnancy.
- A post-dates birth is a live birth after 42 weeks of pregnancy.

Pregnancy is divided into trimesters.
- First trimester = weeks 1 to 12 + 6 (this means 12 weeks + 6 days)
- Second trimester = weeks 13 to 28 + 6
- Third trimester = weeks 29 to 40

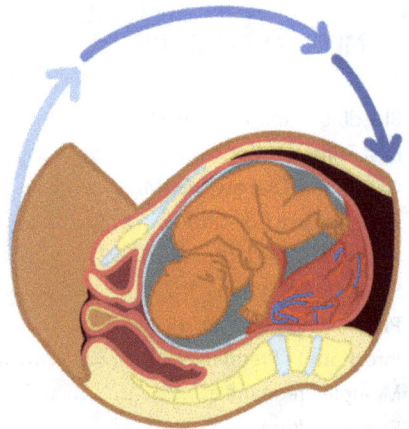

When a woman is pregnant, there are several things she needs to be cautious about.

○ **Alcohol**

UK guidelines state to avoid alcohol throughout the whole pregnancy.
- Alcohol increases the risk of miscarriage in the first trimester.
- Alcohol in pregnancy can result in foetal alcohol syndrome (FAS).

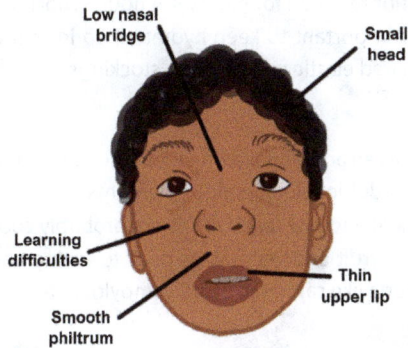

Foetal alcohol syndrome

This refers to the most severe condition within a group of conditions called foetal alcohol spectrum disorders (FASDs).
- It results in developmental problems, including physical abnormalities, delayed speech and language development and learning difficulties.
- Infants have characteristic facial abnormalities, including a smooth ridge between the nose and upper lip, a thin upper lip and small eyes.
- It has no cure and management is supportive.

○ **Smoking**

This increases the risk of miscarriage, intra-uterine growth restriction (low birth weight), pre-term labour, placental abruption and stillbirth.
- Nicotine replacement therapy can be used during pregnancy, but varenicline (Champix) and bupropion (Zyban) are contraindicated.

○ **Exercise**

Moderate exercise is not associated with adverse outcomes.
- Women should avoid scuba-diving and high impact sports which increase the risk of abdominal trauma.

○ **Sexual intercourse**

This is not associated with adverse outcomes.

○ **Air travel**

Flying is not harmful in pregnancy.

- The safest time to fly is < 37 weeks if a singleton pregnancy or < 32 weeks if an uncomplicated twin pregnancy. This is due to the risk of labour after these times.
- Air travel has an increased risk of deep vein thrombosis (DVT) due to the immobility.
- The DVT risk increases with the length of flight.
- Special measures are not required for flights < 4 hours (short haul).
- For longer flights, it is important to keep hydrated, do in-seat exercises, take regular walks and wear graduated elastic compression stockings.

○ **Nutrition**

Carrying the foetus places an additional demand on the nutritional status of the women, and so they should take additional mineral supplements.

- They should ensure meat and raw ready meals are probably cooked.
- It is advised to wash all fruit and vegetables prior to eating and exercise good hand hygiene to avoid bacteria like salmonella and campylobacter.

Supplements

- Folic acid (vitamin B_9) – this is taken in order to reduce the risk of neural tube defects
- The normal dose is 400 micrograms (0.4 mg) taken daily from 4 weeks prior to conception until 12 weeks' gestation
- If the pregnancy has a higher risk of NTD (previous history of NTD, BMI > 30, on anti-epileptic medication or suffer from coeliac disease, diabetes, thalassemia or/and sickle cell disease), then a higher dose of 5 mg daily is recommended
- Vitamin D – 400 IU (10 micrograms) daily and also during breastfeeding
- Iron – recommended if the mother's Hb is < 110 g/dl to prevent anaemia

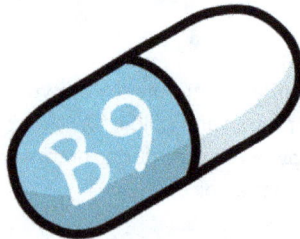

Avoid

- Excess vitamin A – found in foods like liver, as it increases risk of foetal malformations
- Food which may have high levels of listeria – including undercooked meat/eggs, unpasteurised milk (including goat's milk), soft cheeses and raw shellfish/fish

Embryology

The fertilised egg (zygote) enters the uterus 3–5 days after fertilisation.
- It transitions from a morula to a blastocyst which implants into the wall of the uterus.
- The zona pellucida surrounding the blastocyst breaks down so it can attach to the uterine lining (zona hatching).
- Implantation is interstitial, meaning that the entire structure embeds itself into the endometrial stroma.
- The trophoblast layer forms the first syncytiotrophoblast layer of the placenta.

The placenta is a discoid organ which is composed of two plates:
- The chorionic plate covers the foetal surface, and its vessels converge towards the umbilical cord to which it is attached.
- The basal plate is on the maternal side of the placenta. It is composed of decidua (specialised endometrium) and maternal blood enters via spiral arteries.

The placenta is formed in several steps, which are key to its role in achieving efficient nutrient exchange.

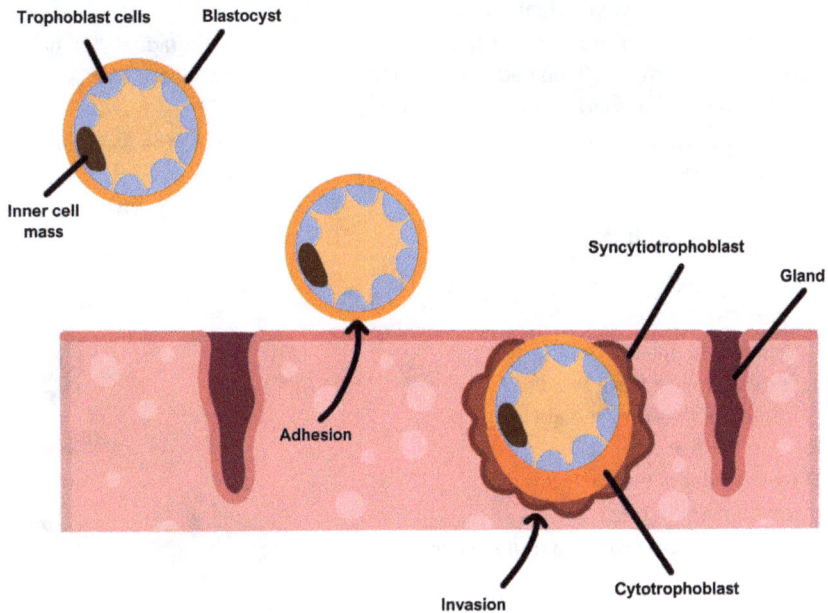

Trophoblast differentiation

The trophoblast (outer layer of blastocyst) differentiates into 2 layers:
- Cytotrophoblasts (CTB) form the inner deeper layer.
- Syncytiotrophoblasts (STB) form the outer multinucleated layer.
- The syncytiotrophoblasts are non-proliferative and are generated by continual fusion of the underlying cytotrophoblast cells.
- They produce the hormone human chorionic gonadotropin (hCG).

Erosion of decidua

The syncytiotrophoblast layer erodes into the decidua (endometrium).
- This breaks the endometrial glands and superficial capillaries.
- Spaces appear within the STB and coalesce to form lacunae, which then fill with glandular secretions and maternal blood (from the uterine spiral arteries).

Formation of villous tree

Cytotrophoblast cells and extra-embryonic mesoderm from the embryo penetrate into the trabeculae of the syncytiotrophoblasts between the lacunae.
- This forms the earliest placental villi.
- Side branches extend from the early villi into the lacunae which gradually branch to become more complex. Repeated branching forms the placental villous tree.
- The lacunae expand to form the intervillous space.
- A vascular network develops in the mesoderm which connects to the foetus via the connecting stalk.

Regression of villi

In early pregnancy, placental villi form over the entire chorionic sac.
- Later however, the villi regress over the superficial pole to leave the discoid placenta (i.e. they only remain in one pole, forming the placenta).
- The remainder of the sac forms the placental membranes.
- These rupture to a provide a route of exit during birth.

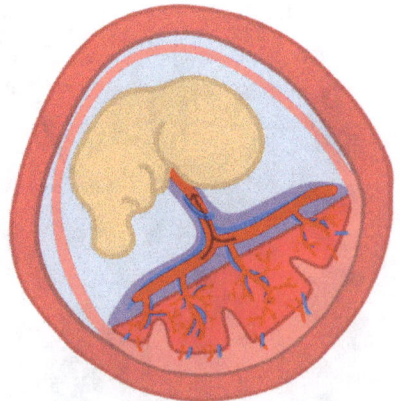

Remodelling of circulation

The general anatomical organisation of the placenta is achieved by 3–4 weeks, but it is not fully functional until maternal circulation has been remodeled by 10–12 weeks.

- CTB cells, known as extravillous trophoblasts (EVTs), invade the maternal spiral arteries which supply the endometrium.
- The EVTs replace the endothelium of the arteries, resulting in vessel dilation and loss of vasoreactivity.
- It results in blood flow to the intervillous spaces that is low pressure and low velocity.
- Failure to convert the spiral arteries is associated with complications like growth restriction and pre-eclampsia.

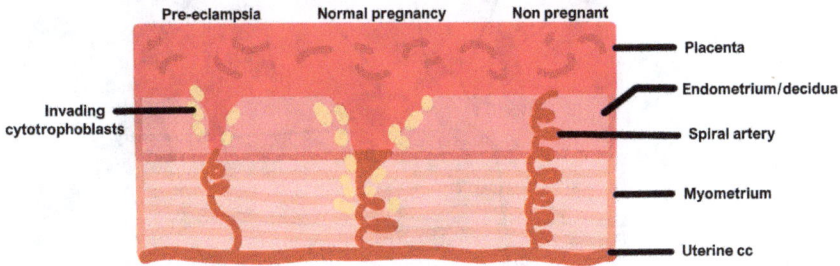

Placental maturation

By the 4th month, the placenta has two components: the decidua basalis (the maternal portion) and the chorion frondosum (the foetal portion).

- During the 4th and 5th months, the decidua form decidual septa.
- These divide the placenta into compartments called cotyledons.
- Cotyledons receive their blood supply through 80–100 spiral arteries.

Full-term placenta

By the end of pregnancy, the placenta has a thickness of about 3 cm, diameter 15–25 cm and weighs about 500–600 g.

- The foetal side is covered by chorionic plate.
- The maternal side is covered by a thin layer of decidua basalis.

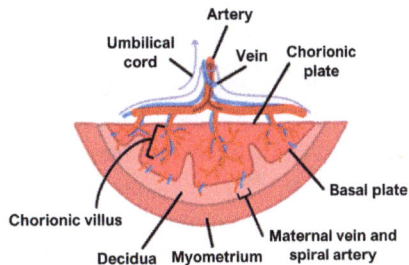

Umbilical cord

The umbilical cord is a connection between the foetus and placenta.
- It is formed from the connecting stalk, vitelline ducts and umbilical vessels.
- It comprises 2 umbilical arteries, which are branches from the internal iliac arteries.
- These carry deoxygenated blood (carrying waste products) from the foetus back to the placenta.
- It also has 1 umbilical vein, which joins the inferior vena cava via the ductus venosus.
- This transports oxygenated blood (with nutrients) from the placenta to the foetus.

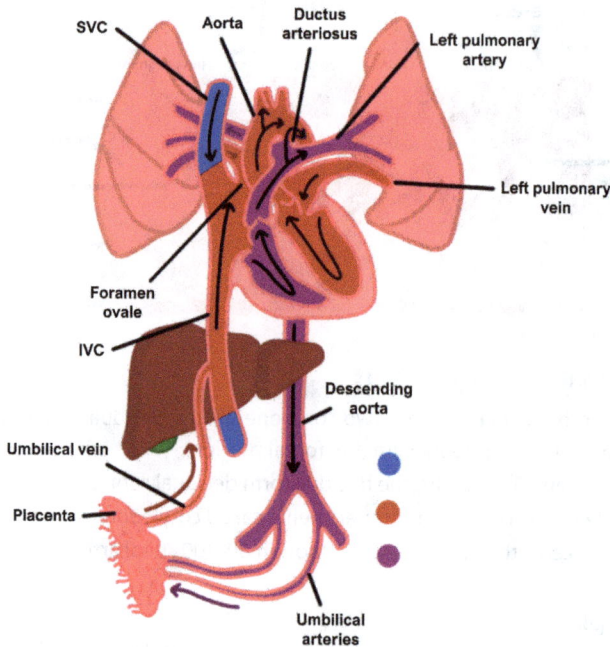

Amniotic fluid

This describes the protective fluid within the amniotic sac that cushions the foetus.
- It also serves as a transport medium for nutrients and metabolites.
- It is formed by maternal plasma diffusing through placenta as well as foetal urine, which is made from approximately 16 weeks.
- The average volume is about 800 mLs at 40 weeks' gestation.
- The amniotic fluid is exchanged every 3 hours towards the end of pregnancy.
- It is eliminated through foetal swallowing (swallows fluid) as well as exchange of fluid at the placenta.
- It contains proteins, electrolytes, vitamins, foetal skin and foetal urine.

Adaptations in Pregnancy

To support the foetus, the mother must undergo several physiological changes to the various tissues and organ systems.

Cardiovascular

Cardiac output increases due to increase in heart rate and stroke volume.
- The heart undergoes left ventricular hypertrophy during pregnancy.
- This displaces the apex beat and can produce an innocent systolic murmur, which disappears after pregnancy.
- The total circulating blood volume also increases in pregnancy due to activation of renin-angiotensin system.

Blood pressure falls in the 1st and 2nd trimester after which it starts to increase.
- This is because progesterone decreases systemic vascular resistance.
- Pre-conception blood pressure levels return by around 36 weeks' gestation.

The enlarged uterus may interfere with venous return. This can lead to ankle oedema, supine hypotension and varicose veins.

Respiratory

In pregnancy, the oxygen capacity needs to increase oxygen to support the foetus.
- This is mediated by hormones as well as physical adaptations which modify the capacity of the thorax.

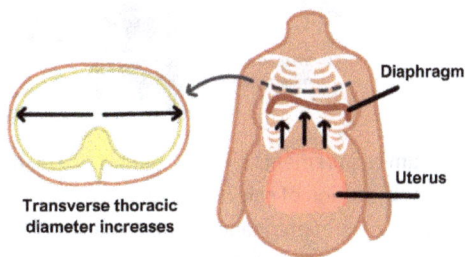

Transverse thoracic diameter increases

Diaphragm

Uterus

- The uterus causes upward displacement of the diaphragm.
- However, there is compensatory increase in the transverse diameter of the thorax.
- This increases the thoracic volume which maintains the vital capacity.

Progesterone is a hormone which stimulates the respiratory centre.
- It increases the tidal volume and hence the minute ventilation (the amount of air that enters the lung per minute = tidal volume × respiratory rate).
- Hyperventilation is common in pregnancy resulting in a physiological, chronic compensated respiratory alkalosis.

Endocrine

Thyroxine is needed for foetal brain development.

- The foetal thyroid does not become functional until the second trimester.
- In the mother total T_3 and T_4 levels rise, whereas free T_3 and T_4 levels remain unchanged. This is because higher oestrogen leads to hepatic production of thyroxine binding globulin which binds more T_3 and T_4.
- The placenta releases thyrotropin-releasing hormone, increasing thyroid-stimulating hormone and T_3 and T_4 production.

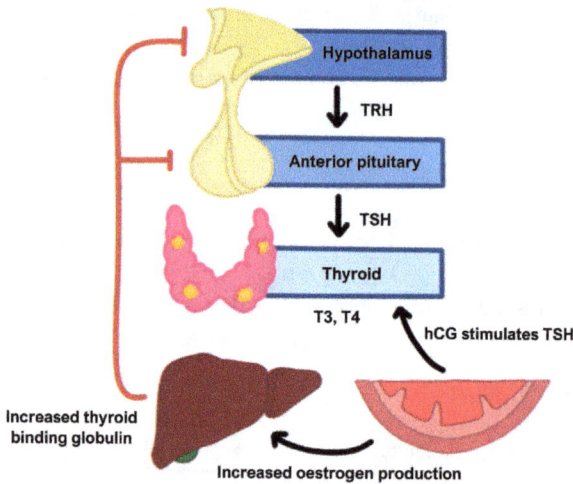

Calcium requirements increase during pregnancy for the baby and for breastfeeding.

- Gut absorption of calcium increases.
- It is advised in pregnancy to take vitamin D supplements to aide calcium absorption.

Metabolic

There is an increase in human placental lactogen, prolactin and cortisol levels during pregnancy which are anti-insulin hormones.

- These hormones increase maternal insulin resistance, thus reducing uptake of glucose by maternal tissues (increasing the risk of gestational diabetes).
- This is needed to ensure that the foetus has a continuous supply of glucose.
- However, it leads to an increased risk of the mother developing gestational diabetes.

Instead of solely glucose, the mother has more dependence on an alternate energy source. This is through free fatty acids (produced by lipolysis) which results in ketosis.

- Diabetic ketoacidosis is an infrequent complication but carries significant risk of morbidity and mortality for both mother and foetus.

Haematological
During pregnancy, there are changes to the components of blood and plasma.
- A physiological dilutional anaemia occurs during pregnancy.
- Blood volume increases more than the red cell mass reducing the haematocrit.
- The WBC count increases (likely due to the physiological stress induced by pregnancy) but platelet numbers fall.
- There is also increased fibrinogen and clotting factors VII, VIII, X, XII, vWF and ristocetin, which reduces the APTT.

Renal

The kidneys are affected by the increase in cardiac output, leading to greater filtration.
- GFR increases due to higher blood flow, decreasing urea and creatinine levels.
- There is relaxation of the ureters, which leads to hydroureter with urinary frequency.
- Relaxation of the bladder increases urinary stasis and predisposes to UTIs.

GI

Anatomically, the foetus can compress the stomach and gut, increasing reflux.
- During pregnancy, smooth muscle relaxes due to increased progesterone.
- This decreases gut motility increasing constipation.
- Relaxation of the gallbladder increases biliary stasis and predisposes to gallstones.
- Progesterone also lower oesophageal sphincter tone, contributing to reflux.

Hepatic

Hepatic blood flow does not change during pregnancy.
- ALP levels increase as it is produced by the placenta.
- The concentration of albumin also decreases, due to the haemodilution during pregnancy.

MSK

The pelvic ligaments relax in preparation for childbirth, which can cause lower backpain.
- There is also increased lumbar lordosis, which helps to maintain the centre of gravity over the hip joints.
- During pregnancy, there is an average weight gain of about 12.5 kg (range = 7–23 kg).

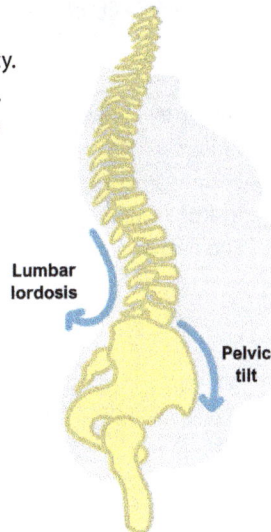

Lumbar lordosis

Pelvic tilt

Lactation and Breastfeeding

During pregnancy the breast tissue develops to prepare for breastfeeding.
- Prolactin promotes growth and development of the mammary tissue during pregnancy. However, milk is not secreted because progesterone and oestrogen block this action of prolactin.
- After delivery of the placenta, the low progesterone levels and high prolactin stimulate milk secretion.
- Oxytocin stimulates milk ejection from the breast as well as uterine contractions.
- Prolactin also disrupts pulsatile GnRH secretion, resulting in the suppression of ovulation and menstruation (natural contraception).

Milk contains the nutrients the infant needs (except vitamin D and K) for the first 6 months of life. It is divided into the colostrum (first milk produced) and mature milk.
- Colostrum refers to milk secreted in the first 2–3 days in small amounts which is rich in proteins and immunoglobulins.
- Mature milk is produced after the first few days and contains proteins, lactose, minerals, trace elements and vitamins as well as fats, some of which are not available in other milks and contribute to neural development.
- It also contains factors protecting against infection: secretory IgA (prevents bacteria from entering cells), white blood cells, lactoferrin and lysozymes.
- It contains bacteria that contribute to the neonates' GI flora.

There are many benefits of breast feeding for mother and infant.

Maternal
- Faster uterine involution
- Aids bonding
- Natural contraception
- Lowers risk of developing type 2 diabetes, osteoporosis, breast and ovarian cancers

Infant
- Lower incidence of diarrhoea and necrotising enterocolitis (NEC)
- Lower incidence of otitis media and respiratory tract infections

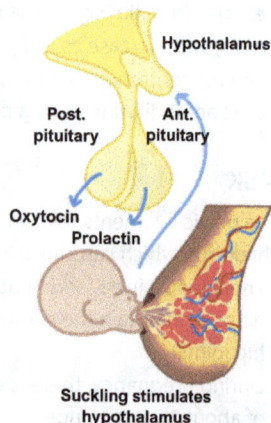

Hypothalamus

Post. pituitary   Ant. pituitary

Oxytocin
Prolactin

Suckling stimulates hypothalamus

Contra-indications to breastfeeding
- Galactosaemia in infant (cannot metabolise galactose)
- Maternal HIV infection – should only breastfeed if an undetectable viral load
- Drug use or excess alcohol consumption

The following drugs are contraindicated in breastfeeding, remembered by the acronym BREAST:

Bromocriptine/benzodiazepines **A**miodarone/amphetamines
Radioactive isotopes/rizatriptan **S**timulant laxatives/sex hormones
Ergotamine/ethosuximide **T**etracycline/tretinoin

Many mothers might struggle with breastfeeding due to technique or latching issues.
- Women can also get additional complications such as infections causing mastitis (see gynaecology chapter) as well as blockage of the milk ducts.

• Engorgement
This refers to the breast becoming swollen with milk.
- It occurs due to compromised milk removal (ineffective suckling, separation of mother or newborn, breast augmentation or less commonly, excess milk production).
- Breast tissue becomes swollen, firm and red, causing difficulty in feeding.
- It causes mild to extreme pain which is typically worse just before feeding.
- It usually occurs in the first few days after birth affecting both breasts.
- If untreated, can lead to blocked milk ducts, mastitis and reduced milk supply.

Management
- Empty the breast by encouraging baby to feed or expression

• Raynaud's disease of the nipple
This is a condition which involves spasm of the arteries which supply the nipple.
- It leads to intermittent pain, which is present before, during or after feeding.
- Blanching of the nipple may be followed by cyanosis and/or erythema.
- The nipple pain resolves when the nipples return to a normal colour.

Management
- Reduce exposure to triggers e.g. minimise exposure to the cold, apply heat packs after breastfeeding, stop smoking
- If symptoms persist, can consider nifedipine

Labour

Labour can be defined as the onset of regular and painful contractions associated with cervical dilation and descent of the presenting part of the foetus.
- The shortening of the uterine myocytes causing contractions is key to labour.
- $[Ca^{2+}]_i$ increases by the influx through calcium channels and by intracellular release of calcium from the sarcoplasmic reticulum (SR).
- Ca^{2+} ions bind to calmodulin, which activates myosin light chain kinase (MLCK).
- MLCK generates ATP which is required for contraction of the filaments.

Uterotonins stimulate uterine contractions. These include:
- Oxytocin – this decreases calcium efflux and increases calcium release from the SR.
- Prostaglandins – these transport calcium ions, increasing intracellular calcium.

Tocolytics on the other hand inhibit uterine contractions. They include:
- Terbutaline and salbutamol – B_2 agonists which increase cAMP levels.
- Nifedipine – this is a calcium channel blocker.
- Atosiban – this is an oxytocin receptor antagonist.
- Magnesium sulphate (weak tocolytic) – this is a MLCK inhibitor.

Labour is divided into 3 stages.

Stage 1

This describes the time from the onset of true labour to when the cervix is fully dilated.
- Uterine contractions start, pulling on the cervix causing it to thin and dilate.
- The cervix dilates to 10 cm allowing the foetus' head to enter the birth canal.
- The latent phase refers to 0–3 cm cervical dilation (slow cervical dilation).
- The active phase is 4–10 cm dilation (faster phase of dilation).
- Primigravida woman usually take about 10–16 hours to complete stage 1, whereas multigravida woman usually less time.

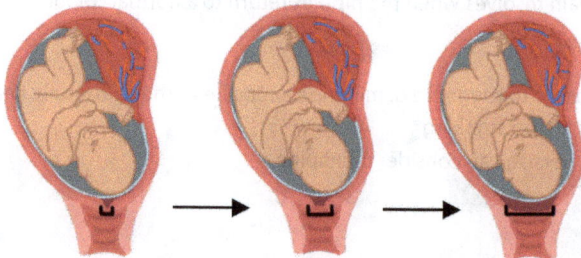

Stage 2

This describes the time from full cervical dilation to the delivery of the foetus.
- It usually can last up to 1 hour.
- The foetal head enters the pelvic inlet with the sagittal suture in the transverse plane.
- It then rotates, so that at the pelvic outlet, the sagittal suture is in the ant-post plane.
- The foetus then rotates again by 90° as the shoulders are delivered.

The ease of stage 2 labour depends a lot on the foetus and its anatomy.
- Size – large foetuses have more difficulty passing through the birth canal.
- Presentation – cephalic (headfirst) presentation is ideal.
- Attitude – refers to foetal flexion (usually foetus is fully flexed, with chin on the chest).

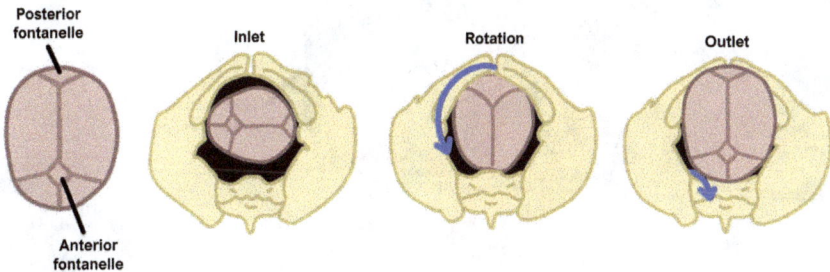

Stage 3

This is the time from delivery of the foetus to delivery of the placenta and membranes.
- After the foetus is delivered, the uterus begins to contract down in size.
- Uterine muscle fibres contract to compress the blood vessels formerly supplying the placenta, which shears away from the uterine wall – it is normal to lose 500 ml of blood.
- This stage is characterised by irregular contractions of low intensity, which forces the placenta out of the vagina.

During labour it is important to monitor both the foetus and mother for complications.

Mother

It is important to check the frequency of the contractions.
- Check BP and temperature to monitor for signs of sepsis.
- Check heart rate as may indicate hypovolaemic shock.
- Vaginal exam is used to check the progression of labour.
- Maternal urine is checked for ketones and protein (risk factors for pre-eclampsia).

Foetus

Foetal heart rate (FHR) is monitored via intermittent auscultation after a palpated contraction at least once every 5 minutes or via continuous electronic foetal monitoring with cardiotocography.

- One of the key things to look out for is decelerations (slowing down) of the heart rate as this can signify reduced blood flow and oxygen to the baby.
- Persistent or severe decelerations may result hypoxic-ischaemic injury and so clinicians may have to take emergency measures like an emergency caesarean.

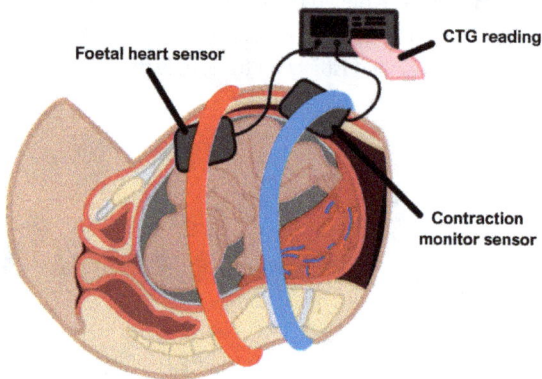

Decelerations refer to temporary decreases in the foetal heart rate.

i) Early deceleration
- This is a symmetrical decrease and increase in the FHR associated with uterine contractions. The timing of these often mirrors that of the contraction.
- They are often caused by compression of the foetal head which results in reduced cerebral blood flow and increased intracranial pressure.

ii) Late decelerations
- This is a reduction in the FHR commencing towards the middle or end of the uterine contraction and finishing after the end of a contraction.
- It occurs when there is reduced blood flow to the placenta, causing reduced blood and oxygen to the foetus. This reverses when the contraction ends.

iii) Variable decelerations
- These are intermittent and periodic reductions in the FHR occurring at variable times in relation to the contraction.
- These are thought to be caused by transient umbilical cord compression.

Whilst the majority of labour in the world occurs naturally, there are times when doctors must intervene to deliver the baby.

- **Induction of labour (IOL)**

This describes the artificial commencement of labour to stimulate delivery of the baby.
- The Bishop score is a tool which guides whether induction of labour may be required.
- It ranges from 0–13. A score of < 5 means labour is unlikely to start on its own soon.
- A score of 9 or more means labour will likely start on its own soon.
- The score takes into account several variables: cervical dilation, effacement, consistency and position as well as foetal station.

Indications

- To avoid prolonged pregnancy (> 42 weeks' gestation)
- Premature prelabour rupture of the membranes
- Maternal health problems (hypertension, pre-eclampsia, diabetes)
- Foetal growth restriction
- Intrauterine foetal death

Contraindications

- Placenta praevia
- Cord prolapse
- Active primary genital herpes
- Vasa praevia
- Breech presentation
- Previous classical C-section

There are 3 main methods of induction.

○ **Amniotomy/artificial rupture of membranes**

This is where the membranes are artificially ruptured using an instrument called an amnihook, releasing prostaglandins.
- It is only performed when the cervix is dilated enough.

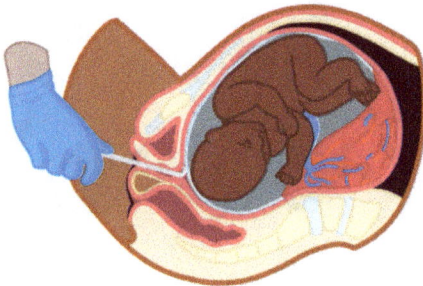

○ **Membrane sweep**

This can be offered at 40–41 weeks for 1st time mothers, and 41 weeks for multiparous women to try to stimulate labour.

- It is done by inserting a finger through cervix and rotating it against foetal membranes.
- This separates the chorionic membrane from the decidua, aiming to release prosta-glandins so natural labour can commence.

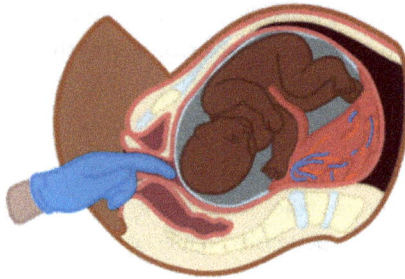

○ **Vaginal prostaglandins**

These are used to ripen the cervix and stimulate uterine smooth muscle.

- They can be given as a gel, pessary or tablet.

Sometimes, there are issues during the labour process, making the delivery more difficult. In such cases, doctors can use instruments or surgically deliver the baby.

● **Instrumental delivery**

This describes a process where the baby is delivered using man-made instruments.

- The decision to perform instrumental delivery is based on the clinical scenario during the 2nd stage of labour. This includes foetal or maternal distress, or failure to progress.
- Contraindications include an incompletely dilated cervix, breech presentation, un-engaged foetal head

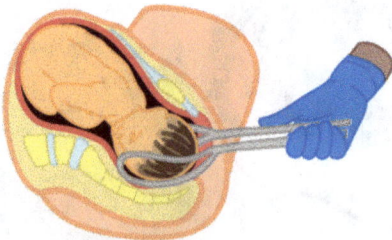

Forceps delivery

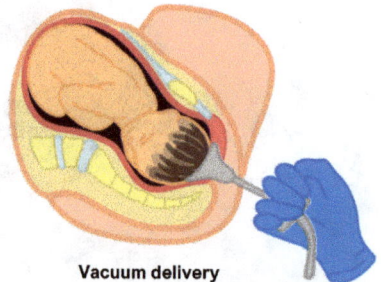

Vacuum delivery

There are 2 main types of instruments used in the UK:
- Ventouse – this attaches a cup to the foetal head via a vacuum.
- Forceps – these are inserted into the vagina and placed around a baby's head.

● **Caesarean section (C-section)**

This is a surgery where an incision is made through abdominal wall and the uterus so that the baby can be delivered.
- Indications include a failure to progress during labour or if there is foetal/maternal compromise during labour.
- The two main types of uterine incision are lower segment caesarean (now 99% of cases) and classical caesarean (longitudinal incision in upper segment of uterus).

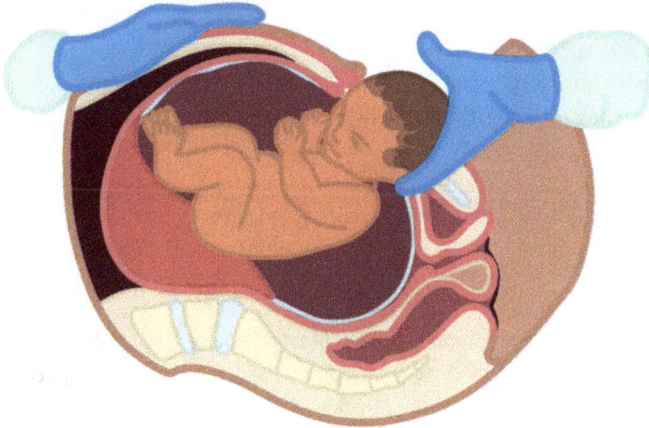

Types

- C-sections are classified based on their urgency
- 1 – immediate threat to the life of woman or foetus
- 2 – maternal or foetal compromise not immediately life-threatening
- 3 – no maternal or foetal compromise but needs early delivery
- 4 – elective (delivery timed to suit the woman/other factors)

Complications

- Foetus – laceration (1–2%)
- Mother – infection, bleeding, pain, blood transfusion, poor wound healing, damage to surrounding structures (bladder, bowel, ureter), emergency hysterectomy
- Future pregnancies – increased risk of uterine rupture, stillbirth, placenta previa and accreta

Antenatal Timeline

When a woman becomes pregnant, there is a schedule of appointments to attend.
- Clinical signs of pregnancy include amenorrhoea (cessation of periods), nausea/ vomiting, breast enlargement and increased urinary frequency and fatigue.
- For uncomplicated pregnancies, NICE recommend women in their first pregnancy to have 10 antenatal visits and 7 for subsequent pregnancies (if previous normal).

Usual route of pregnancy

- **Positive pregnancy test**

Women suspecting pregnancy take a home urine dipstick pregnancy test.

- **GP**

If positive, book an appointment with their GP to discuss folic acid requirements, nutrition and lifestyle. They can book (often online) pregnancy at a chosen hospital.

- **Booking tests**

This is the first major milestone which occurs at 8–12 weeks.
- It comprises of a clinical consultation, investigations and an ultrasound scan.

○ **Consult**

Women are given information on antenatal lifestyle advice.
- Assess the mother's medical history for potential risk factors and complications.
- Take baseline blood pressure, urine dipstick (check for protein) and BMI check.

○ **Booking tests**

Blood tests include FBC, blood group, rhesus status and haemoglobinopathies.
- Screen for infections – HIV, Hepatitis B, syphilis and susceptibility to rubella.
- Urine culture to detect bacteriuria.

○ **Booking scan**

This is an ultrasound scan which is usually done at 11 + 3 to 13 + 6 weeks' gestation.
- It is used to confirm the gestational age and provide an estimated due date.
- Also used to exclude multiple pregnancies.
- It can diagnose early miscarriage (approximately 2%).
- Also assesses risk of Down syndrome and other chromosomal anomalies.

- **16 weeks**

Assess blood pressure, urine dip, anaemia and inform of the screening results.
- Pertussis (whooping cough) vaccine offered anytime from 16–32 weeks' gestation.

- **Anomaly scan**

This is an ultrasound scan which is performed at 20–24 weeks' gestation.
- It is a more detailed scan which reviews each part of the foetal body, specifically the brain, face, spine, heart, stomach, bowel, kidneys and limbs.
- It also determines the position of the placenta.
- It assesses the amount of amniotic fluid and measures foetal growth.

- **25 weeks**

Assess BP, urine dip, symphysis-fundal height (SFH) and discuss foetal movements.

- **28 weeks**

Assess BP, urine dip and measure symphysis-fundal height (SFH).
- Screen for anaemia and red cell alloantibodies (iron supplements are offered if Hb < 105 g/l).
- First dose of anti-D for rhesus negative women.
- Discuss foetal movements and giving vitamin K at the time of birth.

- **31 weeks**

Assess BP, urine dip and measure symphysis-fundal height (SFH).

- **34 weeks**

Assess BP, urine dip and measure symphysis-fundal height (SFH).
- Second dose of anti-D for rhesus negative women.
- Discuss foetal movements and plan for labour and birth options.

- **36 weeks**

Assess BP, urine dip and measure symphysis-fundal height (SFH).
- Discuss foetal movements, palpate the abdomen for foetal presentation.
- Give information on breastfeeding, vitamin K and "baby blues".

At 37 weeks the baby is at term and women may go into labour.
- If pregnancy is prolonged, there may be additional visits required to plan for induction of labour and monitor the foetus.

Termination of Pregnancy

The law regarding termination of pregnancy is based on Great Britain's (England, Wales and Scotland only) 1967 Abortion Act which was amended in 1990.

It states that abortion can be legally provided under the following conditions:

(a) that the pregnancy has not exceeded its twenty-fourth week, and that the continuance of the pregnancy would involve risk, greater than if the pregnancy were terminated, of injury to the physical or mental health of the pregnant woman or any existing children of her family; or

(b) that the termination is necessary to prevent grave permanent injury to the physical or mental health of the pregnant woman; or

(c) that the continuance of the pregnancy would involve risk to the life of the pregnant woman, greater than if the pregnancy were terminated; or

(d) that there is a substantial risk that if the child were born it would suffer from such physical or mental abnormalities as to be seriously handicapped.

In order to conduct an abortion:
- Two doctors must sign a legal document (this requirement for two signatures does not apply in an emergency).
- Only a registered medical practitioner can perform an abortion in an NHS hospital or licensed premise.
- The method of abortion depends on gestational age of the foetus.

Medical methods

- **Mifepristone and misoprostol**

This can be used up to 9 + 6 weeks' gestational age.
- It initially involves giving a tablet mifepristone (progesterone antagonist).
- This causes endometrial decidual degeneration, cervical softening and dilatation, and sensitises the myometrium to the contractile effects of prostaglandins.
- Women are then given the prostaglandin misoprostol 48 hours later (to stimulate uterine contractions) expelling the developing foetus from the uterus.

Surgical methods

- **Vacuum aspiration**

This is used up to 14 weeks' gestation.

- It can be a manual vacuum aspiration (MVA) which consists of evacuating the contents of the uterus through a metal or plastic cannula attached to a vacuum source (handheld aspirator).
- Electric vacuum aspiration (EVA) is similar but employs an electric pump instead.

- **Dilation and evacuation**

This is a technique which is used 14–24 weeks' gestational age.

- It involves preparation of the cervix with osmotic dilators or pharmacological agents pre-operatively.
- The uterus is then evacuated using long forceps and vacuum aspiration.
- This is performed through the vagina and does not require an incision.

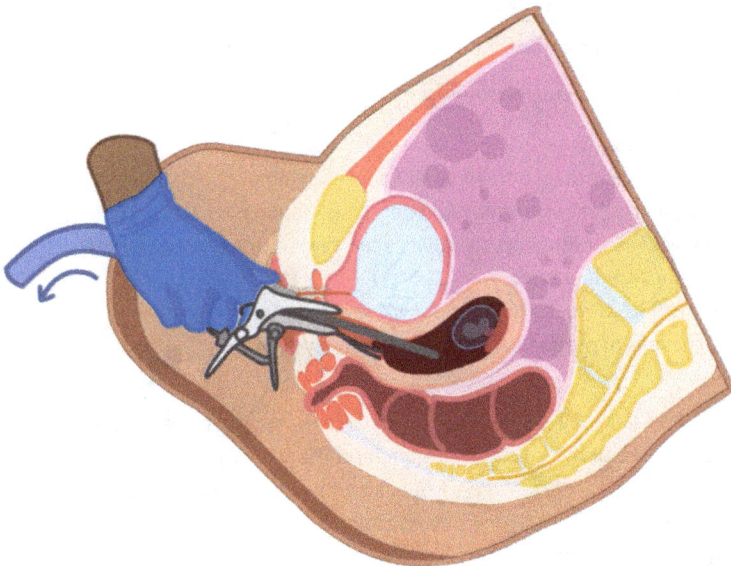

- **Hysterotomy abortion**

This is a technique which removes an intact foetus from the uterus in a process similar to a caesarean section.

- It is not routinely used and instead reserved for cases where other methods are not appropriate e.g. in placenta accreta or if another method of termination has failed.

Tests and Investigations

During the pregnancy, there are some important conditions that the baby and mother are screened for.

Foetus
- Down syndrome (trisomy 21), Edwards' syndrome (trisomy 18), Patau syndrome (trisomy 13)
- Neural tube defects

Mother
- Anaemia, rhesus status, haemoglobinopathies
- Infections – HIV, hepatitis B, syphilis, rubella
- Asymptomatic bacteria in urine
- Pregnancy conditions – pre-eclampsia, gestational diabetes, placenta praevia
- Psychiatric disease
- Domestic abuse
- Those with risk factors or previous disease (e.g. diabetes) may have additional appropriate tests

- **Ultrasound**

Abdominal or transvaginal ultrasound is usual imaging of choice in pregnancy.
- The foetal heartbeat can normally be detected around 6 weeks' gestation.
- At 7–10 weeks of pregnancy, a viability scan can be done to ensure the pregnancy is intra-uterine i.e. not ectopic.
- At 11 + 3 to 13 + 6 weeks of pregnancy, this is called the nuchal scan.
- At 20–24 weeks of pregnancy, this is the anomaly scan.

The nuchal translucency is an important variable that you can measure in pregnancy
- This is a measure of the fluid collected behind the foetus' neck
- Increased nuchal translucency is associated with a range of anomalies:
- Aneuploidy (trisomies and Turner syndrome)
- Congenital heart disease
- Intrauterine infection e.g. parvovirus B19

- **Alpha foeto-protein (AFP)**

This is a screening test used to detect levels of AFP in the maternal serum.
- AFP levels change with gestation (rise from approximately week 14 until week 32).
- Since AFP levels change naturally during pregnancy, an accurate estimate of gestational is required age in order to interpret the results.

Caused of raised AFP: NTDs, abdominal wall defects, twins

Causes of low AFP: Down syndrome, trisomy 18

- **Human chorionic gonadotrophin**

This is a hormone which is produced by trophoblasts, found in the early embryo which become part of the placenta.
- Its main role is to prevent dissolution of the corpus luteum and stimulate production of progesterone by the corpus luteum whilst the placenta is forming.
- This hormone is detected in the urine 14 days after fertilisation and in the serum 6–9 days after fertilisation.
- hCG levels double every 2.5 days, peak at 10 weeks, then gradually decline.
- If low or slow rise, this can indicate an ectopic pregnancy or abortion.
- If high or fast rise, it can indicate b-hCG secreting tumours (e.g. choriocarcinoma).

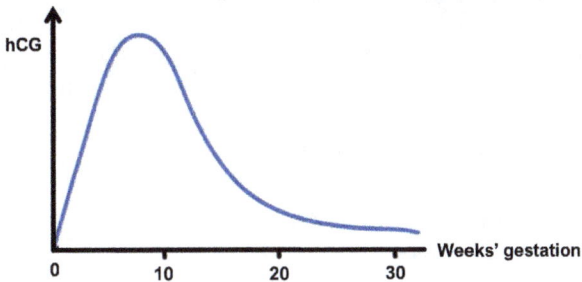

- **Down syndrome screening**

There are two main screening tests used for Down syndrome at different points in the pregnancy. If these indicate a high risk of Down syndrome (> 1 in 150), further investigations are offered.

○ **Combined test**

This is a test which combines ultrasound and a blood test to screen for Down syndrome, Edward's syndrome and Patau syndrome.
- The blood test measures b-hCG and pregnancy-associated plasma protein (PAPP-A) taken at 10–14 weeks.

○   **Quad test**

This test consists of only a blood test to estimate the risk of Down syndrome.

- It is offered in situations where you are unable to measure the nuchal translucency during the nuchal scan or if the first ultrasound scan is > 14 weeks' gestation.
- The blood test is taken between 14–20 weeks' gestation.
- It measures alpha-fetoprotein (AFP), unconjugated oestriol, b-hCG and inhibin A.

Screening which would be indicative of an increased risk of Down syndrome:

Combined test	↑ Nuchal translucency	↑ b-hCG	↓ PAPP-A	
Quad test	↓ Unconjugated oestriol	↑ b-hCG	↓ AFP	↑ Inhibin A

●   **Non-invasive prenatal testing (NIPT)**

This blood test is offered on the NHS in women who have a higher chance result from a combined or quadruple test.

- It screens for Down, Patau and Edward's syndrome.
- The test assesses cell free foetal DNA. This is DNA from placental trophoblast cells which enters the maternal circulation and can be detected samples of maternal blood.
- DNA in placental cells is usually identical to that of the foetus.

Advantages

- There is no increased risk of miscarriage
- Non-invasive
- Earlier diagnosis is possible (from 10 weeks)

Not suitable in the following circumstances:
- For multiple pregnancies (twins)
- If the mother has cancer
- If the mother has a chromosomal or genetic condition e.g. Down's syndrome
- Blood transfusion received in the last 4 months
- Recent transplant surgery

Note that this is still a screening test but the sensitivity for detecting trisomy 21 can be as high as 99% depending on the laboratory. If NIPT suggests a high risk for a genetic condition, further invasive testing can be offered.

- **Chorionic villus sampling (CVS)**

This is a procedure in which a sample of chorionic villi cells are taken transabdominally or transcervically from the placenta under ultrasound guidance needle biopsy.

- It is performed between 11–13 + 6 weeks' gestation.
- Once the maternal material is separated from the placental sample, chromosomal analysis is performed to diagnose chromosomal or genetic disorders.

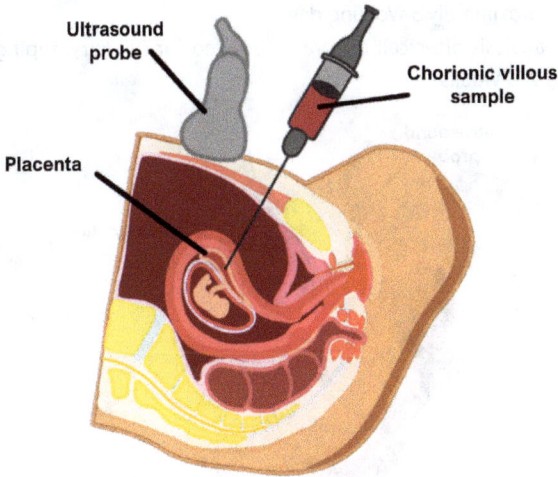

Advantages

- Time of diagnosis – samples taken in the first trimester
- Speed – results within three working days

Risks

- Additional risk of miscarriage following CVS: likely < 0.5%
- Infection
- Amniotic fluid leak
- Maternal rhesus sensitisation
- Sampling failure

In addition, the material sampled is not actually foetal tissue.

- In most pregnancies, this is not a problem as the genetic make-up of the placenta and foetus is the same.
- However, in 1–2% of pregnancies, there is confined placental mosaicism (CPM).
- This is when there is discrepancy between chromosomal makeup of cells in the placenta and cells in the foetus.

- **Amniocentesis**

This is a procedure where amniotic fluid is sampled transabdominally.

- It is performed from 15 weeks' gestation onwards.
- This is used to collect cells from the amniotic fluid and foetal cells within the fluid.
- Amniotic fluid can be tested for different markers (AFP for neural tube defects, enzyme analysis for inborn errors of metabolism).
- Rapid results via PCR on the foetal cells can identify trisomy 21 and other genetic disorders in approximately 3 working days.
- Chromosome analysis after cell culture is required for full karyotyping, which takes approximately 2–3 weeks.

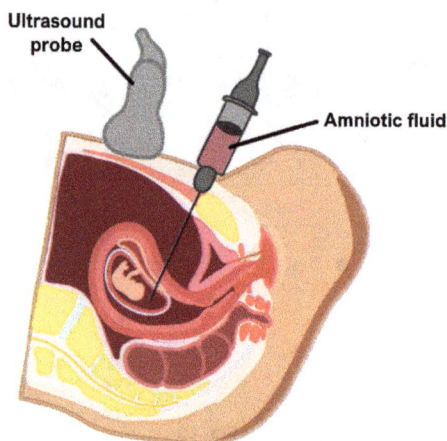

Advantages

- Material sampled – the sample contains foetal material (not extra-embryonic tissue) so CPM is not an issue

Disadvantages

- Speed – full results can take 2–3 weeks
- Time of diagnosis – test is at 15–20 weeks' gestation (or later, at 20 weeks following an abnormal scan)

Risks

- Additional risk of miscarriage following amniocentesis: likely < 0.5%
- Infection
- Amniotic fluid leak
- Maternal rhesus sensitisation
- Failure of cell culture

- **Cordocentesis**

This is known as percutaneous umbilical cord blood sampling.

- It is used to obtain a blood sample from the umbilical cord under ultrasound guidance. It is the only procedure that gives direct access to the foetal circulation.
- It is used to test for foetal anaemia and haematological disorders, chromosomal disorders and congenital infection.
- It can also be used for intra-uterine transfusions and administering medications to the foetus in utero.

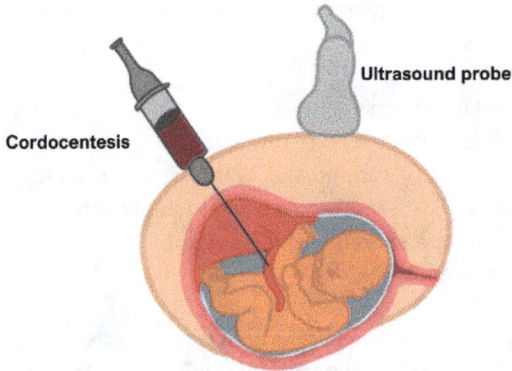

- **Cardiotocography**

This uses transducers to measure the foetal heart rate and contractions of the uterus.

- This can be used antenatally if there are any concerns or during labour (continuously) for higher risk pregnancy.
- It can show bradycardias, tachycardias as well as accelerations and decelerations of the foetal heart rate.
- When reading a CTG, it is classified as either normal, suspicious or pathological.

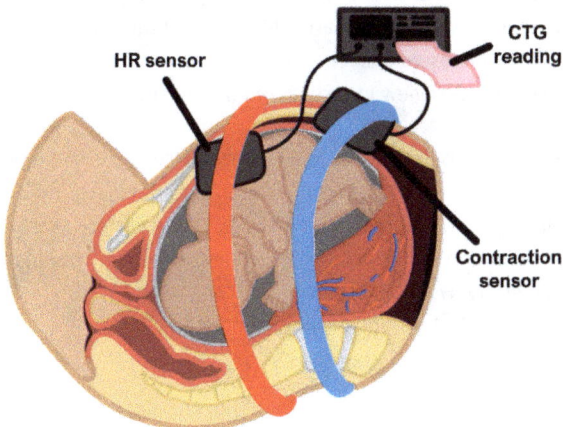

Bleeding in the 1st Trimester

Bleeding in the first trimester of pregnancy is not an uncommon event but is a source of great anxiety for mothers.
- Causes can range from idiopathic to serious conditions like an ectopic pregnancy.
- It can also be due to gynaecological conditions like ectropion, trauma and polyps.

For bleeding, management depends on the gestational age and her symptoms.

If < 6 weeks gestation
- Can offer expectant management.
- Advise the woman to repeat the pregnancy test after 7–10 days.
- If this is positive, contact GP/early pregnancy unit if still concerned.
- If the test is negative this means that the woman has miscarried.
- Alternatively, if there are concerning symptoms (for example, abdominal pain), an ultrasound may be offered.

If > 6 weeks gestation or any pain/tenderness, this requires further assessment
- At assessment, women have blood tests for b-hCG, progesterone +/- routine FBC as well as an ultrasound scan.

Pregnancy of unknown location (PUL)
The term is used to describe when an US scan is inconclusive (i.e. cannot find foetus).
- This usually occurs if the scan is performed < 6 weeks' gestation.
- In this case, take 2 serum hCG measurements 48 hours apart.
- If hCG decreases > 50%, it is most likely is that pregnancy will miscarry.
- Therefore, take urine pregnancy test after 14 days after the second serum hCG.
- If negative, no further follow-up is required.
- If still positive, she needs review in assessment unit again.

If hCG increases > 63%, it is likely is this is a healthy intrauterine viable pregnancy.
- Therefore, offer transvaginal ultrasound between 7–14 days later.
- Consider an earlier scan for women with a hCG ≥ 1500 IU/litre.
- If hCG change is between < 50% and > 63%, review in the early pregnancy assessment service within 24 hours +/- repeat ultrasound scan.
- Serial hCGs are used in PUL alongside ultrasound scans.

- **Miscarriage**

This is a term used to describe a spontaneous loss of an intrauterine pregnancy before 24 weeks' gestational age.
- About 10–25% of diagnosed pregnancies result in miscarriage in the first trimester.
- The most common presenting symptom is vaginal bleeding.

Causes

- 1st trimester – usual cause is chromosomal abnormality (most common trisomy 16)
- 2nd trimester – common cause is an incompetent cervix (risk from cervical surgery)

Miscarriage can be classified into several types:

○ **Threatened miscarriage**

This term means that there is a chance that miscarriage may occur.

Symptoms: Vaginal bleeding, potentially lower abdominal pain

Cervical os: Closed

US findings: Viable intrauterine pregnancy

○ **Inevitable miscarriage**

This term means that miscarriage will definitely occur.

Symptoms: Vaginal bleeding with clots, potentially lower abdominal pain

Cervical os: Open

US findings: Pregnancy still in utero (foetus can be viable or non-viable)

○ **Incomplete miscarriage**

This term means that miscarriage is currently occurring.

Symptoms: Pain and heavy vaginal bleeding. Part of the foetus has been expelled and some remains in the uterus, causing bleeding with clots

Cervical os: Open

US findings: Some products of conception still present in uterus

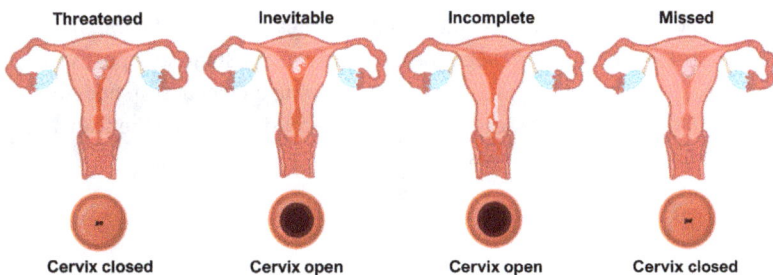

Threatened	Inevitable	Incomplete	Missed
Cervix closed	Cervix open	Cervix open	Cervix closed

○ **Complete miscarriage**

This term means that the miscarriage is fully complete.

Symptoms: History of bleeding +/- pain. Products of conception have passed

Cervical os: Closed

US findings: Uterine cavity empty

○ **Missed miscarriage**

This term means that the foetus has no cardiac activity but is still present in the uterus.

Symptoms: Asymptomatic or light vaginal bleeding/discharge. Had pregnancy symptoms which started to disappear and heavy vaginal bleeding.

Cervical os: Closed

US findings: Non-viable (no cardiac activity) pregnancy within the uterus

○ **Blighted ovum/anembryonic pregnancy**

This term means the gestational sac is present, but the embryo does not develop.

Symptoms: Same as for missed miscarriage

Cervical os: Closed

US findings: Gestational sac mean diameter > 25 mm but no embryo is visible

Key tests

- Transvaginal ultrasound is used, the most important finding is foetal cardiac activity
- If no heartbeat is visualised but there is a visible foetal pole, the crown rump length can be used to estimate the gestational age
- At a CRL of 7 mm, you should normally be able to detect heartbeat
- If CRL < 7 mm, miscarriage cannot be diagnosed at this stage so repeat the scan with a minimum interval of 7 days, then diagnose depending on repeat scan findings
- If CRL ≥ 7 mm and no heartbeat, this suggests that miscarriage has occurred so seek a second opinion on the scan or re-scan with a minimum interval of 7 days

If there is no visible foetal pole, use the gestational mean sac diameter (MSD)
- If MSD < 25 mm, miscarriage cannot be diagnosed at this stage so repeat scan with a minimum interval of 7 days, then diagnose depending on repeat scan findings
- If MSD ≥ 25 mm, diagnose miscarriage so seek a second opinion on the scan or re-scan with a minimum interval of 7 days

Management

Threatened miscarriage
- If there is heavy bleeding admit and observe the patient
- If bleeding is light, reassure and advise to return if worsening bleeding, pain or fevers
- You can take a blood test for hCG (48 hours apart) to check the status of the baby (often if intrauterine pregnancy confirmed but no visible cardiac activity)

Inevitable, incomplete or missed miscarriage
- Can offer expectant/conservative management (watch and wait with a follow up ultrasound scan in 1–2 weeks)
- Medical management is vaginal misoprostol (this contracts and dilates the cervix)
- Surgical options include manual vacuum aspiration or theatre
- This may be recommended if there is persistent heavy bleeding, signs of infection or expectant/medical management is unsuccessful

Complete miscarriage
- Discharge to GP as the miscarriage has already occurred

- **Recurrent miscarriage**
This is the occurrence of 3 or more consecutive first trimester miscarriages.
- Investigations can be split into 3 types used to detect chromosomal abnormalities, underlying haematological issues and anatomical causes.

Investigations
i) Chromosomal abnormalities – these are assessed by karyotyping
- Cytogenic analysis is performed on the products of conception (POC) of the third and subsequent miscarriages. Parental peripheral blood karyotyping is performed when analysis of the POC shows an unbalanced structural chromosomal abnormality.

ii) Blood tests – thrombophilia screen (antiphospholipid syndrome), hormonal profile, TFTs, blood glucose tests.

iii) Imaging – pelvic ultrasound used to detect any structural abnormalities

Management
- This involves managing the underlying condition

- **Ectopic pregnancy**

This is the situation when a fertilised egg cells implants at a site outside of the uterus.

- The most common site is the ampulla of the fallopian tube.
- If it implants in the tube, it usually leads to a tubal abortion or absorption of the embryo, but in some cases, it can lead to rupture.
- Ectopic pregnancy can also occur in the ovary, cervix and peritoneum, or a low caesarean section ectopic (where the ectopic implants in the caesarean scar).

Risk factors

- Damage to the tubes – salpingitis
- Prior ectopic pregnancies
- Inflammatory conditions e.g. endometriosis, pelvic inflammatory disease
- Iatrogenic – IUD, POP (mini-pill)
- Advanced maternal age

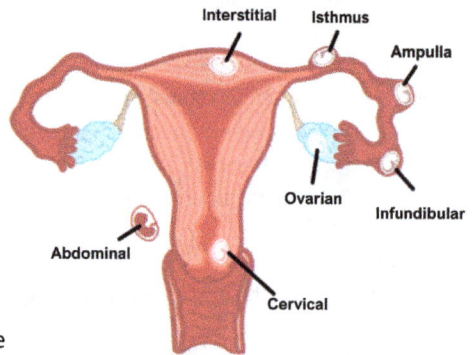

Symptoms

- These occur with a history of a positive pregnancy test or missed period
- Lower abdominal pain, which is usually constant, may be unilateral
- Vaginal bleeding – this is less than a normal period, may be dark brown with clots
- Referred pain to tip of shoulder
- Pain on defecation and urination (due to peritoneal bleeding)
- Dizziness, fainting or syncope if severe with rupture

Key tests

- Positive pregnancy test
- Transvaginal ultrasound is investigation of choice – this is used to detect the size, location and foetal heartbeat (if present)
- Serum b-hCG levels (often serial levels)

Management

Expectant
- This is the preferred method if size < 35 mm, asymptomatic, unruptured, no foetal heartbeat and serum b-hCG < 1000 IU/L
- Monitor patient and repeat serum hCG on days 2, 4 and 7 after the original test

- If the value is dropping by > 15% on each test, repeat weekly until a negative test
- If the b-hCG does not drop by > 15%, re-consider management strategy

Medical management
- This is used if size < 35 mm, no pain, unruptured, no foetal heartbeat and serum b-hCG < 1500 IU/L
- There should also be no co-existing intrauterine pregnancy
- The patient is given methotrexate (this interferes with DNA synthesis killing embryo)
- Repeat serum hCG on days 2, 4 and 7 after the original test and then repeat serum hCG weekly until negative
- A 2nd dose of methotrexate may be required if the hCG levels are not decreasing
- After using methotrexate, couples should wait for at least 3 months prior to conceiving again

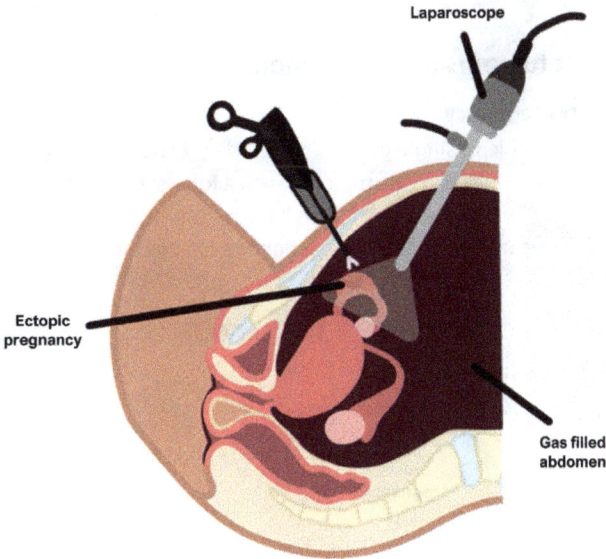

Surgical management
- This is required if size > 35 mm, severe pain, ruptured, there is a visible foetal heartbeat or serum hCG > 5000 IU/L
- In the presence of a healthy contralateral fallopian tube, a (laparoscopic) salpingectomy is usually performed
- If there is contralateral fallopian tube damage or rupture, then an open surgery may be required

First Trimester Conditions

- **Gestational trophoblastic diseases (GTD)**

This refers to a group of pregnancy related intra-uterine tumours which originate from the placenta trophoblast cells.

- They are divided into benign (more common) and malignant conditions.
- These tumours result in very high levels of serum b-hCG which can cause hyperemesis and hyperthyroidism (as b-hCG mimics TSH stimulating thyroid gland).

Risk factors

- Maternal age (< 20 or > 35)
- Use of COCP
- Previous history of GTD

Pre-malignant tumours (more common)

○ **Partial molar pregnancy**

This is a situation in which a single ovum is fertilised by 2 sperm cells.

- This produces a cell which exhibits triploidy, with a total of 69 chromosomes.
- A partial mole may exist with a viable foetus if mosaicism is present (i.e. if the foetus has a normal karyotype and the triploidy is confined to the placenta).

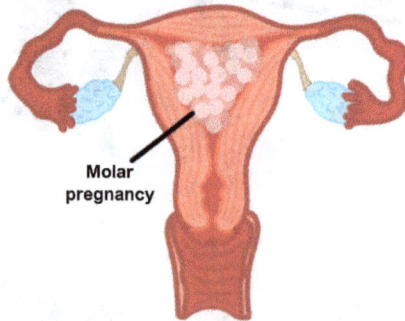

Molar
pregnancy

○ **Complete molar pregnancy**

This is a situation in which one ovum without any chromosomes is fertilised by either one sperm that duplicates (more common) or two different sperm.

- This produces a cell with a total of 46 chromosomes of paternal origin alone.
- On ultrasound, it shows granular/snowstorm appearance with central heterogenous mass surrounding many cystic area/vesicles.

Malignant tumours (rarer)

○ **Invasive moles**

This is partial/molar pregnancy which has become malignant.

○ **Choriocarcinoma**

This is a malignant proliferation of trophoblastic cells of the placenta.

- It commonly co-exists with a molar pregnancy and metastasises to the lungs.

Symptoms

- In early pregnancy, gives vaginal bleeding and abdominal pain
- Soft, boggy uterus
- Hyperemesis, due to very high levels of serum b-hCG
- Can lead to hyperthyroidism (heat intolerance, weight loss, hypertension) as b-hCG mimics TSH
- "Large for dates" uterus, larger than expected for the gestational age

Key tests

- Blood tests show high levels of beta-hCG
- Ultrasound shows an abnormally enlarged uterus which is large for dates
- Histology is performed on the products of conception following their passage to confirm the diagnosis

Management

- This needs urgent referral as the pregnancy is non-viable and needs to be removed
- For molar pregnancies, suction curettage or medical evacuation of the uterus
- It is recommended to avoid becoming pregnant again in the following 12 months

● **Ovarian hyper-stimulation syndrome (OHSS)**

A complication of IVF treatment which occurs after excessive stimulation of the ovary.

- The GnRH and hCG treatment in IVF results in multiple corpus luteum cysts in the ovary which gives rise to high levels of oestrogen, progesterone as well as vasoactive chemicals such as VEGF.
- This results in increased levels of angiogenesis and higher vascular permeability which can cause oedema.

Symptoms

- Oedema – pitting oedema, ascites and pulmonary oedema (giving breathlessness)
- Abdominal pain and bloating
- Dehydration – high risk of venous thromboembolism
- AKI – due to the physical pressure on the kidneys

Key tests

- Measure abdominal girth (used to assess severity of ascites)
- Blood tests show hypoproteinaemia and raised haematocrit

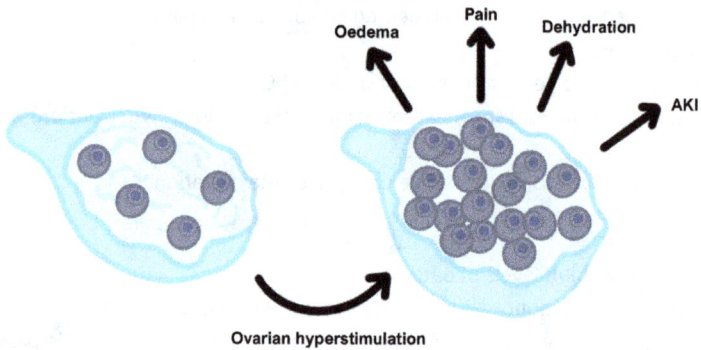

Ovarian hyperstimulation

Management

- This is largely supportive in nature
- Analgesia, titrate fluid balance to reduce fluid shifting into the interstitial space
- Prophylactic low molecular weight heparin to reduce risk of thromboembolism

Prevention

- During IVF, it is suggested to perform single embryo transfer to prevent the risk of OHSS (this also reduces the chance of multiple pregnancies)
- You can also give metformin or cabergoline to help reduce the release of vasoactive substances like VEGF

- **Hyperemesis gravidarum**

This is a condition which causes nausea and vomiting in pregnant women.

- Nausea and vomiting are common during pregnancy, and so the term hyperemesis gravidarum is used if it leads to complications like dehydration or > 5% weight loss.
- This condition is experienced in the first trimester and usually resolves by week 20.
- It is believed to be due to raised beta-hCG sensitising the vomiting centre.
- Severe vomiting leads to dehydration and electrolyte abnormalities in the mother.

Risk factors

- Factors which increase b-hCG – multiple pregnancies, gestational trophoblastic disease
- Hyperthyroidism – TSH is similar to b-hCG
- Obesity

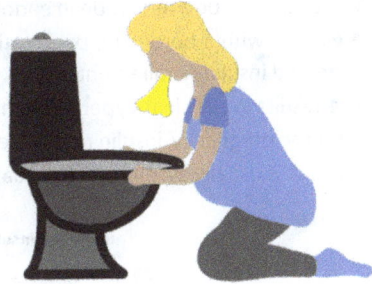

Symptoms

- Severe nausea and vomiting accompanied with weight loss

Complications

- Mechanical – Mallory-Weiss tear of the oesophagus
- Neurological – Wernicke's encephalopathy, central pontine myelinolysis
- Renal – acute tubular necrosis, AKI due to hypovolaemia
- Foetal – preterm birth and intrauterine growth restriction

Key tests

- In addition to the nausea and vomiting, you need additional features such as:
- Weight loss of > 5% pre-pregnancy weight
- Dehydration and electrolyte disturbances (shown on blood tests)
- Check urine for ketones – if these are raised, will likely need to admit the patient

Management

- Anti-emetics – 1st line is usually promethazine or cyclizine
- 2nd line anti-emetics include ondansetron and metoclopramide
- IV fluids (e.g. Hartmann's solution) for rehydration with vitamin B_1 replacement
- VTE prophylaxis – dehydrated patients are at a high risk of venous thromboembolism
- If unresolving, you can give steroids (e.g. IV hydrocortisone)
- Last resort is a termination of the pregnancy

Gestational Diabetes (GDM)

This is a common complication of pregnancy.
- It is defined as any degree of glucose intolerance during pregnancy.
- It most commonly occurs in the 2nd or 3rd trimester.

During pregnancy, women can develop progressive insulin resistance which means a higher volume of insulin is needed to respond to a normal level of blood glucose.
- There can also be a reduction in endogenous production of insulin.
- A woman with a borderline pancreatic reserve is therefore unable to respond to the increased insulin requirement.
- This results in transient hyperglycaemia giving gestational diabetes.
- After the pregnancy, insulin resistance falls and the hyperglycaemia usually resolves.
- Whilst it is usually asymptomatic usually, it can lead to complications for the foetus.

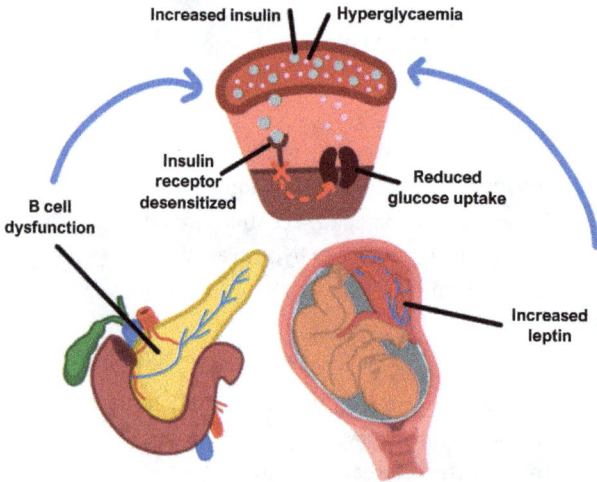

Risk factors

- BMI ≥ 30, PCOS
- Past medical or family history of diabetes, previous gestational diabetes
- Previous baby with a birth weight of ≥ 4.5 kg
- Ethnicity – South Asian, Chinese, African-Caribbean or Middle Eastern

Symptoms

- Usually asymptomatic
- Can give symptoms of hyperglycaemia – polyuria, polydipsia and fatigue

In pregnancy, glucose is transported across the placenta, but insulin is not.
- High levels of glucose in the maternal circulation can cause foetal hyperglycaemia.
- In response, the foetus will increase its own insulin levels, resulting in hyperinsulinemia.

Complications

Antenatal
- Macrosomia (due to the growth stimulating effect of insulin), increasing the risk of shoulder dystocia and labour complications (perineal tears)
- Polyhydramnios
- Pre-term delivery
- Increased likelihood of induction of labour or caesarean section
- Increased risk of stillbirth
- Increased risk of hypertension and pre-eclampsia

Postnatal
- After delivery, the foetus still produces high levels of insulin, but the high glucose environment no longer exists resulting in an increased risk of hypoglycaemia
- Polycythaemia
- Decreased foetal surfactant increasing risk of respiratory distress syndrome
- Increased risk of jaundice
- Increased risk of the baby developing diabetes and obesity in the future
- Increased risk of mother developing type 2 diabetes in the future

Key tests
- Oral glucose tolerance test (measure blood glucose 2 hours after 75 g glucose drink) between 24–28 weeks' gestation
- A positive result is glucose ≥ 7.8 mmol/litre
- Alternatively, it can be diagnosed if fasting glucose ≥ 5.6 mmol/litre

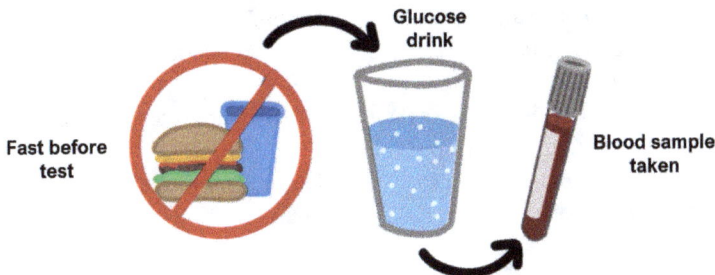

Fast before test   **Glucose drink**   **Blood sample taken**

Screening
- Women are offered screening for gestational diabetes using an OGTT if:
- Previous gestational diabetes, previous macrosomic baby weighing > 4.5 kg
- BMI > 30
- Family history of diabetes (first degree relative)
- Ethnicity with high prevalence of diabetes e.g. South Asian
- If at any point during the pregnancy, urine dipstick shows 2+ glycosuria on one occasion or 1+ glycosuria on two or more occasions, consider screening OGTT

Management

Diabetes
- This involves management of the diabetes and also the pregnancy
- If fasting glucose < 7 mmol/litre on diagnosis, diet control and exercise
- If glucose targets not met within 2 weeks, commence metformin
- If still uncontrolled despite metformin, start insulin
- If fasting glucose > 7 mmol/litre on diagnosis, start insulin +/- metformin
- If 6–6.9 mmol/litre with foetal complications such as macrosomia or polyhydramnios on diagnosis, then insulin +/- metformin is recommended

Pregnancy
- Antenatal – additional growth screen every 4 weeks from week 28 (this frequency can be adjusted depending on the scan results)

- Delivery – the mode of delivery is dependent on estimated foetal weight and other foetal concerns. GDM does not preclude a normal vaginal delivery

- Postnatal – stop all diabetic medications immediately after delivery
- Feed the baby as soon as possible after delivery and at frequent intervals
- Monitor the baby will be monitored for hypoglycaemia
- Test mother's blood glucose in the postnatal period whilst in hospital to exclude persisting hyperglycaemia
- Fasting plasma glucose test 6–13 weeks after delivery (in the community); this is often done at the GP postnatal check
- Annual HbA1C for women with GDM whose blood sugars normalise in the post-natal period to screen for diabetes

Hypertensive Conditions

- **Pregnancy-induced hypertension (PIH)/Gestational hypertension**

This is defined as having high blood pressure which occurs after the 20th week of pregnancy without proteinuria.

- If a woman has a previous diagnosis of hypertension, this is referred to as pre-existing or chronic hypertension.
- If she develops other symptoms such as proteinuria and oedema, this indicates pre-eclampsia on a background of chronic hypertension.
- Gestational hypertension resolves after birth, but women have higher risk of hypertensive disorders in the next pregnancy.
- It is important to be aware of the potential progression to pre-eclampsia.

Hypertension is defined as two separate readings confirming either:
- Systolic > 140 mmHg or diastolic > 90 mmHg
- However, a diagnosis can be considered if there is a significant increase in the patient's BP from the booking BP even if the BP is < 140/90

Key tests

- Monitor BP (once or twice per week depending on BP levels)
- Urine dipstick and protein: creatinine ratio if urine dip 1+ or more proteinuria
- Blood tests – FBC, LFTs, U&Es and coagulation screen

Management

- 1st line is labetalol, 2nd line nifedipine, 3rd line methyldopa
- Monitor BP 1–2 times per week (aim for < 135/85)
- Monitor urine dipstick for proteinuria 1–2 times per week
- Foetal monitoring – CTG only if clinically indicated; ultrasound scans can be repeated every 2–4 weeks if clinically indicated

- **Pre-eclampsia**

This is a disorder during pregnancy which is characterised by the presence of new onset hypertension with proteinuria and maternal organ dysfunction.

- If left untreated it can cause significant problems for both the mother and baby.

Pre-eclampsia is thought to result from poor placental perfusion.
- In normal placentation, trophoblast cells invade the spiral arteries of the uterus.
- Remodelling occurs resulting in spiral arteries that are dilated giving a high flow, low resistance circulation.
- In pre-eclampsia, there is poor remodelling of the spiral arteries resulting in a low-flow and high-resistance circulation.

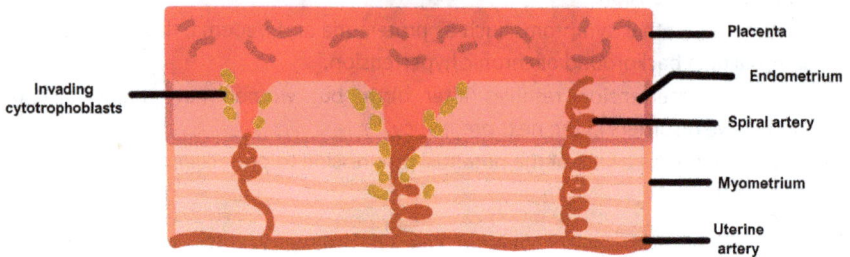

Risk factors

- Chronic hypertension or previous hypertension in pregnancy
- CKD
- Autoimmune diseases (e.g. SLE, antiphospholipid syndrome)
- Type 1 or 2 diabetes or gestational diabetes
- Nulliparity
- Maternal age > 40
- Multiple pregnancy
- Increased pre-pregnancy BMI
- Previous intrauterine growth restriction

Symptoms

- Can be asymptomatic with isolated proteinuria
- Headache with visual disturbances
- Oedema (ankle or pulmonary)
- RUQ/epigastric pain (due to hepatic capsule distension/infarction)
- Oliguria

Complications

- Mother – eclampsia (seizures), HELLP syndrome, haemorrhagic or ischaemic stroke, kidney injury, acute respiratory distress syndrome

- Foetus – prematurity, intrauterine growth restriction, placental abruption, stillbirth

Key tests

- BP measurement, urine dipstick for proteinuria and protein: creatinine ratio
- FBC may show low Hb, low platelets (if there is progression to HELLP syndrome)
- U&Es may show elevated urea and creatinine (different ranges from normal population as plasma is diluted)
- LFTs – look for elevated ALT and AST (used to assess for HELLP syndrome)
- Clotting screen – may show increased APTT

Diagnosis

- For a diagnosis of pre-eclampsia, three criteria should be met:

i) Gestation > 20 weeks

ii) Hypertension: systolic > 140 or diastolic > 90 on two occasions (> 4 hours apart)

iii) Plus one or more of the following:

- Proteinuria – protein: creatinine ratio > 30 mg/mmol or at least 2+ protein on urine dipstick testing
- Maternal organ dysfunction (e.g. seizures, or liver dysfunction)
- Uteroplacental dysfunction such as feta; growth restriction, stillbirth

Grading

- Mild is BP 140/90 – 159/109
- Severe hypertension is BP > 160/110

Management

- It is important to monitor the maternal BP, urine and the foetus regularly
- Antihypertensive medication – labetalol, nifedipine or methyldopa (should be stopped within 2 days of delivery)

Delivery of baby is the only definitive cure for pre-eclampsia
- Plan delivery < 37 weeks if there are foetal or maternal concerns
- If severe pre-eclampsia, the mother should be stabalised pre-delivery
- This will require oral or IV antihypertensives (labetalol, hydralazine)
- Magnesium sulphate to prevent eclamptic fits
- Delivery of baby once mother stabilised
- Monitor mother post-delivery as the mother has still has a high risk of seizures in the 24 hours post-partum

Prevention

- Those who are at high risk of pre-eclampsia are offered a of aspirin 75–150 mg/day from 12 to 36 weeks' gestation. Risk factors include:
- Previous hypertension in pregnancy, or chronic hypertension
- CKD
- Autoimmune disease
- Type 1 or 2 diabetes

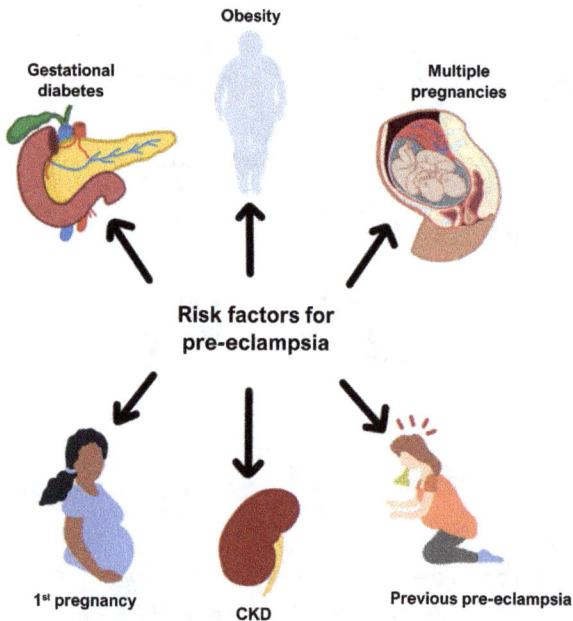

Risk factors for pre-eclampsia

If the patient has more than one of the following moderate risk factors, then it is also advised to take aspirin:

- Nulliparity
- > 40 years of age
- Multiple pregnancy

- BMI $\geq$ 35
- Family history of pre-eclampsia

- **Eclampsia**

This refers to the development of seizures in a woman with pre-eclampsia.

- It is thought to occur due to the failure of cerebral autoregulation and alteration to cerebral blood flow, leading to seizures.
- It can occur any time after the 20th week of pregnancy but typically occurs in the third trimester.

Symptoms

- Worsening pre-eclampsia symptoms, with development of seizures

Management

- Seizures are treated with magnesium sulphate (IV bolus, then infusion)
- Infusion is continued for 24 hours after the last seizure or delivery (whichever is later)
- It can lead to respiratory depression, but this can be reversed with calcium gluconate
- Antihypertensives as per pre-eclampsia to control the BP
- Fluid restriction to prevent pulmonary oedema
- Once mother is stabilised, deliver the baby

● HELLP syndrome

This is a condition which is characterised by haemolysis, elevated liver enzymes and a low platelet count.
- It is a complication or progression of pre-eclampsia or eclampsia.
- However, not all patients may meet the criteria for a pre-eclampsia diagnosis.

Risk factors

- Maternal age > 35
- Obesity, diabetes mellitus
- Chronic hypertension
- Autoimmune disorders
- Migraine
- Previous pre-eclampsia

Symptoms

- Haemolysis – gives anaemia and lethargy
- Elevated liver enzymes – RUQ pain and nausea/vomiting
- Low platelet count – bleeding (e.g. epistaxis)
- Can lead to DIC, placental abruption and kidney failure

Key tests

- Blood tests – show elevated transaminases, low platelet count, low Hb, raised LDH and bilirubin (due to haemolysis)
- Blood smear – schistocytes, burr cells and polychromasia

Management

- Delivery of the baby as soon as possible
- Supportive management for mother, e.g. blood transfusions if bleeding

Placental Disorders

- **Placenta accreta spectrum**

This refers to a spectrum of conditions where all or part of the placenta attaches abnormally to the myometrium.

- There are 3 different grades of abnormal placental attachment depending on the degree of invasion of the myometrium.
- Accreta – chorionic villi attach to the myometrium but do not invade the decidua.
- Increta – chorionic villi invade into the myometrium, down to the serosa.
- Percreta – chorionic villi penetrate through the myometrium and the entire uterine wall and may invade the surrounding pelvic organs such as the bladder.

Risk factors

- Previous caesarean section with the risk increasing per caesarean section
- Previous uterine surgery e.g. endometrial curettage
- Previous placenta accreta

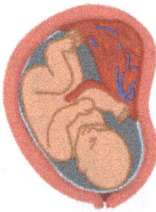

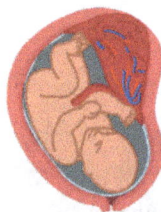

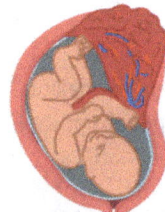

Placenta accreta   Placenta increta   Placenta percreta

Symptoms

- Usually asymptomatic and incidentally found on the ultrasound scan

Key tests

- Ultrasound is the investigation of choice
- MRI can also be used to assess the depth of invasion and lateral extension of myometrial invasion

Management

- Planned delivery via caesarean section between 35–36 + 6 weeks' gestation
- Uterus preserving surgery may be appropriate if the placenta accreta is limited in depth and surface area
- Otherwise, caesarean section hysterectomy with the placenta left in situ is preferable to separation from the uterine wall

- **Placenta praevia**

This is a condition where the placenta lies directly over the internal cervical os.
- If the placenta is < 20 mm from the internal os but not covering the internal os, this is known as a "low-lying" placenta.
- It increases the risk of post-partum haemorrhage if the baby is delivery vaginally.

Risk factors

- Assisted reproductive therapy, multiple pregnancies
- Smoking
- Previous placenta praevia
- Previous endometrial damage e.g. caesarean section, myomectomy
- High parity

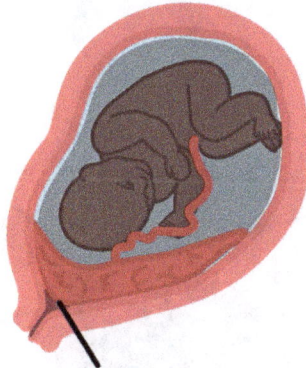

Placenta covering internal os

Symptoms

- These usually occur in the 2nd or 3rd trimester
- Painless vaginal bleeding ranging from spotting or haemorrhage
- Failure of the head to engage

Key tests

- If placenta praevia or a low-lying placenta is suspected at the foetal anomaly scan, a repeat transvaginal ultrasound scan is recommended at 32 weeks' gestation to diagnose persistent placenta praevia or low-lying placenta.

Management

- Caesarean section delivery, the timing is tailored according to symptoms
- If uncomplicated, consider delivery between 36–37 weeks' gestation
- If complicated (e.g. by persistent vaginal bleeding), consider late preterm delivery between 34–36 + 6 weeks' gestation with corticosteroid cover

- **Vasa praevia**

This is a condition where the foetal blood vessels run over or close to the internal os unprotected by placental tissue or the umbilical cord.

- These vessels can rupture in labour or during amniotomy causing bleeding.
- The total foetal blood volume is small so what may appear a small blood loss can be very harmful to the foetus.
- If left undiagnosed, it carries a high mortality risk for the foetus.

Risk factors

- Previous placenta praevia
- Assisted reproductive therapy, multiple pregnancies
- Velamentous cord insertion
- Bipartite placenta

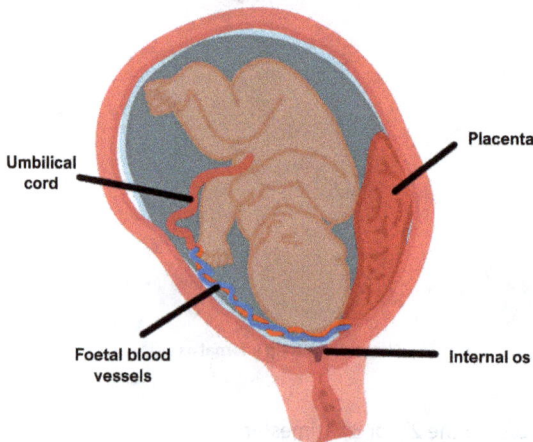

Symptoms

- Painless vaginal bleeding (similar to placenta praevia), usually experienced after the membranes rupture, with associated foetal distress

Key tests

- Ultrasound shows proximity of the foetal vessels to the internal os
- If uncertain, the detection of foetal haemoglobin in vaginal bleeding is diagnostic

Management

- Elective caesarean 34–36 weeks' gestation

- **Placental abruption**

This is a condition where part or all of the placenta prematurely separates from the lining of the uterus prior to the second stage of labour.
- The majority of placental abruption occurs prior to 37 weeks' gestation.
- It can lead to significant bleeding in the space between placenta and uterus, resulting in foetal and maternal compromise if not recognised and treated.

Risk factors

- Smoking
- Cocaine usage during pregnancy
- Maternal age > 35
- Pre-eclampsia, chronic hypertension
- Multiple pregnancies, polyhydramnios
- Short umbilical cord
- Previous history of placental abruption
- Trauma e.g. injury to the abdomen

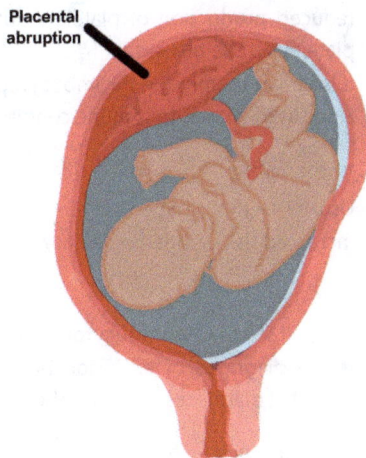

Placental abruption

Symptoms

- Can be asymptomatic
- If severe, causes significant uterine tenderness with sustained contractions (known as a "woody uterus")
- Vaginal bleeding – this is divided into revealed (blood tracks down from the site of placental separation and drains through the cervix) or concealed (bleeding remains within the uterus and typically forms a clot behind the placenta)
- Can cause maternal shock and foetal death

Key tests

- Clinical diagnosis; there are no definitive investigations for diagnosis
- Ultrasound can be used to assess for placenta praevia or haemorrhage, but the latter can be difficult to visualise

Management

- This is dependent on the gestational age and the severity of abruption
- If severe, emergency delivery via caesarean
- If asymptomatic and < 37 weeks' gestation, can monitor

Systemic Conditions

- **Gestational thrombocytopaenia**

This is defined as a drop in the platelet count $< 150 \times 10^9$/L during pregnancy.

- It is the most common cause for low platelets in the third trimester of pregnancy.
- The underlying aetiology is not fully understood but it is thought to be due to a combination of factors, including dilutional due to an increased plasma volume, reduced production of platelets during pregnancy and consumption or pooling of platelets in the placenta.
- It is similar to immune thrombocytopenia (ITP), which is often antibody mediated and associated with autoimmune conditions.

Symptoms

- Usually asymptomatic
- Increased risk of bleeding – easy bruising, petechia, epistaxis etc.

Key tests

- FBC will show a thrombocytopenia
- It is a diagnosis of exclusion based on history, examination and ruling out other potential diagnoses through laboratory testing

Management

- Monitor platelet levels through repeated FBC
- No intervention is usually necessary, and the condition resolves spontaneously 4–8 weeks after pregnancy
- If platelet levels fall $< 70 \times 10^9$/L, steroids and immunoglobulins may be trialled to assess if there is an element of ITP

- **Pulmonary embolism in pregnancy**

VTE is one of the main direct causes of maternal death in the UK.

- The risk of VTE is 4–5 times higher in pregnancy compared to a nonpregnant woman of the same age.
- This is because there are increased levels of fibrinogen, von Willebrand factor and clotting factors VII, VIII, X resulting in a hypercoagulable state.
- These changes become more pronounced as the pregnancy progresses.
- The highest risk is post-partum.
- Women are assessed for thrombosis risk factors at booking.

Risk factors

- Pre-existing conditions – thrombophilia, smoking, BMI > 30, cancer
- Obstetric factors – parity > 3, C-section, preterm delivery, prolonged labour, stillbirth, postpartum haemorrhage
- Transient – dehydration (hyperemesis), infection, OHSS (first trimester only)

Symptoms

- Pleuritic chest pain, haemoptysis, dyspnoea
- May have concurrent symptoms of DVT – unilateral leg pain, swelling (left leg is more common in pregnancy)

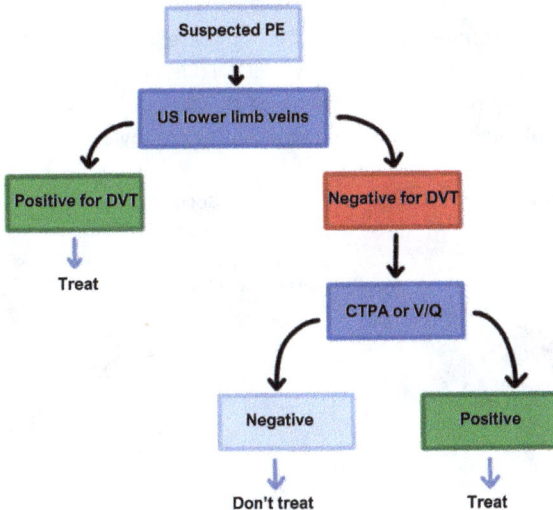

Key tests

- If DVT symptoms present, do a duplex ultrasound of the lower limb veins
- If this is positive, can commence treatment without additional tests
- If US is negative, investigate for PE with ECG, CXR and either V/Q scan or a CTPA
- CTPA increases the risk of maternal breast cancer, whilst V/Q scan increases risk of cancer in the foetus. It also is less sensitive for smaller clots
- D-Dimer testing should not be performed in pregnancy to help diagnose VTE

Management

- If confirmed PE, LMWH for the remainder of the pregnancy and until 6 weeks post-partum until at least a total of 3 months of treatment has been given
- Warfarin and DOACs are teratogenic so are not used in pregnancy

- ● **Haemolytic disease of foetus and newborn (Rhesus disease)**

Haemolytic disease of the foetus and newborn (HDFN) occurs when maternal immuno-globulin antibodies cross via the placenta and induce immune haemolysis of foetal/neonatal red cells (haemolytic anaemia).

- The D antigen is the most important antigen of the Rhesus system which is on RBCs.
- Most mothers are rhesus +ve and so do not produce anti-D antibodies.
- However, if a Rhesus D -ve mother has a Rh +ve foetus, then some foetal RBCs may enter the maternal circulation, causing the mother to produce anti-D IgG antibodies.
- In subsequent pregnancies, the memory B cells produce an immune response destroying foetal RBCs resulting in foetal anaemia.

As anti-D is the most common antibody, "rhesus disease" often refers to the presence of anti-D antibodies. The correct terminology is HDFN due to anti-D antibodies.

- Although previously the most common type of HDFN, this is now preventable with anti-D immunoglobulin injections (known as anti-D prophylaxis).

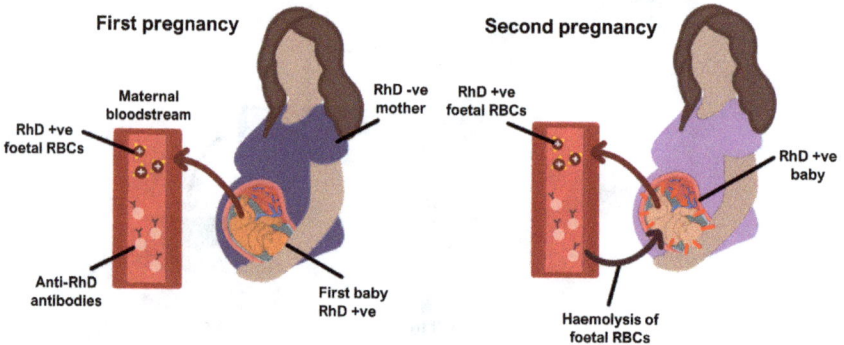

Symptoms

- Anaemia in the newborn – fatigue, lethargy
- Anaemia results in increased immature RBC production
- The liver and spleen enlarge causing portal hypertension
- The liver function is taken over by RBC production, resulting in reduced albumin production and leakage of fluid into body cavities, causing hydrops foetalis
- The heart also compensates by trying to increase cardiac output which can lead to high output cardiac failure
- If untreated, it results in foetal death
- Hyperbilirubinaemia occurs due to destruction of RBCs, leading to jaundice and potentially kernicterus which can result in brain damage or death

Management

- All women have their blood group and antibody status checked at their booking and at 28 weeks' gestation
- If there are maternal antibodies detected that can cause foetal anaemia, then regular ultrasounds are required to monitor the foetus
- If the anaemia is severe, may require intrauterine infusions
- If a woman has clinically significant antibodies, cord blood should be taken at delivery for direct antibody test (direct Coombs test – for antibodies on the surface of the RBCs of baby), haemoglobin and bilirubin

Prevention

- In HDFN due to anti-D antibodies, the goal is to prevent the disease by giving mother anti-D immunoglobin
- Anti-D immunoglobulin binds to any RhD +ve cells that may have passed into the maternal circulation
- It prevents the mother from mounting an immune response against these cells and stops her from generating anti-D IgG antibodies

All mothers are tested for their Rhesus D status at booking
- If positive, no further action is needed
- If negative, give prophylactic anti-D at 28–30 weeks' gestation (one dose treatment) or in week 28 and week 34 (two dose treatment) and within 72 hours of delivery

A sensitising event is an event in which the foetus's blood may enter the maternal bloodstream. In RhD negative mothers, anti-D should be given after these events:
- Ectopic pregnancy
- Miscarriage > 12 weeks
- Abdominal trauma, antepartum haemorrhage
- Invasive obstetric testing e.g. amniocentesis or intrauterine procedures
- Delivery of a rhesus +ve infant (can check by testing umbilical cord blood after birth)

There are 2 main blood tests that should be considered following a sensitising event:
i) Maternal blood group and Ab screen – determines mother's ABO and RhD status
ii) Feto-maternal haemorrhage test – this is known as the Kleihauer test
- It is used to assess how much foetal blood has entered the maternal circulation
- This helps to calculate the dose of anti-D

- **Intrahepatic cholestasis of pregnancy (ICP)**

This is the most common liver disorder in pregnancy, which causes cholestasis (stoppage of normal bile flow and increased level of bile acids) during pregnancy.

- It commonly occurs during the 3rd trimester when hormone levels are at their highest.
- Its aetiology is poorly understood but it is associated with raised hormone levels (oestrogen and progesterone) and genetic factors.

Symptoms

- Classically gives pruritus in the absence of rash or primary skin condition
- Itching that is worse at night, and typically worse on the palms and soles
- Fatigue and nausea
- Jaundice (< 10% of women), dark urine and pale stools
- RUQ pain
- Increased risk of gallstones
- In the foetus, is associated with an increased risk of stillbirth if severe ICP

Key tests

- LFTs show elevated levels of bile acids. ALT and AST may be mildly elevated but not usually > 2× the limit of normal; elevated bilirubin may be present
- Coagulation screen can show a high prothrombin time due to vitamin K deficiency

Management

- Repeat LFTs including bile acids after one week then form an individualised plan depending on results and symptoms
- Topical emollients and ursodeoxycholic acid help to relieve itch and liver function
- Offer earlier induction of labour if moderate (38–39 weeks' gestation) or severe (35–36 weeks' gestation)
- Women do not require additional screening or follow up in the post-partum period

- **Acute fatty liver of pregnancy**

A serious condition which occurs late in pregnancy, which can be fatal for the woman.

- It is thought to be caused by disordered metabolism of fatty acids in the mother leading to an accumulation of fatty acids.
- This can lead to liver and kidney dysfunction and ultimately, death.

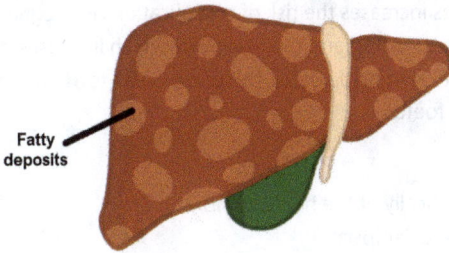

Fatty deposits

Symptoms

- Vague symptoms – abdominal pain, fatigue, malaise, nausea and vomiting
- If untreated, can lead to jaundice, ascites, coagulopathy (bleeding and encephalopathy
- It can overlap with pre-eclampsia/HELLP so may have co-existing symptoms

Key tests

- LFTs show very high ALT and AST; can also include elevated bilirubin
- Blood tests may also show hypoglycaemia, low platelets and coagulopathy
- Liver biopsy can be done for a definitive diagnosis but is usually not necessary

Management

- Supportive care with IV fluids and glucose to stabilise mother
- Prompt delivery of the foetus

Pre-existing Conditions

Pre-existing conditions can alter the course of the pregnancy and often require specific management to minimise the risk to both the mother and the foetus.

- **Diabetes mellitus**

Uncontrolled diabetes increases the risk of complications in pregnancy.
- The placenta secretes cortisol and progesterone which increases insulin resistance.
- For patients with pre-existing diabetes, this predisposes to a higher risk of complications for the mother and foetus.

Complications

- Birth defects – specifically of the heart, spine, and brain
- Increased risk of pre-eclampsia
- Polyhydramnios – can contribute to preterm delivery
- Higher risk of miscarriage, stillbirth, birth injury (due to macrosomia)
- Risk of hypoglycaemia, jaundice and polycythaemia of the baby postpartum
- For the mother, diabetic retinopathy can worsen during pregnancy

Management

- Hyperglycaemia – stop oral antidiabetic medication (except metformin) and switch to insulin. Monitor complications such as retinopathy and nephropathy
- Take higher dose of folate supplements 5 mg/day from pre-conception to 12 weeks'
- Aspirin 75–150 mg daily from 12 weeks to delivery to prevent pre-eclampsia

- **Chronic hypertension**

This is defined as having a history of hypertension (blood pressure of > 140/90 mmHg) before 20 weeks' gestation (without proteinuria or oedema) or the use of antihypertensives prior to pregnancy.
- Normally, blood pressure falls in the first trimester of pregnancy.
- Whilst pre-existing hypertension is asymptomatic, it is a risk factor for the development of pre-eclampsia and HELLP syndrome, and so needs to be controlled.

Management

- BP – stop unsafe drugs (ACEi, ARBs, thiazide diuretics)
- Switch to pregnancy-suitable drugs – labetalol, nifedipine and methyldopa
- If risk factors of pre-eclampsia – take aspirin daily from 12 weeks to delivery

● **Epilepsy**

Anti-epileptic medications can increase the risk of congenital defects.

- However, the evidence shows that it is safer to treat the mother as uncontrolled epilepsy during pregnancy can be fatal.
- Sodium valproate increases the risk of developing neural tube defects, facial clefts and hypospadias.
- Phenytoin is associated with cleft palate and clotting disorders (hence take vitamin K in last month).

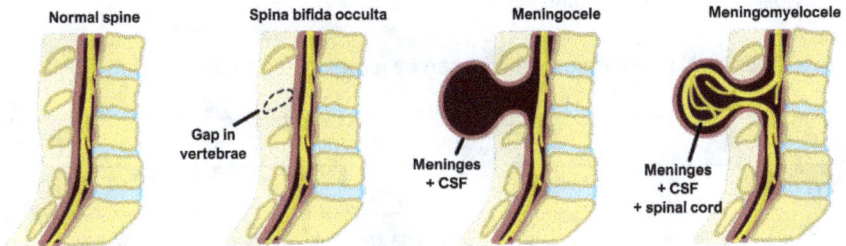

| Normal spine | Spina bifida occulta | Meningocele | Meningomyelocele |

Gap in vertebrae

Meninges + CSF

Meninges + CSF + spinal cord

Management

- Epilepsy – do not use sodium valproate unless necessary
- Ideally switch to lamotrigine or levetiracetam
- Take higher dose of folate supplements 5 mg/day from pre-conception to 12 weeks' gestation to reduce risk of neural tube defects

● **Rheumatoid arthritis**

A lot of women with rheumatoid arthritis notice an improvement in their symptoms during pregnancy.

- This is the because the changes to the hormonal and immune system which protect the unborn baby cause mild immunosuppression which benefits rheumatoid arthritis.
- However, disease activity usually worsens in the post-partum period.
- In addition, many of the medications used are teratogenic so they should be reviewed by an obstetrician and rheumatologist.

Management

- Stop methotrexate 3–6 months before pregnancy for women and men
- This is because it reduces synthesis of folic acid which leads to neural tube defects
- Sulfasalazine, hydroxychloroquine and low dose steroids are safe to use

Infections in Pregnancy

Most infections are unlikely to harm the baby but there are several infections that can be harmful if transmitted from the mother to the foetus (vertical transmission).

Methods of vertical transmission include:
- Transplacental (across placenta in utero)
- Intrapartum (due to contact between maternal and foetal body fluids)
- Postpartum via breastfeeding

Several vertically transmitted infections can be remembered by the acronym TORCH.

T	Toxoplasma gondii		
O	Other		
	Parvovirus B19	Varicella zoster virus	Zika virus
	Syphilis	Chlamydia	HIV
	Coxsackie virus	Hepatitis B	COVID-19
R	Rubella		
C	Cytomegalovirus		
H	Herpes simplex virus 2		

- **Chorioamnionitis (intra-amniotic infection)**

This describes inflammation of the foetal membranes (chorion and amnion), which is usually due to an ascending bacterial infection from the birth canal.

Risk factors

- The major risk factor is preterm premature rupture of membranes
- Prolonged labour, multiple vaginal examinations (after membrane rupture)
- Colonisation of the vagina with Group B Streptococcus

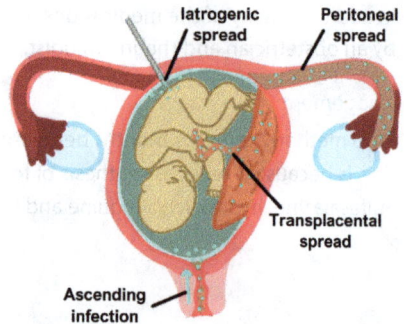

Iatrogenic spread

Peritoneal spread

Transplacental spread

Ascending infection

Symptoms

- Maternal – foul-smelling amniotic fluid from the vagina, uterine tenderness
- Tachycardia, fever
- Foetal – tachycardia

Complications

- Mother – higher risk of caesarean section, post-partum haemorrhage, endometritis
- Baby – death, neonatal sepsis and long-term disability e.g. cerebral palsy

Management

- IV antibiotics to prevent maternal and foetal complications
- Expedite delivery of the foetus

- **HIV**

Human immunodeficiency virus (HIV) destroys CD4+ T cells, leading the individual to become immunocompromised and more susceptible to infection.

Transmission

- Transplacental
- Intrapartum during delivery
- Breastfeeding

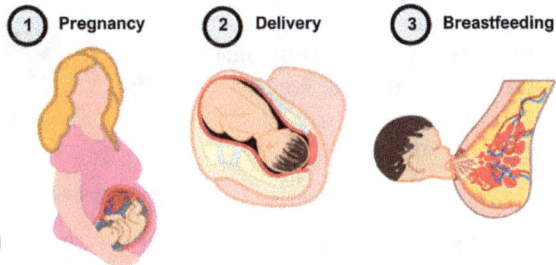

① Pregnancy ② Delivery ③ Breastfeeding

Management

- All pregnant women are screened for HIV at booking
- If positive, treatment with antiretroviral therapy is offered (regardless of CD4+ count)
- Women who conceive on antiretrovirals should continue taking their medication

Mode of delivery depends on the maternal viral load result at 36 weeks
- < 50 HIV RNA copies/ml – vaginal delivery in the absence of obstetric complications
- 50–399 HIV RNA copies/ml – can consider elective caesarean section depending on factors like viral load and obstetric complications
- If ≥ 400 HIV RNA copies/ml – recommend elective caesarean section
- Mothers with HIV can breastfeed if they have an undetectable viral load

Intrapartum zidovudine is recommended for women with viral load of > 1000 HIV RNA copies/ml who present in labour or have spontaneous rupture of membranes (SROM)

- **Group B Streptococcus (GBS)**

This bacterium is the most common cause of neonatal infection.

- It is known as the Lancefield Group B beta-haemolytic Streptococcus infection (Streptococcus agalactiae).
- It is a commensal bacterium, found in the vagina or rectum in up to 40% of women.
- Infants may be exposed to maternal GBS during labour.
- Pregnant women are not routinely screened for GBS in the UK.

Transmission

- Intrapartum (during birth)

Symptoms

- Mother – colonises the rectum/vagina usually giving no symptoms, but can spread to other organs leading to the development of symptoms
- UTI – frequency, urgency, dysuria
- Chorioamnionitis – fever, tachycardia, uterine tenderness, foul discharge
- Neonate – sepsis (fever, floppiness, respiratory distress, cyanosis, hypotension)

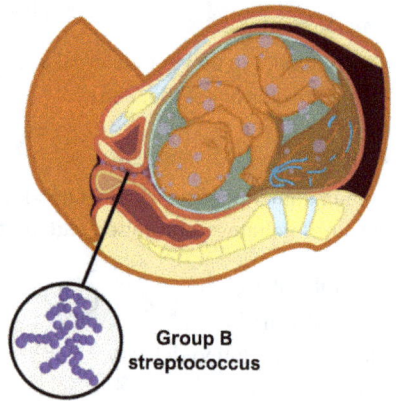

Group B streptococcus

Key tests

- Vaginal/rectal swab and culture

Management

- IV antibiotic prophylaxis with benzylpenicillin is given during labour if:
- Previous infant born with neonatal GBS disease
- Preterm labour
- Known GBS carrier in current pregnancy
- The mother has culture proven GBS bacteriuria in current pregnancy, offer antibiotics to treat the UTI and IV benzylpenicillin during labour (not required if an elective caesarean section)

If woman was GBS positive in a previous pregnancy but the baby was unaffected, she can be offered antibiotics during labour, or tested in late pregnancy (and then given antibiotics if positive).

- **Cytomegalovirus (CMV)**

This is the most common virus transmitted to a foetus during pregnancy.

- CMV may be contracted during pregnancy for the first time (primary infection).
- It can also occur due to re-activation of a prior infection or infection with a new strain.
- During pregnancy, there is a risk of transmission to the foetus.
- Severe foetal infection is most likely during the first trimester.

Transmission

- Transplacental, during birth and postnatally via breastfeeding

Symptoms

Mother

- Usually asymptomatic in immunocompetent individuals
- Can cause myalgia, fatigue, fever, joint pains, cervical lymphadenopathy
- Can also cause pneumonia (less common) and hepatitis

Foetus

- Most babies do not exhibit symptoms that can be detected by clinical examination
- Can be small for gestational age, microcephaly
- Petechial rash, thrombocytopaenia purpura ("blueberry muffin" lesions)
- Jaundice, hepatosplenomegaly
- Later onset symptoms – sensorineural hearing loss and visual impairment
- Psychomotor developmental delay and learning difficulties

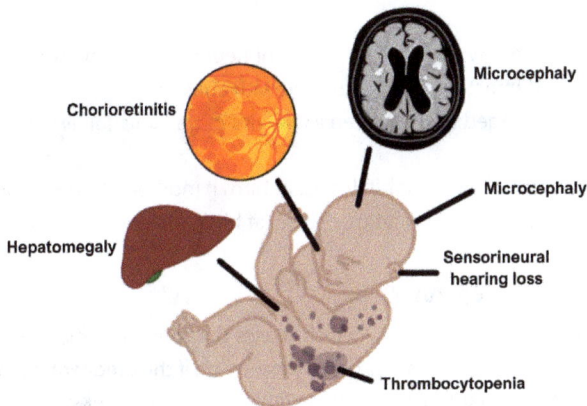

Key tests

- Mother – check for CMV serology
- Foetus – can be diagnosed prenatally by amniocentesis and PCR

Management

- If diagnosed during pregnancy, frequent ultrasounds +/- foetal MRI brain (28–32 weeks' gestation)
- If foetus is asymptomatic, expectant management can be offered
- If there are mild or moderate symptoms such as isolated ultrasound anomalies, consider in utero treatment with antiviral
- If severe symptoms (brain abnormalities), consider termination of pregnancy

- ● **Hepatitis B**

The hepatitis B virus usually causes an acute infection in adults.
- However, in children, it is more common for the virus to persist causing a chronic infection leading to serious liver damage later in life.

Transmission: Transplacental (less common), during delivery (more common)

Symptoms

- Mother – acute jaundice (mixed conjugated and unconjugated bilirubin)
- Fever, tender hepatomegaly, nausea, weight loss and elevated LFTs (ALT > AST)
- May progress to chronic infection, liver cirrhosis and hepatocellular carcinoma

- Foetus – more likely to cause chronic hepatitis infection
- Leads to early onset liver cirrhosis and hepatocellular carcinoma
- Can cause polyarteritis nodosa and glomerulonephritis

Management

- Mother – all pregnant women are screened for hepatitis B at their booking test
- If acute or chronic infection, offer treatment with antivirals
- Mothers are encouraged to breastfeed as the risk of transmission is very low

- Foetus – hepatitis B immunoglobin (HBIG) at birth if mothers are Hep B positive
- All receive full hepatitis B vaccination course (at birth, 4 weeks and 1 year of age)

- ● **Varicella zoster virus (VZV)**

This is a virus from the herpes family which causes the condition chickenpox.
- There is a risk of foetal varicella syndrome developing if the pregnant woman develops chickenpox or has serological conversion within the first 28 weeks.
- Most British women are immune to VZV having had primary VZV during childhood.

Women from tropical or subtropical countries are less likely to have had primary VZV during childhood and are more susceptible to developing primary VZV in pregnancy.

Transmission

- Transplacental or during delivery

Symptoms

- Mother – fever, malaise
- Pruritic rash on head and torso before spreading; develops into maculopapules which become vesicular then crust over prior to healing
- Increased risk of pneumonitis, hepatitis, encephalitis and rarely death

- Foetal – it can lead to foetal varicella syndrome (if infected in first 28 weeks)
- Skin problems – scarring in a dermatomal distribution, hypopigmentation
- Eye defects – chorioretinitis, cataracts, microphthalmia
- Body defects – limb hypoplasia, bowel and bladder dysfunction
- Neurological defects – microcephaly, mental retardation

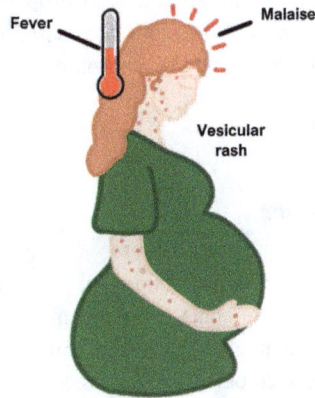

If infected in last 4 weeks of pregnancy, it can lead to varicella infection of the newborn
- The route of transmission is transplacental, ascending vaginal or through direct contact with the skin lesions.

Key tests

- Check maternal blood for immunity status against VZV
- Check IgM and IgG to VZV – if positive, this indicates immunity against the virus

Management

- If the mother has suspected exposure, the first thing to do is check immunity status
- If mother has immunity (natural or vaccination) – no further action is needed
- If no immunity, aciclovir D7–D14 post exposure if > 20 weeks' gestation; consider if < 20 weeks' gestation) or give varicella zoster immunoglobulin (VZIG) within 10 days of contact if there is a contraindication to antiviral therapy
- If chickenpox has developed, a referral to a foetal medicine specialist is required for a detailed scan at 16–20 weeks' gestation or 5 weeks post infection

- ## Congenital rubella syndrome

This is a viral infection known as German measles, which is caused by a togavirus.
- It is transmitted by aerosol droplets, but is now very rare due to the MMR vaccine.
- However, if rubella is contracted during pregnancy, it can pass to the foetus giving congenital rubella syndrome.

Transmission

- Transplacental

Symptoms

- Sensorineural deafness
- Eye problems – congenital cataracts, microphthalmia and glaucoma
- Congenital heart disease – pulmonary stenosis, persistent ductus arteriosus (PDA)
- May also cause skin lesions (blueberry muffin appearance), purpura
- Associated with learning disability and developmental delay

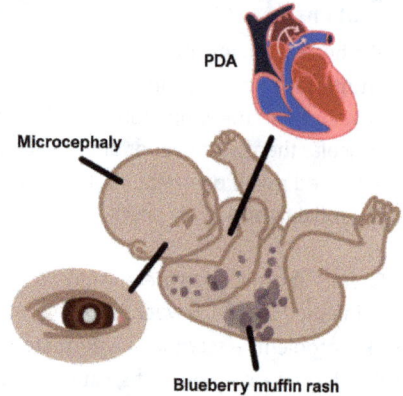

PDA

Microcephaly

Blueberry muffin rash

Key tests

- Viral serology – IgM (in acute infection) and IgG (seen after infection or vaccination)
- Parvovirus B19 serology (done as difficult to distinguish between this and rubella)

Management

- Mother – rubella infection is self-limiting, and no treatment is needed
- Foetus – risk of transmission to is highest in the 1st trimester, so management depends on gestational age
- If < 12 weeks – high likelihood of defects so reasonable to consider abortion
- If 12–20 weeks – requires investigations to see if has caused foetal abnormalities
- If > 20 weeks – no action is required as there is a very low risk of vertical transmission from the mother to the foetus

There is no screening programme for rubella.
- If woman is tested and no immunity is shown, then avoid contact with anyone who may have rubella.
- Get the MMR vaccine in the postnatal period.
- It is a live vaccine so it is not given during pregnancy.

- **Toxoplasmosis**

This is an infection due to the parasite Toxoplasma gondii, found in cats.
- Cats acquire the infection by eating cysts in infected tissue.
- These then grow and release trophozoites and form tissue cysts.
- The trophozoites release gametes which form oocysts, which are released in faeces.
- The faeces are eaten by rats and birds, which are then consumed by cats again.

The problem is that humans acquire oocysts via the GI tract (infected animals and water) or through breaks in the skin which can spread to organs.
- In pregnant women, then can also cross the placenta to enter the foetus.

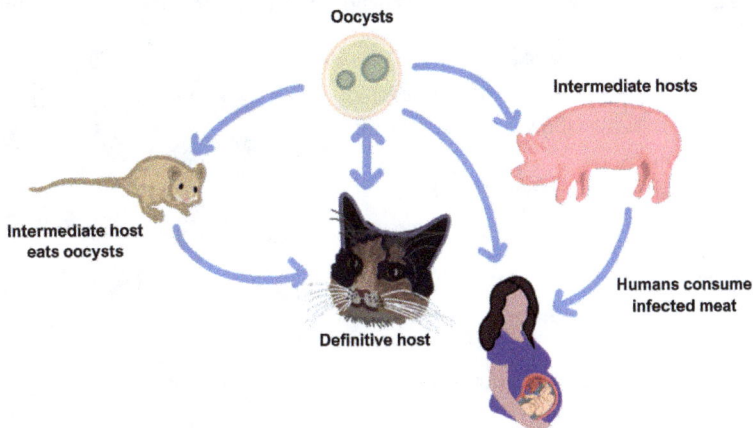

Oocysts

Intermediate hosts

Intermediate host
eats oocysts

Humans consume
infected meat

Definitive host

Transmission
- Transplacental, breastfeeding (less common)

Symptoms
- Mothers – most immunocompetent patients are asymptomatic
- Can resemble infectious mononucleosis (fever, lymphadenopathy, fatigue)
- Meningoencephalitis – this is usually seen in HIV-infected patients

Foetus – encephalitis and calcifications of the cerebral hemispheres
- Increases risk of learning disability, seizures, hearing loss
- Can cause eye inflammation (necrotising retinochoroiditis) and cataracts
- Can also give nasal malformations (rarer)

Management
- Antibiotics e.g. spiramycin and sulphonamides

Multiple Pregnancies

The probability of having twins is just under 1%.
- There are two main types of twins, depending on whether one or two egg cells have been fertilised.

- **Monozygotic (MZ) twins**

This refers to twins that develop from a single zygote which undergoes mitotic division.
- Sharing of the amniotic sac and placenta depend on the exact time the zygote divided into two separate zygotes.
- There is a higher rate miscarriage in monochorionic twins compared to dichorionic.

○ **Dichorionic, diamniotic (DCDA)**

This is when the zygote divides before day 3.
- Each twin has its own individual amniotic sac and placenta.
- These twins account for about 1/3 of monozygotic pregnancies.

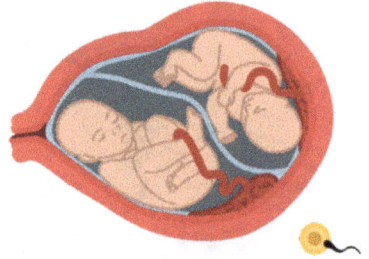

○ **Monochorionic, diamniotic (MCDA)**

This occurs when the division occurs between days 4–8.
- These twins share a placenta but have individual amniotic sacs.
- These accounts for about 2/3 of monozygotic pregnancies.

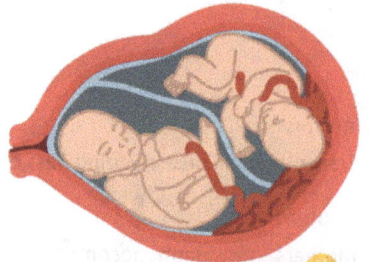

○ **Monochorionic, monoamniotic (MCMA)**

This is where the division occurs between days 9–13.
- The twins share both the placenta and amniotic sac.
- These are the rarest type of monozygotic pregnancies.

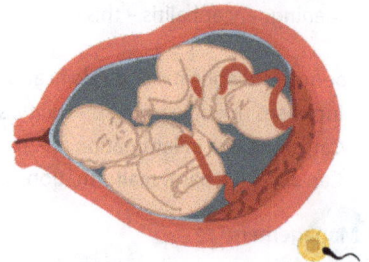

If there is incomplete division of the zygote, this will result in conjoined twins.

- **Dizygotic (DZ) twins**

This describes twins that develop from two separate eggs cells fertilised by two different spermatozoa. The majority of twins deliver prior to term (37 weeks).
- The twins share the same gene proportions as normal siblings.
- All dizygotic pregnancies are dichorionic and diamniotic.
- There is a higher chance of dizygotic twins in older mothers, assisted conception (IVF) as well as those with a positive family history.

Twin pregnancies have increased risk of complications for both mother and twins:
- All obstetric risks are increased in multiple pregnancies
- Antepartum – twin-twin transfusion (if MZ twins), prematurity, IUGR
- Intrapartum – higher risk of malpresentation, cord prolapse and PPH
- Mother – anaemia, pre-eclampsia, gestational diabetes
- Foetus – increased risk of mortality (due to preterm labour) and disability

Management

- Mothers require more supplements (iron and folate)
- Early ultrasound to assess for chorionicity and regular ultrasound surveillance

Twin-twin transfusion syndrome

This is one of the biggest complications of sharing a placenta (monochorionicity), which occurs when the blood supply can become connected between foetuses.
- This allows blood to pass from one twin to the other.
- Blood may be transferred from one twin (the donor) to the other (the recipient).
- For the donor, reduced blood volume results in IUGR, anaemia and oligohydramnios.
- For the recipient, excess blood can result in volume overload, polycythaemia, cardiac failure and polyhydramnios, which causes distension of the uterus.
- It results in a high risk of death in utero or very preterm delivery.

Key tests

- Ultrasound – polyhydramnios around one twin and oligohydramnios around other and an imbalance of blood flow across the placental vessels from one foetus to other

Management

- Selective reduction, endoscopic laser ablation of the communication vessels

Foetal Position

In the uterus, there are 3 variables that we monitor regarding the baby's position.

Lie

This is the relationship between the long axis of the foetus and that of the mother.
- Can be longitudinal – head and bottom are palpable at each end.
- Transverse – the pelvis is empty and the foetus is across the uterus.
- Oblique – head or bottom are palpable in an iliac fossae.

Presentation

This refers to the part of the foetus's body that leads the way out through the birth canal (presenting part). It is the part of the foetus that is in the lower part of the uterus.
- Cephalic (head-first), breech (bottom-first) and empty pelvis (if transverse lie).

The attitude of the head describes the degree of flexion.
- When cephalic, vertex presentation refers to maximum flexion of the head, which keeps the head bowed; this is ideal for delivery.
- When cephalic, extension of the head increases the presenting diameter, making delivery more difficult.
- Extension of 90 degrees of the head is a brow presentation.
- Extension of 120 degrees of the head is a face presentation.

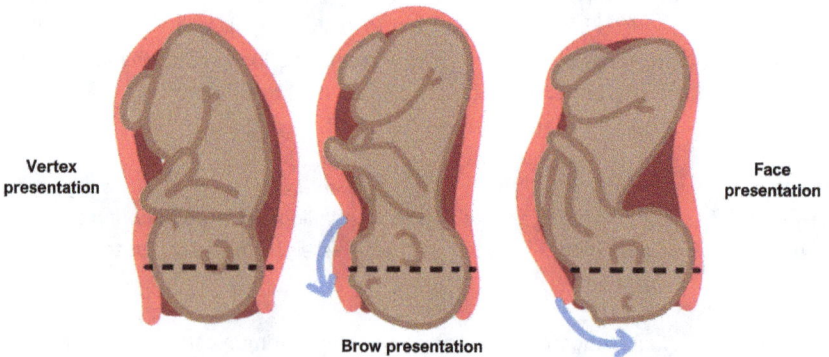

Vertex presentation   **Brow presentation**   **Face presentation**

Position

This describes the rotation of the foetal head.
- It can be described as occipito-anterior (OA, this is ideal), occipito-posterior (OP) or occipito-transverse (OT).

Abnormal lies, presentations and positions may be secondary to other conditions during the pregnancy or labour, for example, polyhydramnios (more room to turn), placenta praevia (can result in abnormal lie).

○ **Transverse lie**

This describes a foetal position where the baby is lying horizontal across the uterus.
- There may be an identifiable cause e.g. polyhydramnios.
- Usually, no action needed until 37 weeks of gestation.
- It is recommended for an elective admission at 37 weeks of gestation due to the risk of premature rupture of membranes and cord prolapse.

Management

- External cephalic version (ECV) – this is an attempt to manually turn baby into cephalic presentation, however this may be unsuccessful
- If the foetus spontaneously switches position to cephalic and this persists for 48 hours, the mother can be discharged
- C-section if persistently transverse at term

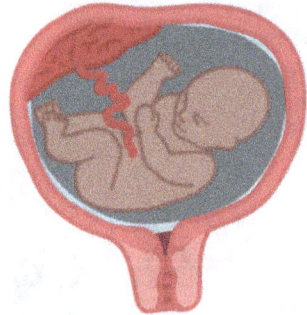

○ **Breech presentation**

This refers to presentation of the bottom part rather than the head of the foetus.
- It is associated with an increased risk of maternal and foetal complications.

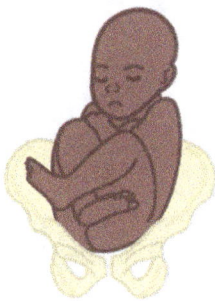

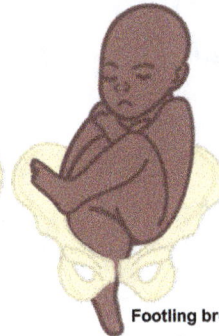

| Complete breech | Frank breech | Footling breech |

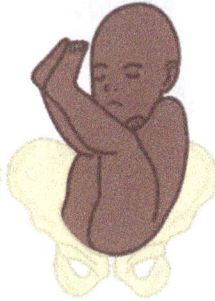

Types of breech presentation:
- Extended – both legs are extended (at the knee)
- Flexed – both legs flexed (at the knee)
- Footling – one or both feet below the bottom (more common in preterm deliveries)

Risk factors

- Usually no underling cause although prematurity is the most common association
- Prevention of movements e.g. multiple pregnancy, uterine abnormalities
- Prevention of head engagement e.g. placenta praevia
- Pelvic deformity

Complications

- Cord prolapse
- Entrapment of the foetal head

Key tests

- Ultrasound is the investigation of choice

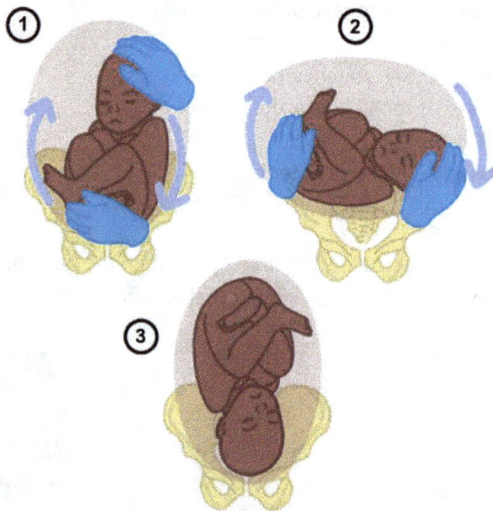

Management

- If < 36 weeks, no action is required yet as many foetuses will turn spontaneously to cephalic presentation
- If > 36 weeks, 1st line is external cephalic version (ECV)
- It is offered at 36 weeks for nulliparous women and 37 weeks for multiparous women
- However, it is not offered if there are multiple pregnancies or ruptured membranes
- In addition, do not perform if there is concern about the foetus with abnormal CTG
- If unsuccessful, can offer a repeated attempt, elective caesarean section or vaginal breech delivery
- In reality, most mothers nowadays will opt for an elective caesarean section rather than attempt a vaginal breech delivery

Foetal Size

During pregnancy, it is important to monitor the size of the baby, as both small and large babies are associated with adverse outcomes.

- Babies are measured during the antenatal scans using ultrasound.
- We use variables like abdominal circumference, head circumference and femur length to calculate estimated foetal weight (EFW) usually using the Hadlock formula.
- In addition, you can use Doppler ultrasound to measure the flow through the vessels such as the umbilical artery.
- The EFW is plotted on a growth chart to see the trend and assess if the baby is following a steady trajectory. You can also measure the EFW percentile in comparison to other foetuses of the same gestational age.

- **Small for gestational age (SGA)**

This is used to describe a foetus which is small for its age compared to the average.
- SGA describes a foetus < 10th centile EFW for its gestation.

SGA can be divided into 2 subtypes:

o **Constitutionally small**

These infants are small without a pathological reason.
- This is usually due to inherited genes and characteristics from the parents.
- Therefore, their size is what is expected of them, and they usually grow consistently.

o **Intrauterine growth restriction (IUGR)**

A term used to describe pathological restriction of the genetic growth potential.
- Foetal or maternal features stop the foetus achieving its genetic growth potential.
- It is this subtype which has higher risk of postnatal complications.

Causes

- Maternal – conditions affecting pregnancy (e.g. pre-eclampsia), chronic medical conditions (e.g. hypertension), placental dysfunction and maternal substance abuse
- Foetus – chromosomal abnormalities, intrauterine infection, errors of metabolism

Types

- Growth restriction can be divided into asymmetrical and symmetrical

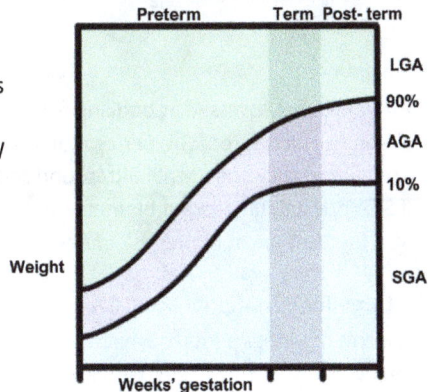

i) Asymmetrical – this is a type of restriction where the head grows normally out of proportion of the body, and it is normally seen in the third trimester.
- It is due to a compensatory mechanism to preserve blood flow to important organs like the brain and heart at the expense of less important tissues like muscle and fat.
- It is usually due to placental factors such as chronic hypertension.

ii) Symmetrical – this is called global growth restriction as the head circumference is proportional to the rest of the body.
- It occurs if the baby is affected at an early stage and so always develops slowly.
- These babies are more likely to have permanent neurological damage.
- This is usually due to foetal factors (intrauterine infections, genetic disorders) but also chronic maternal issues (e.g. substance abuse).

Management
- All women are assessed at booking for risk factors for SGA
- If high risk factors for SGA, perform uterine artery doppler at the anomaly scan and if a normal anomaly scan, serial ultrasound scans at 32 weeks of gestation
- If SGA present, ultrasound biometry and umbilical artery doppler every 2 weeks
- SGA foetuses are at higher risk of needed emergency caesarean sections

- **Large for gestational age (LGA)**
This term describes a foetus which is large for its age compared to the average.
- Infant LGA is an infant born with a weight > 90th centile.
- Foetal LGA refers to a foetus with estimated foetal weight (EFW) or abdominal circumference (AC) > 90th centile.

Causes
- Maternal diabetes (pre-existing or gestational)
- Genetics – associated with conditions like Beckwith-Wiedemann syndrome

Complications
- Increased complications during delivery e.g. shoulder dystocia
- Polyhydramnios

Management
- Monitor growth, if very large, may induce early or need elective caesarean section

Amniotic Fluid

- **Oligohydramnios**

A term used to describe an abnormally low level of amniotic fluid during pregnancy.
- It is characterised by having less than < 500 ml at 32–36 weeks and amniotic fluid index (AFI) < 5th percentile.
- It can lead to abnormal foetal presentations and underdevelopment of foetal parts.

Causes

- Low production of foetal urine – renal agenesis (Potter's syndrome), dysplastic kidney, obstructive uropathy
- Poor placental diffusion – due to conditions like hypertension and pre-eclampsia
- Leakage of amniotic fluid – premature rupture of membranes
- Congenital infections – CMV
- Twin-to-twin transfusion syndrome – leads to oligohydramnios for one and poly-hydramnios for the other

Complications

- Abnormal lie and development
- Poor respiratory development – amniotic fluid is needed for maturation of the alveoli, so infants are born with respiratory distress
- Foetal muscle contractures (amniotic fluid allows the foetus to move its limbs in utero)

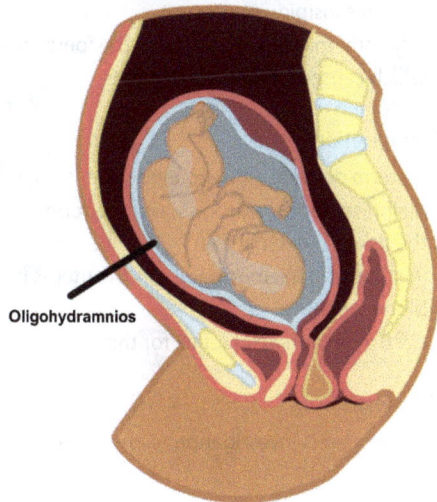

Oligohydramnios

Key tests

- Ultrasound is investigation of choice (shows fluid level < 5th centile)

Management

- Increase maternal hydration (+ amniofusion during labour to stop cord compression)
- Management of the underlying condition

- **Polyhydramnios**

This refers to an abnormally high level of amniotic fluid during pregnancy.
- It is used when the amniotic fluid index is above the 95th centile for gestational age.
- It causes over-distension of the uterus which can lead to preterm labour as well as other complications.

Causes

- Idiopathic in the majority of cases
- Congenital infections
- Decreased foetal swallowing of fluid – foetal oesophageal/duodenal atresia or CNS abnormalities
- Increased production of fluid – due to macrosomia (big babies produce more urine)
- Maternal lithium ingestion (leads to foetal diabetes insipidus)
- Adenomatoid malformation of the foetal lung which causes high lung secretions

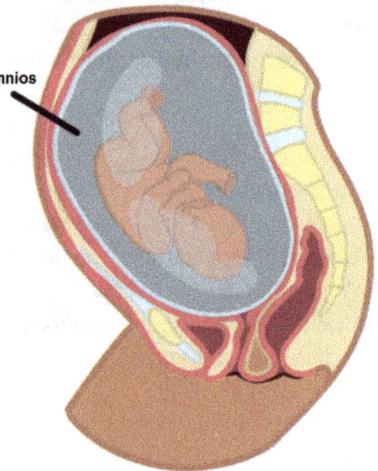

Polyhydramnios

Complications

- Preterm delivery – due to over-distension of the uterus
- Malpresentation – foetus has more room to move within the uterine cavity increasing the risk of breech delivery
- Post-partum haemorrhage – as the uterus must contract more to compress the dilated blood vessels
- Gastro-oesophageal reflux for the mother

Key tests

- Ultrasound is investigation of choice (shows fluid level > 95th centile)

Management

- Antacids to relieve heartburn for the mother, monitor complications for foetus

Labour Complications

- **Post-partum haemorrhage (PPH)**

This refers to blood loss of > 500 mls from the genital tract after delivery and it is divided into two subtypes:

○ **Primary**

This refers to blood loss which occurs within 24 hours of delivery.
- The causes can be remembered by thinking of the 4 T's.
- Tone (uterine atony most commonly), trauma (laceration), tissue (retained placenta) and thrombin (coagulopathy).

Management
- Resuscitate (IV fluids, crossmatch blood and blood transfusion if required)
- Vaginal examination is necessary to review for lacerations, rule out rare uterine inversion and provide bimanual compression of the uterus if required
- Identify and treat the cause of bleeding

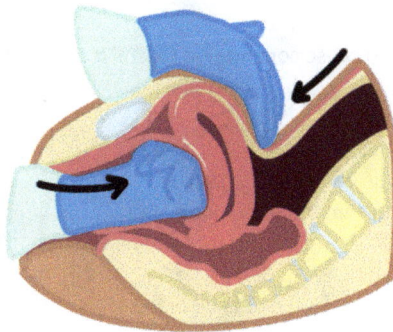

Bimanual uterine compression massage

Uterine atony can be managed in the following way:
- Vaginal examination for removal of clots and bimanual compression
- Medical management involves giving uterotonins to cause uterine contractions
- IM oxytocin is usually given prophylactically
- IM ergometrine and IM carboprost – these activate prostaglandin receptors which stimulate uterine contractions and are given should the atony persist
- An IV oxytocin infusion can also be given along with the IM dose
- Tranexamic acid can also be given in combination with these medications to reduce bleeding (inhibits fibrinolysis)

If pharmacological management fails, consider surgical management:
- Intrauterine balloon tamponade
- Haemostatic suturing (B-lynch suture) or uterine artery embolisation
- Stepwise uterine devascularisation (ligation of uterine and ovarian arteries) and then internal iliac artery ligation
- The last resort is a hysterectomy

○ **Secondary**

This is blood loss which occurs 24 hours – 12 weeks after delivery.
- The most common causes are retained products of conception (RPOC) or infection of the uterus (endometritis).

Management

- Treat underlying condition (surgical evacuation for RPOC, antibiotics if endometritis)

● **Cord prolapse**

This is when the umbilical cord comes out of the cervix before the presenting part of the foetus. It can lead to cord compression, as the foetus compresses cord occluding blood flow to foetus.
- Exposure to cold can also cause cord arterial spasm, reducing blood flow to the foetus resulting in hypoxia.

Risk factors

- General – preterm labour, abnormal lie, polyhydramnios
- Procedures – artificial rupture of membranes

Symptoms

- Cord is palpable vaginally or visible outside of the vagina
- Foetal distress – abnormal heart rate patterns on CTG

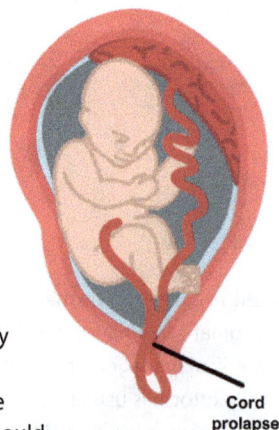

Cord prolapse

Management

- The definitive management is immediate delivery, usually by C-section
- In the meantime however, procedures are used to reduce pressure on the cord and handling of the cord directly should be avoided:
- Elevating the presenting part of the foetus (manually or by filling the bladder)
- Place mother in knee-chest or left lateral positions to relieve pressure on the cord
- Tocolytics (terbutaline) can be used to pause/reduce uterine contractions

- **Amniotic fluid embolism**

An obstetric emergency in which amniotic fluid enters the blood stream of the mother.

- The embolism travels to the lungs where foetal cells in the amniotic fluid react with maternal blood cells triggering a hyper-immune reaction.
- This results in cardiorespiratory collapse (heart and lung) and disseminated intravascular coagulation (DIC).
- Most cases occur during labour, but they can also occur during a C-section or immediately after vaginal delivery.

Symptoms

- Disseminated intravascular coagulation – profuse bleeding
- Respiratory collapse – tachypnoea, shortness of breath, cyanosis
- Cardiovascular collapse – tachycardia, hypotension, loss of consciousness

Key tests

- Blood tests show raised APTT, PT and low fibrinogen
- It is a clinical diagnosis of exclusion

Management

- Supportive management of symptoms to stabilise mother, then delivery of the foetus

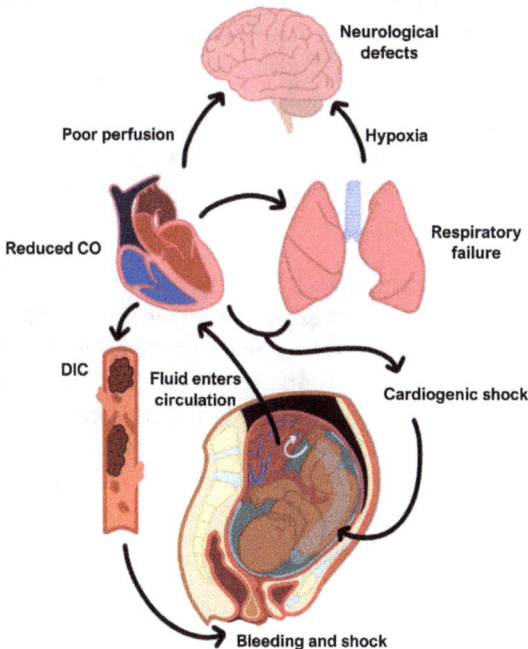

- **Shoulder dystocia**

This is an obstetric emergency where there is inability to deliver the body of the foetus after the head is delivered out of the vagina.

- During labour, the foetal head is delivered first via extension out of the pelvic outlet.
- This is followed by rotation of the foetus so that the foetal shoulders now lie in an anterior-posterior position.
- Shoulder dystocia occurs when there is either impaction of the anterior foetal shoulder behind the maternal pubic symphysis (more common) or the posterior shoulder on the sacral promontory (less common).
- This delay in delivery can lead to complications for the foetus including hypoxia.
- Additionally, applying excessive force can cause physical damage to the foetus.

Risk factors

- Maternal diabetes (most significant risk factor), macrosomia, previous shoulder dystocia, induction of labour, maternal obesity

Symptoms

- Failure of restitution – the foetal head remains in the occipital anterior position after delivery whereas the body remains in the vaginal canal
- Turtle neck sign – the foetal head retracts towards the perineum after its delivery

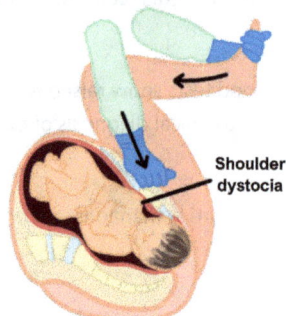

Shoulder dystocia

McRobert's manoeuvre

Complications

- Foetus – hypoxia, brachial plexus injury, humerus fractures
- Mother – perineal tears, risk of postpartum haemorrhage

Management

- This involves performing manoeuvres to aid delivery
- 1st line is McRoberts' manoeuvre – flex and abduct the maternal hips, bringing thighs towards abdomen with application of suprapubic pressure. This straightens the lumbo-sacral angle and increases the anterior-posterior diameter of the pelvis
- If this fails, 2nd line manouevers include positioning the patient on all-fours or attempting internal rotational manoeuvres (Rubin or Wood's screw manoeuvre)
- 3rd line manoeuvres comprise of vaginal replacement of the head (Zavanelli's manoeuvre) followed by an emergency caesarean section

- **Perineal tears**

A laceration/tear of the skin and soft tissues which separate the vagina from the anus.
- As the baby is expelled out of the vagina, the pressure causes the tissue to tear away. It is the most common form of injury caused by childbirth.

Risk factors

- Maternal – Asian ethnicity, nulliparity
- Foetus – macrosomia, occipito-posterior position
- Labour – prolonged second stage of labour, instrumental delivery, shoulder dystocia

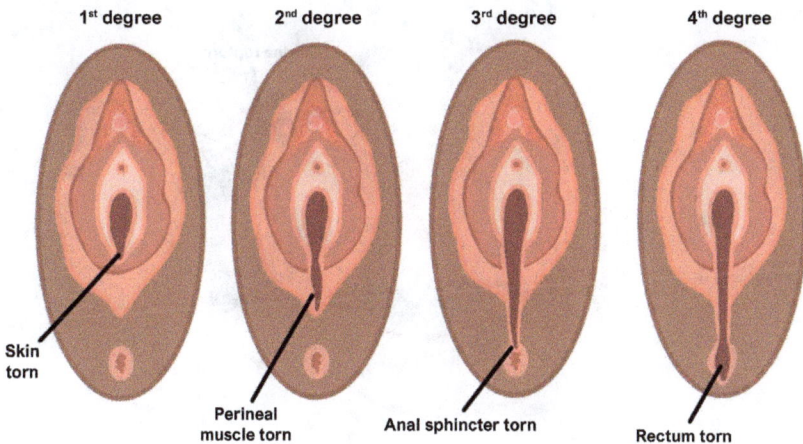

1st degree — Skin torn

2nd degree — Perineal muscle torn

3rd degree — Anal sphincter torn

4th degree — Rectum torn

Types

1st degree – there is damage to the skin and subcutaneous tissue, but no muscle

2nd degree – injury to the pelvic floor muscles but does not involve the anal sphincters

3a – there is a < 50% thickness tear of the external anal sphincter
3b – there is a > 50% tear of the external anal sphincter
3c – the tear extends to the internal anal sphincter

4th degree – injury to both sphincters and the mucosa of the rectum

Management

- 1st degree tears do not usually require treatment and heal spontaneously
- 2nd degree tears can usually be repaired under local anaesthetic with sutures
- If there is sphincter damage (3rd degree and above), this requires surgical repair

- **Uterine rupture**

This describes a full thickness disruption of all three layers of the uterus.
- It most commonly occurs during labour, due to the pressure caused on the wall as the woman tries to deliver the baby.
- However, it can occur anytime during the third trimester of pregnancy.
- It is divided into incomplete (peritoneum over uterus intact) and complete (peritoneum also torn allowing uterine contents into the peritoneal cavity).

Risk factors

- Previous uterine surgery (C-section, myomectomy), labour augmentation, obstructed labour

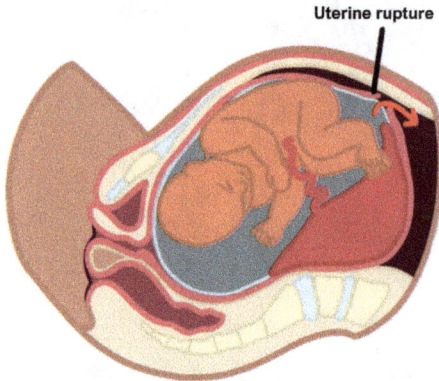

Uterine rupture

Symptoms

- Can give non-specific symptoms of shock and abdominal pain
- Abdominal pain which persists in-between the contractions, with a feeling that something "gave-way"
- Vaginal bleeding
- Referred chest/shoulder pain due to blood in the peritoneum irritating the diaphragm
- Maternal hypovolaemic shock – tachycardia, hypotension
- May cause foetal distress

Key tests

- Ultrasound can show rupture of the uterus
- Foetal distress on CTG – late decelerations, reduced variability, bradycardia

Management

- Emergency C-section +/- exploratory laparotomy

- **Preterm prelabour rupture of membranes (PPROM)**

This refers to the rupture of membranes (chorion and amnion) which occurs < 37 weeks' gestation. The membranes normally weaken at term in preparation for labour.

- When the membranes rupture, amniotic fluid is released which contains prostaglandins and this stimulates the uterine muscle to contract.

Risk factors

- Maternal – smoking, short cervical length, infections, low BMI, bleeding during pregnancy
- Foetal factors – polyhydramnios, twins

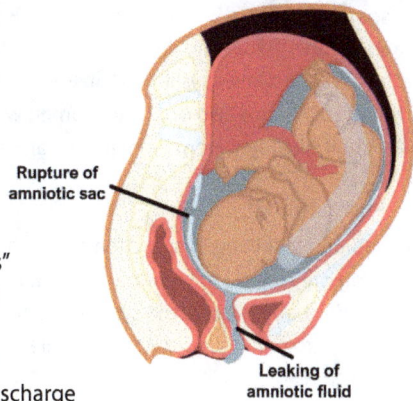

Rupture of amniotic sac

Leaking of amniotic fluid

Symptoms

- The classic dramatised "breaking of waters" (painless "popping" sensation followed by gush of watery fluid from vagina)
- Painless leakage of fluid out of the vagina
- Change in colour/consistency of vaginal discharge

Key tests

- Perform a sterile speculum exam to assess for amniotic fluid
- If pooling of fluid is visualised, this is diagnostic and no need for further tests
- If no pooling is visualised, there is need to sample the vaginal fluid using a swab
- Vaginal fluid sampling tests for insulin-like growth factor binding protein-1 – this is a protein made by cells lining the uterus and leaks prior to delivery
- Also test for placenta alpha-microglobulin-1 (PAMG-1) – this is found in very high concentrations in amniotic fluid (and low concentrations in vaginal discharge)
- If these are positive, it confirms a diagnosis of PPROM

Management

- Admit the patient to hospital as the highest risk of labour is in the first 24–48 hours
- Antibiotics e.g. erythromycin 10 days or until patient is in labour (whichever sooner)
- Antenatal corticosteroids reduce the risk of respiratory distress syndrome
- If in established labour or having a planned preterm birth, recommend IV magnesium sulphate for foetal neuroprotection if 24–29 + 6 weeks' gestation
- If there are no contraindications, offer expectant management until 37 weeks' gestation; patients can be discharged and be reviewed regularly

Postpartum Complications

After giving birth, women may experience a variety of symptoms.
- Urinary – incontinence which decreases in the days and weeks after delivery.
- GI – constipation and increased risk of haemorrhoids.
- Vaginal bleeding – known as lochia (this is vaginal discharge containing blood, mucous and uterine tissue) and it can continue for up to 6 weeks after delivery. It usually slows and darkens a few days after delivery.
- Breast pain – this also occurs in women who are not breastfeeding.
- Psychological symptoms – increased anxiety and low mood.

● **Postpartum thyroiditis**

A condition involving dysfunction of the thyroid gland in the year after giving birth.
- During pregnancy, the immune system is in a partial state of immunosuppression.
- Once the baby is born, the system rebounds which can lead to autoimmune damage of the thyroid gland. As thyroid cells are attacked and destroyed, this causes leakage of T_4 which leads to hyperthyroidism.
- However, it can then progress to hypothyroidism after as there are fewer functioning thyroid follicle cells.

Symptoms

- Hyperthyroid phase – irritability, palpitations, heat intolerance (from 2–6 months)
- Hypothyroidism – low energy, cold intolerance, weight gain, impaired concentration
- Normal thyroid function is usually restored after 1 year

Management

- Hyperthyroid phase – propranolol to stabalise the heart (most require no treatment)
- Hypothyroid phase – levothyroxine

● **Postpartum (baby) blues**

This is a very common condition which refers to the development of mild and transient depressive symptoms which normally start a few days after birth, lasting 1–2 weeks.

Symptoms: Anxiety, low mood, crying, difficulty sleeping, irritability

Management: No formal treatment is required
- Most mothers have complete resolution of symptoms by 2 weeks

- **Perinatal depression**

This is a mood disorder during pregnancy or within the first 12 months after childbirth.
- It develops later than baby blues, but the symptoms persist for months.
- Risk factors include previous episodes of postnatal depression, mental illness, complications of childbirth.

Symptoms

- Classic features of depression – low energy, low mood and anhedonia
- Emotional – persistent sadness, low self-esteem, guilt, thoughts of self-harm
- Behavioural – sleep disturbance, changes in appetite, irritability with a negative attitude towards the infant

Key tests

- Edinburgh postnatal depression scale is a tool used to aide diagnosis

Management

- Psychotherapy (CBT), support groups and medication e.g. SSRIs (sertraline is used in breastfeeding mothers); if untreated, this can lead to a chronic depressive disorder

- **Puerperal psychosis**

This is a psychiatric emergency where the mother exhibits symptoms of mania, depression, hallucinations and delusions after giving birth to her child.
- A large proportion of women who experience it may have no preceding risk factors.
- Postpartum bipolar disorder (characterised by bouts of depression and mania) is the most common subtype in high income countries.

Risk factors

- Previous postpartum psychosis, mental illness, childbirth complications

Symptoms

- Severe mood swings (like bipolar disorder) with periods of mania and depression
- Psychotic symptoms – hallucinations, delusions and bizarre ideas (about the baby)
- Agitation and distress
- Suicidal ideation and thoughts about harming the baby

Management

- Mental health assessment, may require sectioning to a psychiatric hospital
- Psychotropic medication (e.g. antipsychotics if psychotic symptoms)

Paediatrics

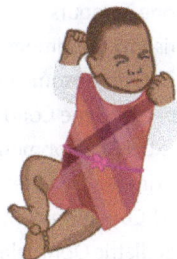

BACKGROUND

MEDICAL CONDITIONS

Neonatal Background

After birth, several physiological adaptations occur to allow neonates to transition from intrauterine to extrauterine life.

In utero, the foetal lungs are filled with fluid and are not involved in gas exchange.
- Pulmonary vessels are constricted, leading to high pulmonary vascular resistance.
- Most of the blood from the right side of the heart bypasses the lungs via two foetal shunts: the ductus arteriosus and the foramen ovale.

There are several changes that occur in the period just before and during labour.
- Production of lung liquid decreases.
- The infant's chest is compressed as it moves through the birth canal, helping to expel some fluid from the lungs.
- Breathing is triggered by several factors, including exposure to cooler temperatures and a surge in adrenaline.
- Catecholamines stimulate alveolar fluid reabsorption into the pulmonary circulation.
- Once the baby takes its first breath (typically within 6 seconds), remaining lung fluid is rapidly absorbed, and functional residual capacity is established.
- Regular breathing is usually achieved within 30 seconds of delivery.

After birth, there are several steps that are performed by medical professionals to optimise outcomes for the baby.

- **Cord clamping**
After the baby is born, the umbilical cord is clamped and cut.
- In term infants, delayed cord clamping (by 2–5 minutes) is recommended.
- This helps increase the neonate's circulating blood volume and reduces the risk of anaemia later in infancy.

- **Neonatal assessment – APGAR score**
The APGAR score assesses the baby's condition at 1, 5, and 10 minutes after birth.
- It may be repeated every 5 minutes if the condition remains poor.
- If the infant appears unwell, immediate drying and assessment should begin and the clock is started.

The APGAR score assesses the baby according to 5 criteria, each scored from 0–2.
- The five criteria are appearance (skin colour), pulse, grimace (reflexes), activity (muscle tone), and respiration.
- Scores are interpreted as follows, good condition is 7–10, moderately depressed is 4–6, severely depressed is 0–3.
- A low or decreasing APGAR score signals the need for urgent intervention and may require more intensive support.

Score	0	1	2
Heart rate	Absent	< 100 bpm	> 100 bpm
Respiratory effort	Absent	Gasping or irregular	Regular, strong cry
Activity	Flaccid	Some flexion of limbs	Well flexed, active
Reflex irritability	None	Grimace	Cry, cough
Appearance	Pale/blue	Body pink, extremities blue	Pink

● **Vitamin K injection**
This is given shortly after birth to prevent vitamin K deficiency bleeding (VKDB).
- This is a condition that can cause serious bleeding in newborns due to low levels of vitamin K-dependent clotting factors.

● **Newborn hearing screening**
All babies in the UK are offered an otoacoustic emission (OAE) test shortly after birth.
- If the result is abnormal, the baby is referred to a paediatric audiologist for further assessment (e.g. auditory brainstem response test).

● **Pulse oximetry screening**
This is performed in some hospitals across the UK within the first 24 hours of life.
- It measures oxygen saturation which can help detect critical, duct-dependent congenital heart disease.
- If oxygen saturations are abnormally low or there is a significant difference between pre- and post-ductal measurements, further assessment is needed including medical review and echocardiography.

- **Newborn and infant physical examination (NIPE)**

This is a screening examination which is performed on babies within 72 hours of birth, and then once again between 6 to 8 weeks.

- The purpose of the examination of the newborn is to screen for congenital abnormalities that will benefit from early intervention.
- It also helps to make referrals for further tests or treatment as appropriate as well as providing reassurance to the parents if the examination is normal.
- The main organs and tissues tests are the eyes, heart, hips and testes.

- **Newborn blood spot screening (Heel prick test)**

This is performed between days 5–8 of life.

- A small blood sample is taken from the baby's heel and screened for 9 conditions.
- You can divide the 9 conditions into groups to help remember them.

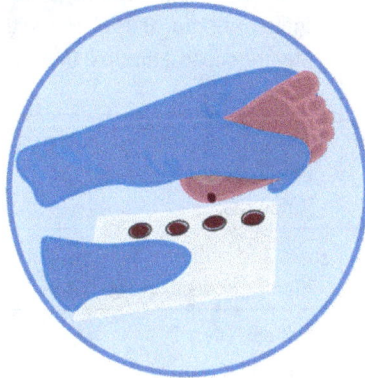

Blood disorder
- Sickle cell disease (SCD)

Congenital conditions
- Cystic fibrosis (CF)
- Congenital hypothyroidism

6 metabolic disorders
- Medium-chain Acyl-CoA dehydrogenase deficiency (MCADD)
- Maple syrup urine disease (MSUD)
- Phenylketonuria (PKU)
- Homocystinuria (HCU)
- Isovaleric acidaemia (IVA)
- Glutaric aciduria type 1 (GA1)

Vaccinations

Maternal antibodies begin to transfer to the foetus during the last trimester.
- However, at birth, this transfer stops, making infants susceptible to infections.
- Breast milk, particularly colostrum (the first milk), is rich in antibodies (mainly IgA).
- These IgA antibodies are transferred to the baby's digestive system.
- These antibodies help protect the baby's gut and fight infections.
- While maternal antibodies provide crucial early protection, a baby's own immune system gradually develops, becoming fully functional around 2–3 months of age.

In the UK, infants have a set vaccination schedule to help prevent various infections.

Age	Diseases protected against
8 weeks	- 6 in 1 (diphtheria, tetanus, pertussis, polio, Haemophilus influenzae type B (Hib), Hepatitis B) - Meningococcal group B (Men B) - Rotavirus
12 weeks	- 6 in 1 (diphtheria, tetanus, pertussis, polio, Hib, Hep B) - Pneumococcal (13 serotypes) - Rotavirus
16 weeks	- 6 in 1 (diphtheria, tetanus, pertussis, polio, Hib, Hep B) - Meningococcal group B (Men B)
1 year old (12 months)	- HiB and Men C - Pneumococcal - Measles, mumps, rubella (MMR) - MenB
3 years 4 months*	- 4 in 1 booster (diphtheria, tetanus, pertussis, polio) - MMR (2nd dose)
12–13 years old	- Human papillomavirus (HPV) types
14 years old	- 3 in 1 booster (diphtheria, tetanus, polio) - Meningococcal groups A, C, W and Y

*For children born after 1st July 2024, at 18 months, they get a 4th dose of the 6-in-1 vaccine and 2nd dose of the MMR vaccine (rather than at 3 years 4 months).

**From January 2026, a chickenpox vaccine is being offered on the NHS. The vaccine is a MMRV jab, protecting against measles, mumps, rubella, and chickenpox.
- It is given in two doses as part of the routine immunisations at 12 and 18 months.

Developmental Milestones

Developmental milestones are a set of functional skills or age-specific tasks that most children can do at a certain age range.
- They are used by paediatricians to assess a child's growth and development across several domains. Certain diseases can lead to delays in one or more of the domains.

There are 4 main domains used to assess development.
- Gross motor skills – this refers to large movements using the arms, legs, or the whole body (e.g. crawling, walking, jumping).
- Fine motor skills – this refers to small movements using hands and fingers (e.g. grasping, drawing, using utensils).
- Speech and language – this refers to an ability to understand and use language to communicate (e.g. babbling, saying words, following instructions).
- Social – this refers to a child's interaction with others, including caregivers, other children and their ability to express feelings and develop relationships.

The main developmental milestones and key ages are summarised below.
- Failure to reach these milestones at the correct age should be taken seriously as it can be an early sign of a disease and warrants referral to a paediatrician.

6 weeks
Gross motor: Stabilises head in sitting position

Fine motor: Can track object/face

Speech: Startles at loud noise

Social: Smiles

6 months
Gross motor: Can sit up briefly/with support, and roll over from prone to supine

Fine motor: Develops palmar grasp, reaches for objects

Speech: Babbles two syllable sounds, turns to their name

Social: Shakes rattles, reaches for bottle and puts objects to mouth

9 months

Gross motor: Sits up steady, attempts crawling, stands up holding on

Fine motor: Index finger poke, learns object permanence

Speech: Responds to their name, understands "no", imitates sounds

Social: Finger feeds, apprehensive to strangers

12 months (1 year)

Gross motor: Can stand alone and starts walking (anytime 9–18 months)

Fine motor: Develops pincer grip, casts bricks (should disappear by 18 months)

Speech: Can say 3 words, shows an understanding of nouns (e.g. mummy)

Social: Waves "bye-bye", claps, expresses desires with pointing

18 months

Gross motor: Can run and jump

Fine motor: Can draw to and fro, builds tower of 4 blocks

Speech: Can say 1–6 different words, understands nouns

Social: Imitates activities

2 years

Gross motor: Runs tiptoe, walks upstairs both feet each step, throws ball

Fine motor: Draws a vertical line, builds tower of 8 blocks

Speech: Shows understanding of verbs, uses 2 words joined together

Social: Eats with fork/spoon

3 years

Gross motor: Hops on one foot, starts doing stairs one foot per step

Fine motor: Copies drawing a circle, builds a bridge with blocks

Speech: Understands adjectives and negatives

Social: Uses knife and fork, shares toys with friends, plays alone without parents

4 years

Gross motor: Can walk upstairs and downstairs in adult manner

Fine motor: Cuts paper in half, copies cross, draws man with 3 parts

Speech: Counts to 10, understands complex instructions

Social: Shows concern for others hurt, has a best friend

Cardiology Introduction

During embryological development, there are three main foetal circulatory features which undergo changes shortly after birth.

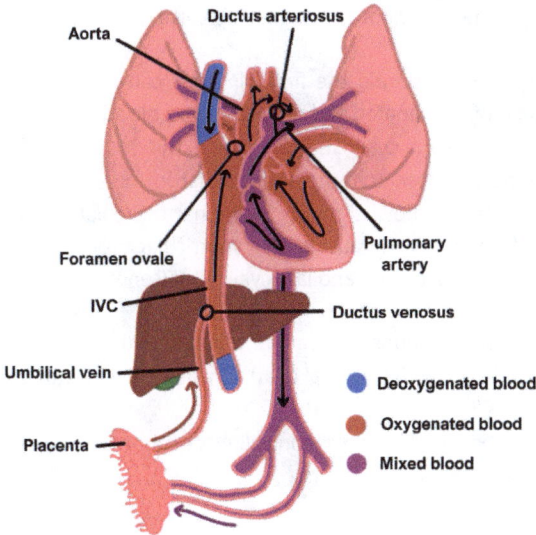

Ductus arteriosus

This connects the pulmonary artery to the aorta allowing blood to bypass the lungs.
- After birth, a drop in maternal prostaglandins causes it to close.

Ductus venosus

This is a temporary foetal blood vessel that allows oxygenated blood from the umbilical vein to bypass the liver and flow directly into the IVC to the heart.
- It closes functionally within minutes to hours after birth and structurally within a few days, eventually becoming the ligamentum venosum, a fibrous cord in the liver.

Foramen ovale

In the foetus, left atrial pressure is low as little blood returns from the lungs.
- Right atrial pressure is high as it receives all the systemic venous return (including blood from the placenta).
- Therefore, the flap valve of the foramen ovale is held open and blood flows from the right atrium to the left atrium.

When the baby starts breathing after birth and the lungs expand full of air, resistance to pulmonary blood flow falls.
- The volume of blood flowing through the lungs increases, causing a rise in left atrial pressure, whilst the volume of blood returning to the right atrium falls as the placenta is excluded from the circulation.
- This change in pressure gradient causes the flap valve of the foramen ovale to close.

Defects in embryogenesis during the first trimester can cause defects in the heart, allowing the mixing of oxygenated and deoxygenated blood.
- Right-to-left shunts result in cyanosis soon after birth.
- Left-to-right shunts are often asymptomatic at birth.
- However, the increased flow through pulmonary circulation causes pulmonary hypertrophy and hypertension, causing right ventricular hypertrophy and the eventual formation of a right-to-left shunt and late cyanosis (Eisenmenger syndrome).

Many paediatric heart conditions cause a murmur, due to the turbulent flow of blood.
- However, many children with a normal heart can also present with a murmur.
- This is known as an "innocent" murmur.
- Murmurs may also be heard during a febrile illness or anaemia due to increased cardiac output, which are called flow murmurs.

Features of an innocent murmur include the 4 S's:
- **A**symptomatic
- **S**oft blowing murmur
- **S**ystolic only (never diastolic)
- Heard along the left **S**ternal edge
- These murmurs will also have no added sounds like thrills or clicks, no radiation and may vary with posture.

There are different types of innocent murmurs that are seen in children.
- Ejection murmurs occur due to turbulent flow of blood experienced at the outflow locations of the heart.
- Venous hums occur due to turbulent blood flow in the IVC/SVC which return blood to the heart. These sound like a continuous blowing noise, usually heard just under the clavicles.
- Still's murmur is a low-pitched sound which is heard at the lower left sternal edge.

Heart Failure

This is defined as a cardiac output which is inadequate for the body's requirements.
- In children, the causes of heart failure are significantly different from adults.
- Many cases are due to congenital malformations which cause high output cardiac failure.

Causes

- Neonates (immediately after birth) – conditions which impair outflow from the heart, e.g. severe aortic stenosis, interrupted aortic arch, transposition of the great arteries
- Infants (within 1st year of life) – conditions which lead to mixing of oxygenated and deoxygenated blood, e.g. large patent ductus arteriosus, VSD
- Older children – typically due to acquired conditions, e.g. rheumatic fever, cardiomyopathy, Eisenmenger syndrome

Symptoms

- Can be very non-specific, making it harder to diagnose
- Shortness of breath
- Inability to gain weight, poor growth
- Predisposition to recurrent chest infections
- Hepatomegaly
- Signs of the underlying cause – murmurs, cardiomegaly, cyanosis

Key tests

- Chest X-ray may show cardiomegaly or an abnormal heart shadow
- ECG can show ischaemic changes as well as congenital arrythmias
- Echocardiogram is used to diagnose structural disease and quantify cardiac function

Management

- Treat the underlying cause
- Medical management, such as diuretics, can be used to reduce cardiac afterload (reducing the work the heart has to do)
- Surgical management is required in some cases
- If unresolving, consider heart transplant

Left-to-right Shunts

These shunts do not cause cyanosis at birth, as the pressure in the left circulation is more than the right, meaning deoxygenated blood from the right side does not enter the main systemic circulation.

However, if left untreated, the increased pressure in the pulmonary circulation over time leads to remodeling and pulmonary hypertension.
- This causes right ventricular hypertrophy and eventually a right-to-left shunt.
- This is called **Eisenmenger's syndrome** which occurs about 10–15 years after birth.
- It is a progressive condition which causes heart failure, typically around age of 40.
- This gives symptoms such as cyanosis, clubbing as well as right sided heart failure (hepatomegaly, peripheral oedema, ascites).
- Definitive management is a heart and lung transplant.

- **Atrial septal defect (ASD)**

This is a condition where a hole remains between the left atrium and right atrium.
- During embryogenesis, the septum primum grows downwards from the roof of the common atrium toward the endocardial cushions, separating the left and right atria.
- A gap called the ostium primum remains, allowing blood to shunt between the atria.
- The septum primum fuses with the endocardial cushion closing the ostium primum.
- A second opening called the ostium secundum is formed to allow blood flow.
- Thereafter, a second, thicker wall called the septum secundum develops to the right of the septum primum.

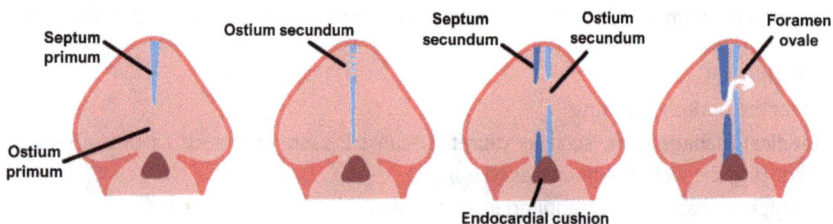

The septum secundum partially covers the ostium secundum, leaving a curtain-like opening called the foramen ovale, which functions as a right-to-left shunt.
- At birth, the septum primum and septum secundum fuse to close the foramen ovale.
- A failure of this fusion results in a patent foramen ovale (PFO).
- As the left-sided heart pressure is higher in the neonatal heart, a PFO results in blood being shunted from the left to the right atrium.

There are two main types of atrial septal defects:

i) Ostium primum
- This is a defect at the bottom of the atrial septum. It occurs when the septum primum fails to fuse with the endocardial cushions.

ii) Ostium secundum
- This is a defect in the centre of the atrial septum.
- It is more common than ostium primum defect.
- This occurs either when the septum primum is excessively resorbed, or if the septum secundum is underdeveloped.

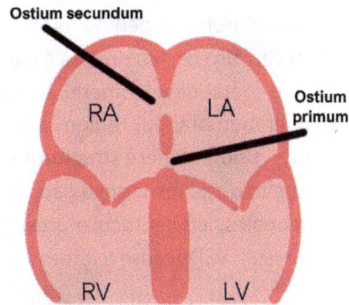

Symptoms
- Most are asymptomatic and go undetected for many years
- Symptoms can begin to appear in adulthood – shortness of breath on exertion
- Arrythmias, tiredness and swelling of the legs
- Risk of paradoxical emboli – emboli from the venous system can pass through an ASD to the left side of the heart, entering the systemic circulation and causing a stroke

Signs
- Fixed splitting of S2 (due to a delay in the closing of the pulmonary valve)
- Ejection systolic murmur, loudest at the upper left sternal edge

Key tests
- Echocardiogram detects defects in the atrial septum (ostium secundum ASD) or near the atrioventricular valves (ostium primum ASD)
- Bubble contrast study – microbubbles injected into a peripheral vein may be seen passing from the right to the left atrium via an ASD, good for assessing small ASDs
- ECG – may show RBBB with axis deviation and right atrial enlargement
- CXR – can show cardiomegaly and enlarged pulmonary arteries

Management
- Small ASDs may close on their own and so many only require monitoring
- ASDs large enough to cause symptoms or right ventricular dysfunction will require surgery or cardiac catheterisation for closure

- **Ventricular septal defect (VSD)**

A ventricular septal defect (VSD) is the most common congenital heart defect, occurring when an abnormal opening forms between the ventricles.

- VSDs can also be acquired as a complication of myocardial infarction.
- During foetal development, a muscular ridge grows upward from the apex, while a thinner membranous region extends downward from the endocardial cushion.
- Proper fusion of these structures is essential.
- Failure to do so results in a gap, leaving a defective ventricular septum.
- In neonates, left ventricular pressure is higher than right ventricular pressure.
- As a result, VSDs cause a left-to-right shunting of blood.

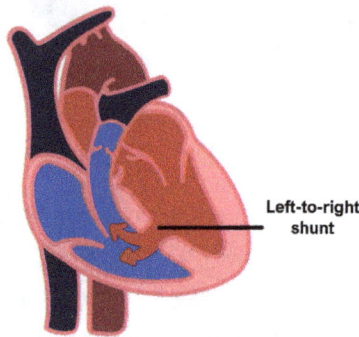

Left-to-right shunt

Symptoms

- Most small VSDs are asymptomatic
- If large, they can give symptoms of heart failure (breathless, poor growth)
- Predisposes to recurrent chest infections
- Pansystolic murmur at lower left sternal edge with a loud P2
- The louder the murmur is, the narrower the hole and less severe the disease
- If left untreated, will progress to Eisenmenger's syndrome

Key tests

- Echocardiogram identifies the septal defect, turbulent left-to-right blood flow on Doppler, and chamber enlargement
- ECG – may show left or right ventricular hypertrophy and signs of volume overload
- CXR – may show cardiomegaly and increased pulmonary vascular markings due to excess pulmonary blood flow

Management

- Medical management of heart failure followed by surgery to close defect if large

- **Patent ductus arteriosus (PDA)**

A condition where the ductus arteriosus fails to close within a few days after birth.

- This results in a left-to-right shunt between the aorta and the pulmonary artery, as the pressure is higher in the aorta than pulmonary artery.
- It is associated with prematurity and maternal rubella infection.

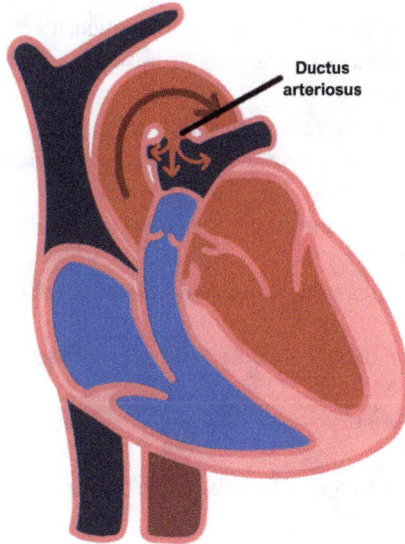

Ductus arteriosus

Symptoms

- Usually asymptomatic at birth
- Continuous "machine-like" murmur described as "rolling-thunder" with a left subclavicular thrill
- If left untreated can lead to Eisenmenger syndrome and heart failure later in life
- Wide pulse pressure
- Heaving apex beat
- Poor growth

Key tests

- Echocardiography shows continuous left-to-right shunting, ductal flow, left heart enlargement, hyperdynamic circulation

Management

- Ibuprofen or indomethacin – these inhibit prostaglandin E synthesis causing closure of the ductus arteriosus
- If very large or persistent, requires surgical repair

Right-to-left Shunts

These conditions lead to the mixing of deoxygenated blood from the right side of the circulation with oxygenated blood in the left side of the circulation.
- This results in cyanosis, a bluish-purple discoloration of the tissues.

Cyanosis is not always due to arterial oxygen desaturation. It's divided into two types:
- Peripheral cyanosis occurs in the extremities such as feet and hands and is very common in the first 24 hours of life.
- It is most commonly secondary to increased oxygen extraction in these tissues.
- It can also occur when the child is crying, cold or unwell from any cause, and is usually less serious that central cyanosis.
- Central cyanosis is seen when there is increased concentration of reduced haemoglobin in the blood.
- This is serious as it indicates an oxygen deprived state, which can be fatal.

In order to differentiate between cardiac and non-cardiac causes of cyanosis, the hyperoxia test can be used.
- The infant is given 100% oxygen (via a headbox/ventilator) for ten minutes and an arterial blood gas is taken.
- A pO_2 of less than 15 kPa suggests a cardiac cause of cyanosis.

When treating cyanotic heart disease, the child should be given the following:
- Supplemental oxygen – this dilates pulmonary vessels, decreases pulmonary vascular resistance and enhances systemic oxygen delivery.
- Prostaglandin E1 – this maintains a patent ductus arteriosus in ductal-dependent congenital heart defects.
- The ductus arteriosus gives a connection between the pulmonary artery and aorta.
- By keeping it open, oxygenated blood is able to pass from the pulmonary artery into the systemic circulation which is required to maintain life in ductal-dependent congenital cardiac defects.
- This buys time so the patient can be transferred to a tertiary centre for heart surgery.

- **Tetralogy of Fallot (TOF)**

This is the most common cyanotic congenital heart disorder, defined by 4 issues:
- Aorta overriding the VSD (accepting right heart blood)
- Right ventricular hypertrophy
- Pulmonary outflow stenosis
- Ventricular septal defect

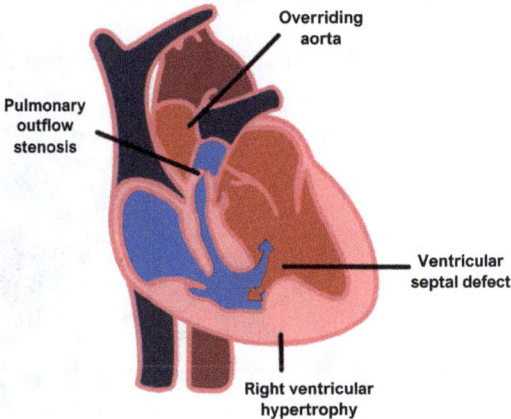

Overriding aorta

Pulmonary outflow stenosis

Ventricular septal defect

Right ventricular hypertrophy

Symptoms
- Cyanosis, which usually occurs around 1–2 months after birth
- Tet spells – sudden spells of cyanosis, breathlessness and loss of consciousness which often occur when children cry or have bowel movements
- Squatting in toddlers – this is a compensatory mechanism used by children with cyanotic spells. Squatting increases peripheral vascular resistance, decreasing the right-to-left shunt and allowing more blood to reach the lungs to get oxygenated
- Clubbing
- Harsh ejection systolic murmur at the left sternal edge (due to pulmonary stenosis)
- If left untreated, it can lead to heart failure (dyspnoea, poor growth, poor feeding)

Key tests
- Echocardiogram – shows 4 classical issues (above) and a right-to-left shunt
- Chest X-ray – classic finding is a "boot"-shaped heart which may be small in size
- ECG – usually normal at birth, but right ventricular hypertrophy as child grows

Management
- If acute cyanosis at birth, treat with oxygen and prostaglandin infusion
- Medical management – Tet spells can be treated with beta blockers and morphine
- Total surgical repair is curative, usually performed after 6 months of age

- **Transposition of great arteries (TGA)**

This is a condition where the pulmonary artery arises from left ventricle and the aorta from the right ventricle.

- This results in oxygenated blood being stuck in a closed loop between the heart and the lungs, and deoxygenated blood stuck in a loop between the body and the heart.
- This means that there are 2 parallel circulations which do not mix.
- Unless there is mixing of blood between them (a shunt), the condition is incompatible with life, and the child will die.
- Fortunately, TGA often occurs in association with anomalies that allows this mixing such as a VSD, ASD and/or PDA.

Symptoms

- Cyanosis shortly after birth (on day 2 when the ductus arteriosus closes)
- The more mixing of blood there is, the less severe the presentation
- A loud single S2 but no murmur
- If left untreated, it leads to heart failure and ultimately death

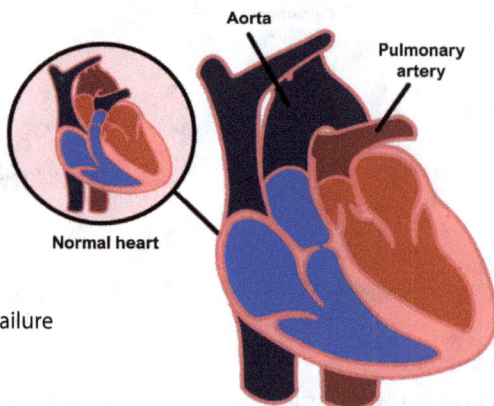

Aorta

Pulmonary artery

Normal heart

Key tests

- Echocardiogram is diagnostic – shows aorta arising from right ventricle, pulmonary artery arising from left ventricle, parallel great vessels (instead of usual crisscrossing)
- Pulse oximetry shows reverse differential cyanosis (SpO_2 in legs > SpO_2 in the right arm), as the legs can receive some oxygenated blood through the PDA (post ductal)
- In contrast, the branches to the right arm occur before the PDA (preductal) so they only get deoxygenated blood
- CXR shows a narrow upper mediastinum with an "egg on side" appearance of the cardiac shadow

Management

- Prostaglandin infusion and oxygen to manage acute cyanosis
- Surgical correction, arterial switch procedure is the definitive treatment

Common Mixing Conditions

These conditions lead to the mixing of deoxygenated and oxygenated blood in a chamber, which leads to progressive cyanosis. These conditions are rarer in comparison to septal defects.

- **Atrioventricular septal defect (AVSD)**

This is a condition where there is a defect in the middle of the heart with a single 5-leaflet valve between the atria and ventricles, which occurs due to poor fusion of the endocardial cushion with the atrial and ventricular septum.

- This 5-leaflet valve stretches across the AV junction but tends to leak allowing the mixing of blood (left-to-right shunt).
- It is associated with Down's syndrome.

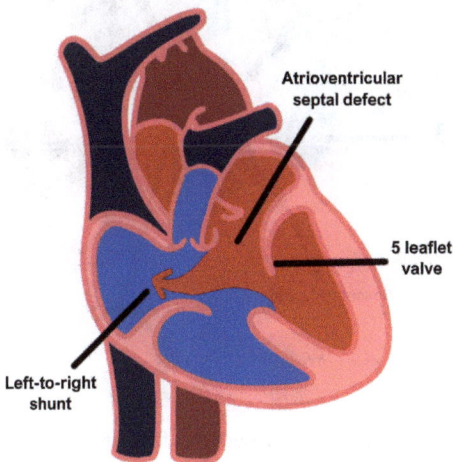

Atrioventricular septal defect

5 leaflet valve

Left-to-right shunt

Symptoms

- If severe can give cyanosis at birth
- Heart failure – dyspnoea, poor growth, oedema, fatigue
- Leads to pulmonary hypertension as blood backs up into lungs due to weakened LV

Key tests

- Echocardiogram shows common AV valve, atrial and ventricular septal defects, left-to-right shunting. This may be detected antenatally with foetal cardiac ultrasound

Management

- Medical treatment of heart failure followed by surgery to correct the defect

- **Tricuspid atresia**

This is when the tricuspid valve orifice fails to develop.

- This means that the right ventricle is small, hypoplastic and non-functional leaving only one effective ventricle.
- It leads to the mixing of systemic and pulmonary venous return in the left atrium.
- Because of a lack of a connection, an atrial or ventricular septal defect must be present to allow blood from the pulmonary vein to pass into the pulmonary artery.

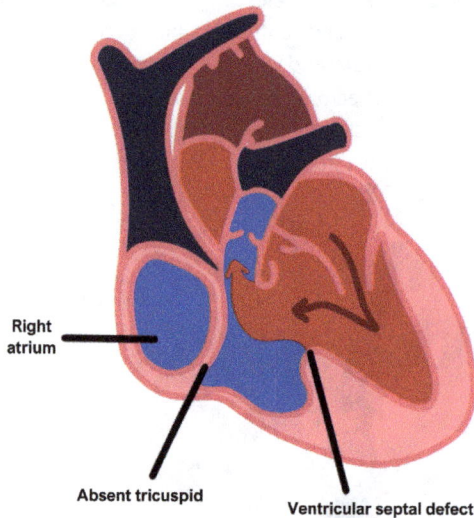

Right atrium

Absent tricuspid   Ventricular septal defect

Symptoms

- Progressive cyanosis
- VSD murmur
- Heart failure – dyspnoea, poor growth, oedema, fatigue

Key tests

- Echocardiogram shows an absent tricuspid valve, hypoplastic right ventricle, ASD, VSD, pulmonary flow abnormality

Management

- Prostaglandin infusion to maintain the ductus arteriosus
- Surgical management is performed in stages
- Glenn procedure is a surgery which connects the superior vena cava to the pulmonary artery
- Fontan procedure channels inferior vena cava flow straight into the pulmonary artery, bypassing the non-functional right side of the heart

- **Ebstein's anomaly**

This is a rare congenital heart defect where the tricuspid valve is improperly formed.
- The valve is abnormally low, leading to a large right atrium and small right ventricle.
- This is called "atrialisation" of the ventricle.
- It is associated with Wolff-Parkinson-White syndrome and maternal lithium use in the 1st trimester of pregnancy.
- 50% of affected individuals also have an associated atrial septal defect (ASD) or patent foramen ovale (PFO), creating a right-to-left shunt allowing deoxygenated blood from the large right atrium to enter the left.

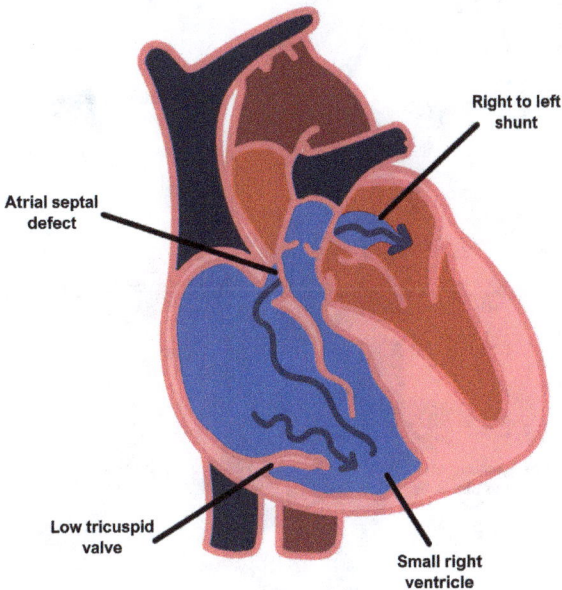

Right to left shunt

Atrial septal defect

Low tricuspid valve

Small right ventricle

Symptoms
- Cyanosis and breathlessness
- Systolic murmur due to tricuspid regurgitation
- Can lead to congestive heart failure due to valve incompetence
- Associated with Wolff-Parkinson-White syndrome and other arrhythmias

Key tests
- Echocardiogram shows an apically displaced tricuspid valve, "atrialised" right ventricle, enlarged right atrium, tricuspid regurgitation, right-to-left shunt

Management
- Medical management includes anti-arrhythmics
- Surgical correction is the definitive management

- **Persistent truncus arteriosus**

During embryological development, the truncus arteriosus gives rise to the aorta and the pulmonary trunk.

- Persistent truncus arteriosus occurs due to failure of the truncus arteriosus to divide into the pulmonary trunk and aorta, which allows deoxygenated and oxygenated blood to mix.
- It occurs due to problems in the cardiac neural crest cells which are responsible for forming the aorticopulmonary septum dividing the two main blood vessels.
- It is associated with chromosome 22q11 deletion syndrome (DiGeorge syndrome).

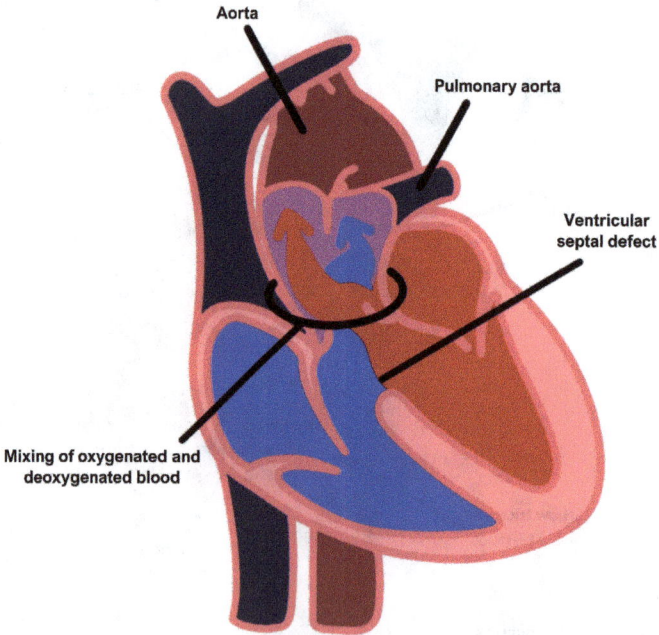

Aorta

Pulmonary aorta

Ventricular septal defect

Mixing of oxygenated and deoxygenated blood

Symptoms

- Neonatal cyanosis due to mixing of blood
- Systolic ejection murmur at left sternal border
- Heart failure will occur within weeks giving cardiomegaly

Key tests

- Echocardiogram shows a single great artery, VSD, overriding vessel, abnormal valve, mixed blood flow, increased pulmonary circulation

Management

- Surgical repair

Outflow Obstruction

These conditions impair the flow of blood into the circulation. As such, many of these will give rise to a murmur due to turbulent flow created at the site of constriction.

- **Aortic stenosis**

This is a condition where the aortic valve leaflets become partly fused together, narrowing the aortic valve orifice restricting the exit of blood from the left ventricle.

- This defect often occurs in association with mitral stenosis and aortic coarctation.

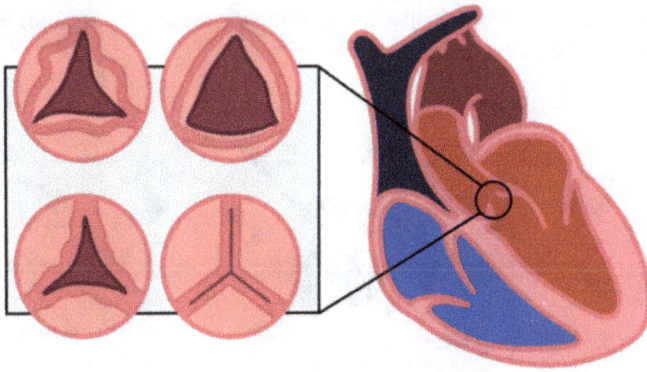

Symptoms

- Many are asymptomatic
- Ejection systolic murmur which radiates to the carotids and a carotid thrill
- If severe, causes reduced exercise tolerance, chest pain on exertion, syncope
- If critical, it causes severe heart failure leading to shock
- Narrow pulse pressure with slowly rising pulse

Key tests

- Echocardiogram is diagnostic

Management

- Regular clinical monitoring with echo to determine whether they need intervention
- Balloon valvotomy if symptoms on exercise or high resting pressure gradient
- Children with significant aortic valve stenosis will eventually require aortic valve replacement later in life

- **Coarctation of aorta**

This refers to narrowing of the aorta, which is divided into infantile and adult forms.

- It occurs due to arterial duct tissue encircling the aorta at the point of insertion of the ductus arteriosus. When the duct closes, the aorta constricts, causing a severe left ventricle outflow obstruction.

○ **Infantile coarctation of aorta**

The infantile form is a congenital narrowing of the aorta.

- It is associated with a persistent ductus arteriosus (PDA) and Turner's syndrome.
- The coarctation occurs distal to the aortic arch but before the PDA.
- It can cause collapse of the circulation when the ductus arteriosus closes leading to heart failure and poor systemic perfusion.

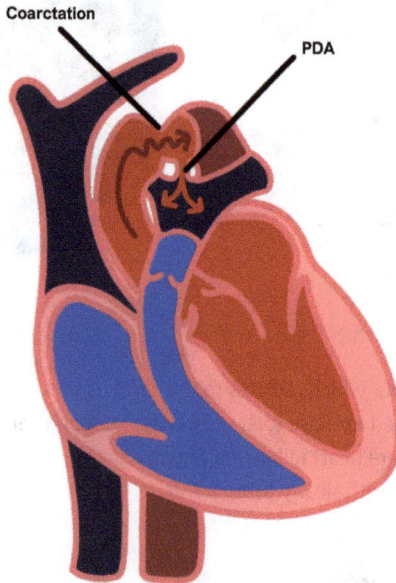

Symptoms

- Mid systolic murmur which radiates to the back
- Decreased or absent femoral pulses
- Systolic hypertension in the upper extremities and low or unobtainable arterial blood pressure in the lower extremities

Key tests

- Echocardiogram shows aortic narrowing, left ventricular hypertrophy, turbulent flow and possible PDA

Management
- Prostaglandin E1 to stop closure of the ductus arteriosus
- Surgery is the definitive management

○ **Adult coarctation of the aorta**

This refers to narrowing of the aorta that gradually becomes more severe over a period of years.
- Blood bypasses the obstruction via collateral vessels in the chest wall.
- It is not associated with a PDA and the coarctation lies distal to the origin of left subclavian artery.

Symptoms
- Over time causes hypertension in upper limbs and hypotension in lower extremities
- Radio-femoral delay
- Systolic murmur which radiates to the back
- Weak femoral pulse and cold feet
- Collateral circulation develops across intercostal arteries to reach lower bodies, causing these blood vessels to dilate

Key tests
- Chest X ray shows "notching" of ribs due to engorged collateral arteries
- Echocardiogram can show the discrete narrowing in the thoracic aorta
- CT aorta is a useful adjunct to echocardiography to fully define the anatomy of the aortic arch

Management
- May require stenting or surgery depending on the severity

- **Interruption of aortic arch**

This is a heart condition in which there is no connection between the proximal ascending and the descending aorta.

- This prevents blood from the left ventricle from entering the systemic circulation.
- The interruption occurs before the origin of the left subclavian artery, meaning oxygenated blood can still go to the right side of the body and head and neck, but not the left arm and legs.
- Flow of blood into the systemic circulation distal to the interruption is dependent on right-to-left shunting via the ductus arteriosus from the pulmonary artery into the descending aorta.
- A ventricular septal defect is also usually present allowing oxygenated blood into the descending aorta.

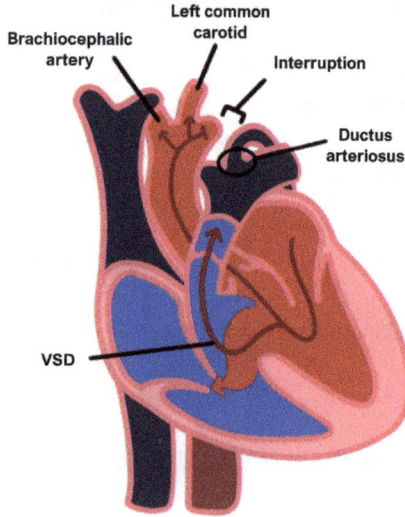

Symptoms
- Acute circulatory collapse around 2 days of age (when the ductus arteriosus closes)
- This leads to cyanosis and heart failure
- Absent femoral pulses and left brachial pulse

Key tests
- Echocardiogram shows aortic discontinuity, ventricular hypertrophy, patent ductus arteriosus, abnormal flow patterns

Management
- Prostaglandin E1 to stop closure of the ductus arteriosus
- Surgery is the definitive management

Respiratory Infections

- **Acute epiglottitis**

This refers to inflammation of the epiglottis, which typically has been caused by the bacterium Haemophilus influenzae type B.

- It should be recognised and treated quickly as it can lead to airway obstruction.
- It usually presents in children, but Haemophilus influenzae type B vaccination has meant that it is rare in children and now increasingly seen more in adults.
- Care should be taken when assessing a patient's throat due to risk of airway obstruction.

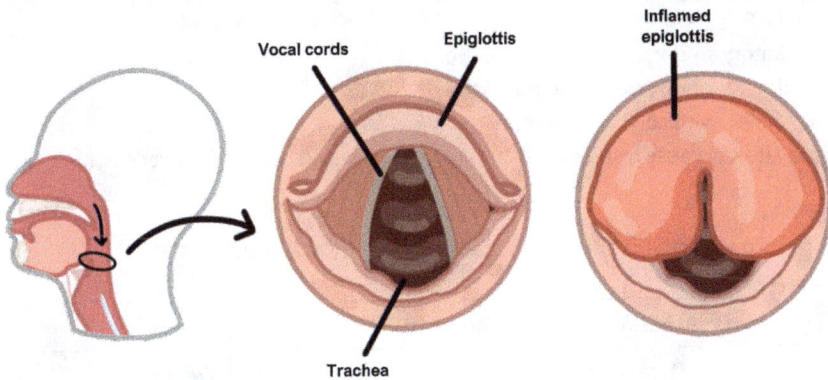

Symptoms

- Rapid onset of high fever and malaise
- Drooling of saliva
- Muffled voice due to very sore throat
- Inspiratory stridor, a high-pitched sound due to turbulent air flow in the upper airway
- Tripod position – this is a compensatory position where a child leans forward, extends the neck, supports themselves with hands or knees. This position helps maximise airway patency and ease breathing in severe upper airway obstruction

Key tests

- Clinical diagnosis after visualising throat (should only be done by experienced physician or ENT specialist)

Management

- This is a medical emergency as there is a high risk of upper airway obstruction
- Anaesthetics involvement to secure airway if signs of compromise
- Management includes IV fluids, antibiotics and oxygen

- **Croup (laryngotracheobronchitis)**

This is an infection of the upper airway seen in infants and toddlers less than 3 years old.

- It causes inflammation and swelling in the larynx, trachea, and bronchi.
- It is common particularly in the autumn months.
- It is usually due to a virus, with parainfluenza virus the most common cause.

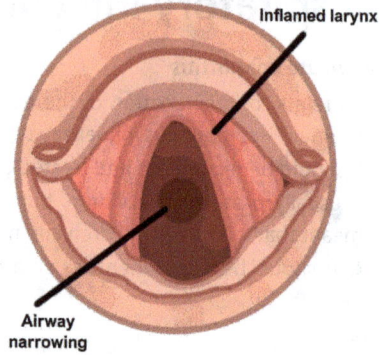

Inflamed larynx

Airway narrowing

Symptoms

- Inspiratory stridor and hoarseness of voice
- Barking cough (worse during the night)
- High fever, with coryzal symptoms
- If severe can cause respiratory distress e.g. chest wall recession (Hoover's sign)

Grading

- The following criteria are used to grade the severity of croup

	Mild	**Moderate**	**Severe**
Cough	Occasional	Frequent	Frequent
Stridor	None at rest	Easily audible at rest	Prominent at rest
Recession	None/mild	Suprasternal and sternal retraction at rest	Marked sternal retraction
Behaviour	Happy, eats, drinks and plays	Little distress or agitation Interested in surrounding	Significant distress and agitation Lethargy

Key tests

- It is diagnosed clinically

Management

- As presentation can be similar to epiglottis, it is necessary to rule this out
- Steroids (oral dexamethasone) are the mainstay of management
- If severe, < 6 months of age or known upper airway abnormality, then admit to hospital, may need to administer oxygen and nebulised adrenaline

- **Whooping cough**

A condition which is caused by the Gram-negative bacterium Bordetella pertussis.

- It is a notifiable disease, which means that it is required to report confirmed cases to the government authorities.
- Although pregnant mothers are immunised during pregnancy and infants are vaccinated during childhood, these vaccines do not provide lifelong protection.
- Symptoms can last up to 10–14 weeks and are more severe in infants.

Symptoms

- Few days of coryzal symptoms initially
- Sudden coughing attacks with a distinctive inspiratory whoop, caused by forced inspiration against a closed glottis
- Coughing episodes which are followed by vomiting, more frequent at night and following meals
- Complications include rib fractures and pneumothorax
- Subconjunctival haemorrhages
- Apnoea, which can lead to cyanosis, syncope and seizures if severe

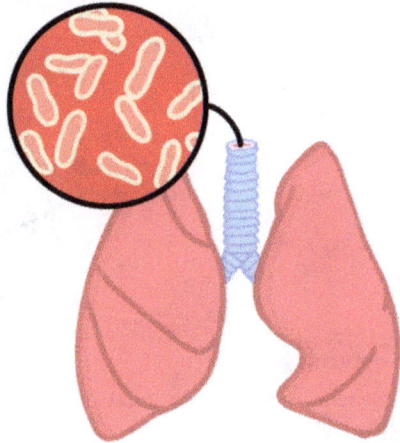

Key tests

- Nasopharyngeal aspirate or swab – this is sent for culture and PCR
- Serological testing for antibodies – a serum anti-pertussis toxin antibody concentration of > 100 IU/mL is suggestive of infection
- Blood tests show elevated white cell count and lymphocytes

Management

- 1st line treatment is an oral macrolide (azithromycin or clarithromycin) if onset of cough is within previous 21 days
- If patient is less than 6 months old, will usually require hospital admission
- Prophylactic antibiotics should be given to household contacts
- School exclusion for 48 hours after starting antibiotics

- **Bronchiolitis**

A respiratory tract infection which leads to the blockage of small airways in the lungs.

- It can lead to significant respiratory distress, especially in infants or children with comorbidities such as prematurity, congenital heart disease or immunodeficiency.
- It is most commonly seen in children < 2 years of age.
- Cases usually spike in the autumn and winter.
- Respiratory syncytial virus is the most common cause, rhinovirus is second.

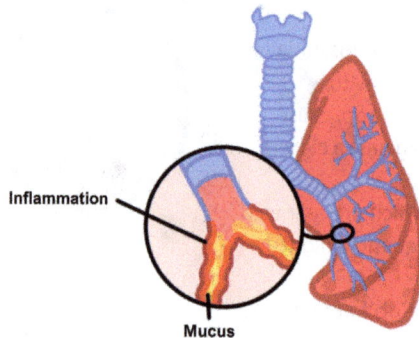

Inflammation

Mucus

Symptoms

- General – coryza, fever, irritability, poor feeding
- Dry cough
- Respiratory distress – chest wall recession, nasal flaring
- Apnoeic episodes may occur
- Wheeze and crackles on auscultation

Key tests

- Diagnosis is usually made based on clinical symptoms
- Chest X-ray can be used to exclude pneumonia
- Immunofluorescence of nasopharyngeal secretions may show RSV, but this has little influence on management

Management

- This is largely supportive with fluids, oxygen, nutrition as most cases self-resolve
- If apnoeic episodes, cyanosis, RR > 70 breaths/minute, SpO_2 < 92%, will require admission to hospital

Palivizumab is a monoclonal antibody which can prevent serious respiratory illness caused by respiratory syncytial virus (RSV) in high-risk infants and young children, such as those with underlying heart and lung disease and premature babies.

- **Pneumonia**

This refers to a lower respiratory tract infection which often occurs when normal defenses are impaired. The causative pathogen varies according to age.

Causes

- Neonates – organisms from the maternal genital tract (Group B streptococci, bacilli, gram negative enterococci)
- Children (< 5 years) – respiratory viruses are most common
- Children (> 5 years) – Strep pneumoniae (most common), mycoplasma, chlamydia

Symptoms

- Fever, cough, chest pain and lethargy
- Tachypnoea (most sensitive sign)
- Nasal flaring and recession (signs of respiratory distress)
- Bronchial breathing, focal coarse crackles on auscultation

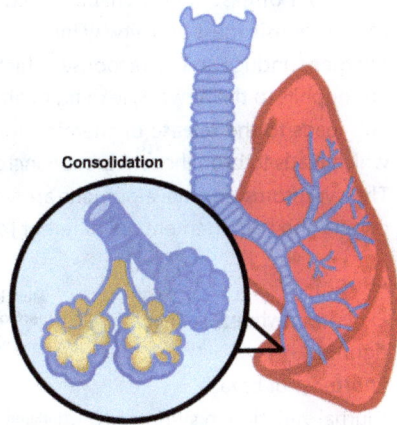

Consolidation

Key tests

- Blood tests show raised inflammatory markers
- CXR can be used to confirm diagnosis but cannot differentiate between viral and bacterial infection. Also useful to assess for a parapneumonic pleural effusion
- Pleural ultrasound/fluid analysis – if an effusion is present then an ultrasound will further define the fluid, and a pleural aspiration can be performed to analyse the fluid
- Sputum sample – sent for culture to help determine antibiotic sensitivity

Management

- 1st line is antibiotics e.g. amoxicillin
- If mycoplasma or chlamydia pneumonia, give macrolides
- Chest drain in case of empyema

Respiratory Conditions

- **Asthma**

Asthma is a disease that is characterised by reversible bronchoconstriction, bronchial hyper-responsiveness and airway inflammation.
- Allergens induce a Th_2 response which stimulates production of IgE and attracts eosinophils to the airways, leading to airway inflammation.
- This leads to the release of chemical mediators (such as histamine and leukotrienes) which leads to bronchoconstriction increasing airway resistance.
- The symptoms and development are very similar to adults; however, the diagnostic criteria and management are different for children.

Symptoms

- Expiratory wheeze, chest tightness
- Shortness of breath
- Diurnal variation in symptoms (worse in morning and night)
- Cough with mucous production
- Reduced peak flow rate

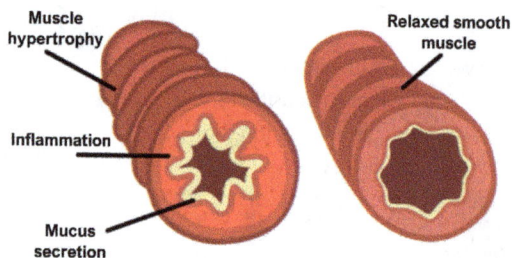

Muscle hypertrophy

Inflammation

Mucus secretion

Relaxed smooth muscle

Key tests

Patients < 5 years
- Diagnosis based on clinical judgement

Patients 5–16 years
- Spirometry shows an obstructive pattern (FEV1/FVC < 0.7)
- Bronchodilator reversibility (BDR) test – positive if improvement in FEV1 $\geq$ 12%
- Fractional exhaled nitric oxide (FeNO) is the measurement of nitric oxide levels in exhaled breath, which reflects eosinophilic airway inflammation
- FeNO is only requested if spirometry is normal or BDR test is negative
- A level of $\geq$ 35 parts per billion (ppb) is considered positive

Grading

- Acute asthma severity is divided moderate, severe and life threatening
- The cut-off thresholds are lower for children than adults as asthma can rapidly become fatal in children

Severe	Life-threatening
SpO$_2$ < 92%	SpO$_2$ < 92% with one of:
PEF < 33–50% predicted	PEF < 33%
HR > 140 bpm (1–5 years) HR > 125 bpm (5+ years)	Cyanosis
RR > 40/min (1–5 years) RR > 30/min (5+ years)	Confusion
Can't complete sentences in one breath	Silent chest
Use of accessory neck muscles	Hypotension

Acute management

- If moderate, give salbutamol inhaler one puff every 60 s up to 10 puffs via spacer or a fitting mask and spacer (if < 3 years)

- If severe or life-threatening, oxygen therapy to maintain SpO$_2$ ≥ 94%
- 1st line is nebulised salbutamol with oral or IV corticosteroid
- If no response, add ipratropium to the nebuliser
- If still symptomatic, consider IV salbutamol and magnesium sulphate
- Further measures include IM adrenaline and intubation and ventilation in ICU

Chronic management

Age < 5 years
- Start with short acting B$_2$ agonist (SABA) for symptomatic relief
- If symptoms > 3 times/week or at night
- Step 1 is SABA + very low paediatric dose inhaled corticosteroid (ICS)
- Step 2 is SABA + paediatric low-dose ICS + leukotriene receptor antagonist (LTRA)
- Step 3 is to consider increasing dose of the ICS
- If still unresolving, refer the patient for specialist care

Ages 5–16
- Start with SABA for symptomatic relief
- If symptoms > 3 times/week or at night
- Step 1 is SABA and low dose ICS
- Step 2 is SABA + low-dose ICS + leukotriene receptor antagonist (LTRA)
- Step 3 is SABA + low-dose ICS + long-acting beta agonist (LABA)
- If still unresolving, refer patient for specialist care

- **Cystic fibrosis (CF)**

This is an autosomal recessive condition that is caused by a mutation in the cystic fibrosis transmembrane conductance regulator (CFTR) gene on chromosome 7.
- In the UK, most common mutation is the δF508 mutation (deletion of phenylalanine).
- This gene encodes the CFTR protein, a Cl^- channel.
- The mutation causes misfolding of the CFTR protein, impairing chloride secretion, leading to production of thick, sticky mucus which clogs airways and exocrine ducts.
- It affects 1 per 2500 births and the carrier rate is 1 in 25.

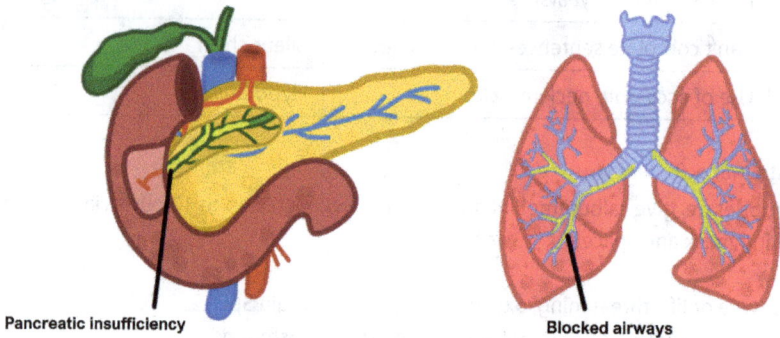

Pancreatic insufficiency   Blocked airways

Symptoms

Neonates
- Typically presents as meconium ileus, which is bowel obstruction that occurs due to abnormally thick and sticky meconium (first bowel movement)

Young children
- Failure to thrive
- Steatorrhea (fat in faeces)
- Prolonged neonatal jaundice
- Recurrent chest infections (often due to S. aureus and Pseudomonas)
- Rectal prolapse
- Nasal polyps, sinusitis

Adolescents
- Respiratory – recurrent infections, bronchiectasis, nasal Polyps
- GI – pancreatic insufficiency, rectal prolapse, liver disease
- Endocrine – CF-related diabetes, delayed puberty
- Reproduction – male infertility

Key tests

- Newborns in the UK are screened for CF as part of the heel prick test
- The sweat test measures Cl^- in sweat, which is elevated in cystic fibrosis (> 60 mEq/L)
- This is because defective CFTR in sweat glands causes less Cl^- to be reabsorbed causing it to be accumulated in sweat

Management

- This uses an MDT approach
- Respiratory – chest physiotherapy, acapella device to aide airway clearance
- Frequent antibiotics (oral and nebulised) for recurrent infections and aggressive treatment of Pseudomonas aeruginosa infection
- GI – pancreatic enzyme replacement, high calorie/fat diet, liver transplant

New medications such as **Orkambi** (Lumacaftor/Ivacaftor) or **Kaftrio** (Elexacaftor/Tezacaftor/Ivacaftor) are used to treat patients which are homozygous for the δF508 mutation, and can sometimes be indicated for some heterozygous.
- Lumacaftor increases the number of CFTR proteins transported to the cell surface.
- Ivacaftor potentiates opening of the CFTR channels to promote less viscous mucus.

- **Primary ciliary dyskinesia (PCD)**

This is a rare autosomal recessive disorder where there is a genetic defect in the cilia which lines the respiratory tract, the fallopian tubes, and the flagella of sperm cells.
- Mutations disrupt ciliary and flagellar proteins, impairing their function.
- This prevents effective mucous clearance, leading to chronic respiratory infections.
- If untreated, it leads to chronic inflammation of the respiratory tracts leading to severe bronchiectasis.
- In addition, dysfunction of cilia during embryological development mean that transcription factors may not flow in the right direction.
- This can lead to organs being developed in the opposite direction.
- This can lead to dextrocardia/situs inversus (known as Kartagener syndrome).

Symptoms

- Recurrent productive cough
- Purulent nasal discharge
- Chronic ear infections
- Infertility due to poor sperm mobility
- Dextrocardia/situs inversus seen in half of patients with PCD

Key tests

- Microscopy of the cilia of nasal epithelial cells brushed from the nose, genetic testing

Management

- Chest physiotherapy to clear secretions
- Proactive treatment of recurrent infections with antibiotics, similar to cystic fibrosis

Developmental Conditions

- **Tracheo-oesophageal fistula (TEF)**

TEF is a congenital anomaly characterised by an abnormal connection between the oesophagus and trachea.

- During early embryonical development, the oesophagus and trachea originate from a common foregut tube.
- Under normal circumstances, this structure undergoes division into two distinct tubes during the first trimester of gestation.
- Failure of proper separation results in a persistent communication between the trachea and oesophagus, permitting the passage of food and secretions into the respiratory tract.
- The most prevalent subtype of TEF is Type C, which involves proximal oesophageal atresia with the distal oesophagus abnormally connected to the trachea.

Symptoms

- Drooling, coughing and choking during feeding
- Recurrent aspiration pneumonias

This condition is associated with a type of disorder that affects many body systems, called the VACTERL association:
- Vertebral defects
- Anal atresia
- Cardiac defects
- Tracheo-oesophageal fistula
- Renal anomalies
- Limb anomalies

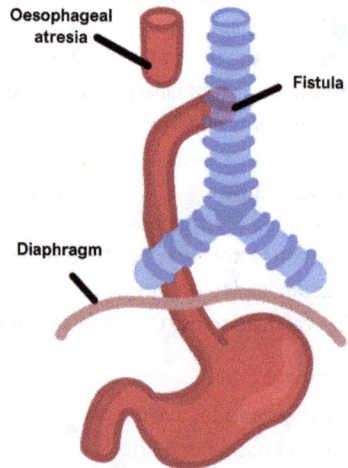

Key tests

- Antenatal ultrasound shows polyhydramnios (excess amniotic fluid in utero as baby cannot swallow fluid) and an absent stomach bubble
- After birth, a trial of NG tube insertion with CXR and abdominal XR is used to assess if it can reach the stomach. If it cannot, this suggests oesophageal atresia

Management

- Surgical correction is the definitive management

- **Pyloric stenosis**

This is a narrowing of the opening between the stomach and the duodenum.
- It occurs due to congenital hypertrophy of the pyloric sphincter.
- It presents in the first month of life, is more common in males, usually affects the first born and is associated with a positive family history.

Symptoms
- Projectile non-bilious vomiting, about half an hour after feeding
- Constipation and dehydration
- Olive-like mass in the abdomen

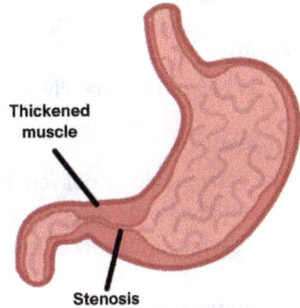

Thickened muscle

Stenosis

Key tests
- Ultrasound shows a thickened pyloric muscle and elongated canal

Management
- Supportive management with fluids and correcting electrolyte abnormalities
- Surgical correction (e.g. Ramstedt pyloromyotomy) is the definitive management

- **Gastroschisis**

This is a congenital malformation of the anterior abdominal wall just lateral to the umbilical cord, which results in herniation of the bowel and stomach out of the abdominal wall without a protective sac.
- If left untreated, it can lead to severe dehydration and protein loss.

Symptoms
- Exposure of the abdominal organs out of the abdomen

Key tests
- Can be seen antenatally on the foetal anomaly scan

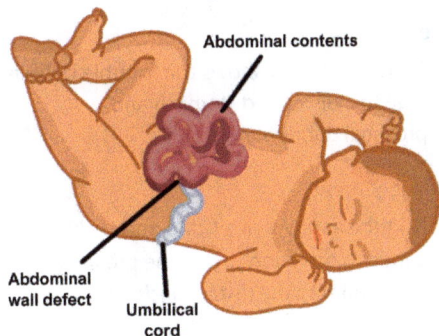

Abdominal contents

Abdominal wall defect

Umbilical cord

Management
- The baby can be delivered vaginally as the exposed bowel tolerates labour well
- The abdomen is covered in clear occlusive wrap to minimise fluid/heat loss
- Urgent surgical correction is required

- **Exomphalos**

This is a condition similar to gastroschisis; however, the herniating abdominal contents are covered by the amniotic sac.
- The amniotic sac membrane is protective against dehydration and protein loss.
- It is associated with disorders which lead to the overgrowth of organs, such as Beckwith-Wiedemann syndrome.

Key tests

- It can be seen antenatally on the foetal anomaly scan

Management

- The baby should be delivered via Caesarean section as this can minimise trauma to the amniotic sac and preserve its integrity, preventing rupture and infection
- Surgical repair (usually in stages) is the definitive management

- **Duodenal atresia**

A condition in which the duodenum ends blindly, disconnecting from the distal bowel.
- This blocks the flow of food and secretions, resembling small bowel obstruction.
- It is associated with Down's syndrome.

Symptoms

- Polyhydramnios in utero
- Bilious vomiting and abdominal distension a few hours after birth

Key tests

- Abdominal X-ray shows the "double bubble sign" (due to a distended stomach and proximal duodenum)

Management

- NG tube and IV fluids ("drip and suck")
- Surgical correction to join the proximal duodenum to the distal duodenum

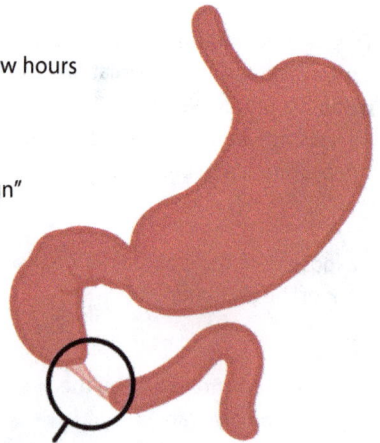

Duodenal atresia

- **Meckel's diverticulum**

This refers to an outpouching of the ileum which occurs due to failure of the vitelline duct to involute.
- It follows the rule of 2s: seen in 2% of people, usually 2 inches long, is located within 2 feet of ileocecal valve, is twice as prevalent in males than females
- It is seen in young children around the age of 2.
- It contains remnants of gastric and pancreatic tissue and can secrete stomach acid.

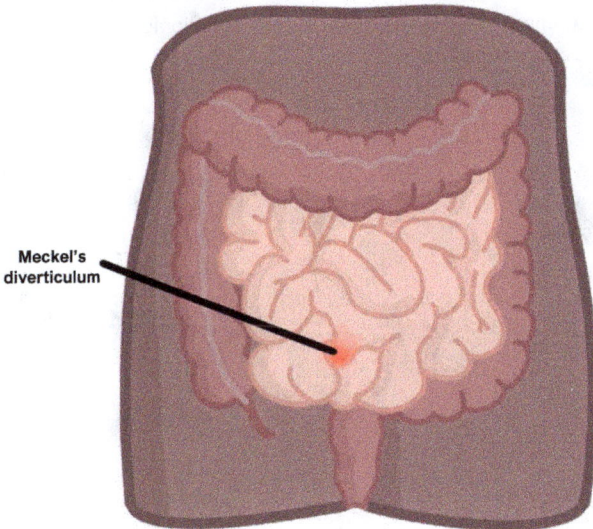

Meckel's diverticulum

Symptoms
- Most cases are asymptomatic but can cause a variety of presentations
- Bleeding – acute, painless rectal bleeding
- Small bowel obstruction – the diverticulum acts as a lead point for intussusception
- Meckel's diverticulitis – clinically similar to appendicitis

Key tests
- If bleeding is the presenting symptoms, a technetium-99 scan (demonstrates increased uptake by ectopic gastric mucosa)
- If suspected small bowel obstruction or Meckel diverticulitis, CT abdomen is usually investigation of choice

Management
- Surgical removal

- **Hirschsprung disease**

This is a condition caused by a problem in the development of neural plexuses supplying the distal large bowel.
- It is caused by poor migration of the crest cells to this area.
- This results in an aganglionic segment of large bowel.
- Without these nerve cells, there is no innervation of the smooth muscle resulting in ineffective peristalsis.
- This abnormal segment is therefore left narrow and contracted, causing obstruction.
- The normal segment of bowel proximal to the aganglionic segment will be dilated as food and secretions collect here.

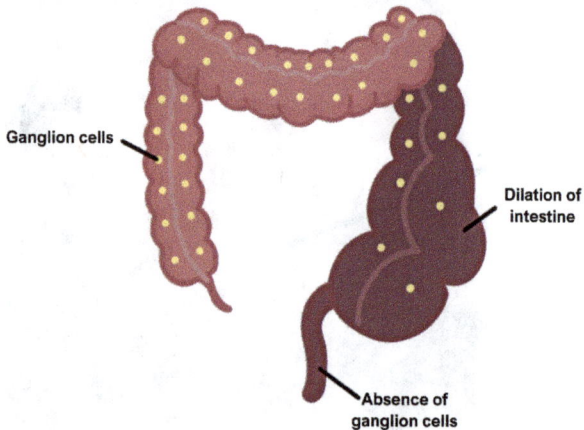

Symptoms
- Delayed passage of meconium (> 48 hours after birth)
- Signs of bowel obstruction – abdominal distension, bilious vomiting
- Poor growth
- Chronic constipation in childhood

Key tests
- Rectal examination reveals a narrowed segment followed by a gush of liquid stool/ flatus on withdrawal of the examining finger
- Suction rectal biopsy – this shows the absence of ganglion cells and presence of large acetylcholinesterase-positive nerve trunks

Management
- In the acute setting, bowel irrigation
- Surgery – an anorectal pull through is where the aganglionic segment is removed followed by anastomosis of the bowel to the anus

- **Malrotation**

This is a condition which is caused by a failure of the normal sequence of rotation of the bowel during development.

- The caecum remains high in the midline and fixed to the posterior abdominal wall.
- This can lead to duodenal obstruction in 2 ways: small bowel volvulus (which can lead to SMA compromise) or extrinsic compression from Ladd's bands (peritoneal bands that cross the duodenum anteriorly).
- It usually presents in the first week of life.

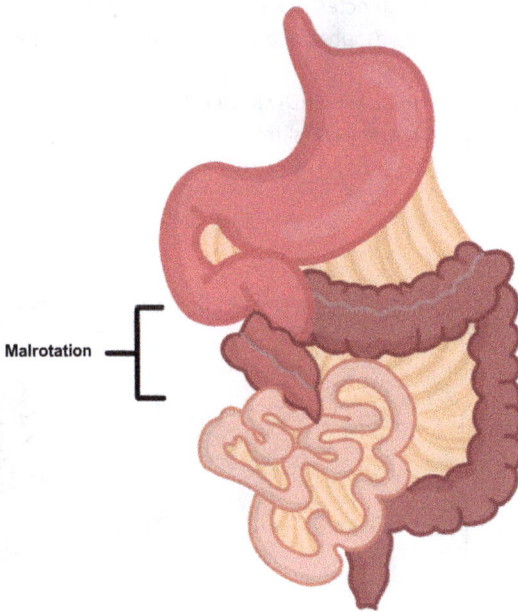

Malrotation

Symptoms

- Obstructive symptoms – bilious vomiting, distension
- Can give bowel ischaemia causing abdominal pain and tenderness

Key tests

- Upper GI contrast study shows abnormal intestinal positioning, corkscrew appearance and delayed passage of contrast

Management

- Surgical correction (Ladd's procedure) – this treats malrotation by smoothing out twisted intestines and cutting through Ladd bands that block the baby's intestines

Digestion Conditions

- **Gastro-oesophageal reflux disease (GORD)**

Reflux refers to the passage of gastric contents into the oesophagus.
- Reflux is a common event and is self-limiting, with nearly all cases resolving spontaneously by 12 months of age.
- It is characterised by vomiting/reflux after feeds with normal weight gain and growth.
- Reflux is common in children due to a host of factors, such as inappropriate relaxation of the lower oesophageal sphincter (LOS) because of functional immaturity, a short intra-stomach length of the oesophagus and a predominantly fluid-based diet.

Gastro-oesophageal reflex disease (GORD) specifically refers to reflux that causes symptoms severe enough to merit medical treatment or with complications.

Risk factors

- Prematurity
- Oesophageal atresia
- Congenital diaphragmatic hernia
- Neurological conditions

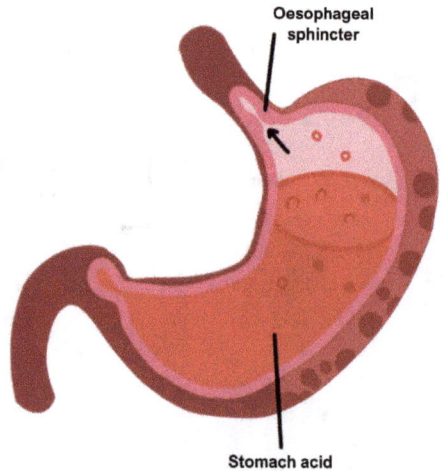

Oesophageal sphincter

Stomach acid

Symptoms

- Vomiting and regurgitation of food after meals
- Faltering growth
- Oesophagitis – pain on feeding, haematemesis, anaemia
- Pulmonary aspiration – recurrent pneumonia, cough, or wheeze
- Dystonic neck posturing – Sandifer syndrome, a very rare movement disorder that causes head, neck, and back arching spasms
- Frequent otitis media

Key tests

- In most cases, it is diagnosed clinically
- If diagnostic doubt, can do a pH impedance study (measure pH in oesophagus)
- Other tests include OGD, upper GI contrast study or manometry

Management
- Give advice to parents about keeping the baby's head up during feeding
- If breast fed, a breastfeeding assessment should be conducted, second line is alginate therapy (e.g. Gaviscon)
- If formula fed, 1st trial thickened formula or smaller more frequent meals, second line is alginate therapy
- If unresolved despite above, trial of PPI (e.g. omeprazole) or histamine receptor antagonist (e.g. ranitidine) for infants
- If still persistent, refer to gastroenterology for possible endoscopy

• Constipation
Constipation is a common issue in children, especially around the ages of 2–3 when they are being potty trained.
- Common reasons include not eating high-fibre foods, not drinking enough fluids or feeling anxious about something such as starting nursery or school.
- However, it can also be due to serious medical conditions.
- Therefore, it is important to differentiate between benign and more sinister causes.

Symptoms
- Less than 3 complete stools/week
- Hard, stool like rabbit dropping (type 1 according to Bristol Stool chart)
- Difficulty passing stool – straining, abdominal pain that is relieved by defecation
- Anal fissures
- Soiling of underwear with diarrhoea, which can be a sign of overflow

In addition, there are some red flag symptoms which may point towards a more sinister cause:
- Constipation since birth
- Delayed passage of meconium (> 48 hours after birth)
- Poor weight gain and growth
- Neurological symptoms e.g. leg weakness

Management
- First line is an osmotic laxative like Movicol (add polyethylene glycol if faecal impaction is present)
- If persistent, then add in a stimulant laxative
- If red flag symptoms, refer to specialist for further investigation

- **Gastroenteritis**

This is a condition which refers to acute inflammation of the gut due to an infective cause, most commonly rotavirus in children.

- Whilst it usually self-resolves without antibiotics, the child's hydration status must be closely monitored to prevent dehydration and serious complications.

Symptoms

- Diarrhoea (usually stops within 2 weeks) and vomiting (usually stops within 3 days)

Key tests

- It is a clinical diagnosis
- If child has been abroad, has blood in stool or signs of sepsis, send a stool culture
- Blood tests such as U&Es, FBC are usually only required if the child appears severely dehydrated or has signs of sepsis

Management

- The first step is to assess the hydration status of the child
- Signs of dehydration include reduced urine output, lethargic, sunken eyes, however the child will be haemodynamically stable (normal BP, normal capillary refill time)
- Signs of shock include reduced consciousness, pale skin, appears unwell and they may have signs of haemodynamic compromise (low BP, high HR, long CRT, cold)

The mainstay of management is to treat the dehydration according to severity:
- If no evidence of dehydration, continue usual feeding and monitor closely
- If clinical dehydration, give oral rehydration salts and continue usual feeding
- If in shock, will require admission to hospital for IV fluid rehydration

- **Toddler diarrhoea**

A chronic, non-specific diarrhoea, which is usually seen in children aged 1–5 years.
- It is possibly due to gut dysmotility and fast-transit diarrhoea.
- One of the most common causes is cows' milk intolerance.

Symptoms

- Chronic diarrhoea in an otherwise well child
- Stools of variable consistency which may contain undigested food

Key tests

- It is a diagnosis of exclusion (rule out other causes of chronic diarrhoea)

Management

- Dietary management is the mainstay of treatment, avoid precipitating cause
- Reduce refined sugar (juice, fizzy drinks, sweets, chocolate)
- Increase dietary fat intake and avoid excessive fluid intake

- **Cow's milk protein (CMP) intolerance and allergy**

This is a relatively common condition which is caused by an intolerance to a protein found in cow's milk.
- Children can either be allergic to the protein, which is characterised by an immediate, IgE-mediated response.
- On the other hand, they can be intolerant to the protein, which is characterised by a delayed, non-IgE-mediated response.

Symptoms

- GI – regurgitation, vomiting, diarrhoea, colic
- Skin – urticaria, atopic eczema
- General – irritability, crying, failure to thrive
- In rare cases, can lead to angioedema and anaphylaxis

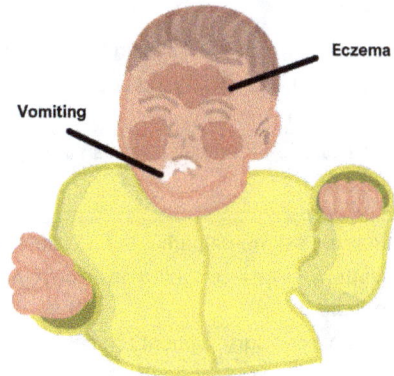

Key tests

- Clinical diagnosis by seeing symptom improvement after excluding cow's milk
- If suspicion of true allergy, further investigations include skin prick testing, total IgE and specific IgE (RAST) for cow's milk protein

Management

- This depends on whether the baby is formula or breast-fed
- If breastfed, continue breastfeeding and eliminate cow's milk from the maternal diet
- Switch to extensively hydrolysed formula (eHF) milk when breastfeeding stops

For formula fed infants, if mild or moderate symptoms, use extensive hydrolysed formula (eHF) milk (this contains a small amount of CMP).
- If severe symptoms, use amino-acid based formula (AAF) milk.

Intestinal Conditions

- **Acute appendicitis**

This refers to inflammation of the appendix.
- It is the most common cause of abdominal surgery, occurring at any age.
- It typically results from luminal obstruction, commonly due to lymphoid hyperplasia (in children) or a faecolith (adults).
- Obstruction allows gut organisms to invade the appendix wall, causing oedema, ischaemia, and necrosis.
- Initial visceral irritation progresses to localised peritoneal inflammation in the right iliac fossa.

Symptoms

- Migrating periumbilical pain to right iliac fossa
- Mild fever (37.5–38°C) and anorexia
- Infrequent vomiting
- Constipation (but diarrhoea can also occur)

Signs

- Rovsing's sign – palpating the LIF causes pain in the RIF
- Dunphy's sign – coughing gives pain in the right lower quadrant
- Hamburger sign – patient refuses to eat, as anorexia is a strong sign for appendicitis

Faecolith

Key tests

- Blood tests show raised inflammatory markers (WCC and CRP)
- If diagnostic doubt then do ultrasound, or CT scan if diagnosis is still unclear

Management

- Laparoscopic appendectomy, IV antibiotics

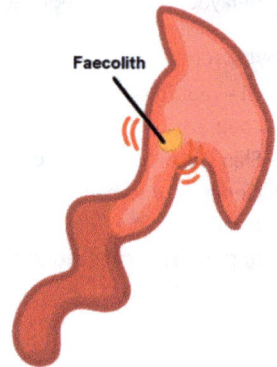

- **Mesenteric adenitis**

This refers to inflammation of the mesenteric lymph nodes, often secondary to an viral (URTI) infection, but can also be due to a bacterial infection.

Symptoms

- Symptoms of a concurrent URTI
- Diffuse abdominal pain (can mimic appendicitis)
- Nausea, vomiting, diarrhoea
- Non-localised abdominal tenderness
- Extra mesenteric lymphadenopathy
- Fever

Key tests

- It is a diagnosis of exclusion
- Many are diagnosed during an appendectomy for suspected appendicitis

Management

- Reassurance and pain control (usually self-resolves)

- **Infantile colic**

A common condition causing colicky spasms in early infancy, with an unknown cause.
- It is defined by crying episodes > 3 hours/day, > 3 days/week, for at least 3 weeks.
- Despite this, the infant remains otherwise healthy.
- It typically starts in the first few weeks of life and ends by 4–5 months of age.
- Food allergy may play a role in the pathogenesis.

Symptoms

- Paroxysmal, inconsolable crying, screaming
- Drawing up of the knees
- Passive of excessive flatus

Key tests

- It is a diagnosis of exclusion once other more sinister causes have been ruled out

Management

- Reassure parents as the condition self-resolves by 6 months of age

- **Intussusception**

This is a condition where a proximal segment of bowel telescopes into the lumen of the adjacent distal bowel, which usually affects infants less than 2 years old.
- It usually involves the ileum passing into the caecum through the ileo-caecal valve.
- No underlying cause is typically found, but in children < 2 years, an identifiable lead point is more likely to be present (e.g. polyp, Meckel diverticulum).

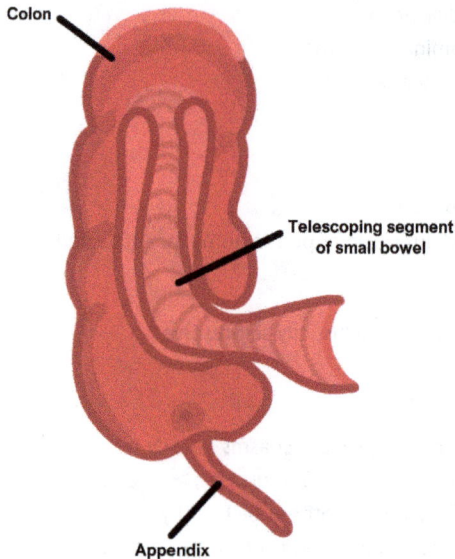

Colon

Telescoping segment of small bowel

Appendix

Symptoms
- Abdominal pain during which the infant characteristically will pull their legs up to the chest area
- Vomiting (which can be green in colour due to bile)
- Blood-stained stool (red-currant jelly stool)
- Sausage-shaped mass in RUQ
- Can cause venous obstruction giving bowel necrosis and perforation

Key tests
- Abdominal ultrasound is imaging of choice and shows a target-like mass
- A CT scan can also be performed if there is diagnostic uncertainty

Management
- 1st line is fluid resuscitation and contrast enema reduction
- If unsuccessful or if bowel perforation is suspected, surgery is required

Liver Conditions

Jaundice occurs due to elevated levels of bilirubin in the blood. While neonatal jaundice is common, jaundice within the first 24 hours of life is always pathological.
- There are a variety of causes for jaundice, including haemolysis, infection, as well as metabolic disorders like Crigler-Najjar syndrome.
- As unconjugated bilirubin is fat-soluble, it can cross the blood-brain barrier.
- Unconjugated bilirubin is highly neurotoxic, risking irreversible neurological damage.

● **Genetic liver diseases**

This refers to a group of autosomal recessive disorders which lead to errors in bilirubin conjugation, uptake, or excretion by the liver.
- The ones which lead to unconjugated hyper-bilirubinaemia are more serious as unconjugated bilirubin can cross the BBB, causing neurological problems.

○ **Gilbert's syndrome**

This is an autosomal recessive condition due to a mutation in the gene UGT1A1.
- This results in a mild deficiency of UDP-glucuronosyltransferase, an enzyme that conjugates bilirubin.
- It is a mild condition which is usually asymptomatic and only gives jaundice in times of stress e.g. illness, exercise or fasting.
- Blood tests show raised unconjugated bilirubin.

○ **Crigley-Najjar syndrome**

This is an autosomal recessive condition due to a mutation in the gene UGT1A1.
- Type 1 causes a complete deficiency of UDP-glucuronosyltransferase, whereas type 2 causes a significant but not complete deficiency of this enzyme.
- This gives a very severe neonatal jaundice which can lead to kernicterus.
- Blood tests show raised unconjugated bilirubin.
- It is treated with phototherapy and may require a liver transplant.

○ **Dubin-Johnson syndrome**

This is an autosomal recessive condition due to a mutation in the gene MRP2.
- This results in defective hepatic excretion of bilirubin.
- It is more common in the Iranian Jewish population.
- It is usually asymptomatic but gives a black pigmented liver.
- Blood tests show raised levels of conjugated bilirubin.

○ **Rotor syndrome**

This is an autosomal recessive condition due to a mutation in the gene SLCO1B1/3.

- This results in defective hepatic uptake and storage of bilirubin.
- It is similar to Dubin-Johnson syndrome but does not give a black liver.
- Blood tests show raised levels of conjugated bilirubin.

● **Biliary atresia**

This is a condition causing progressive fibrosis and obliteration of the biliary tree.

- This obstructs bile flow, resulting in bile stasis giving a cholestatic picture.
- As hepatocytes are still able to conjugate bilirubin, it causes a conjugated hyper-bilirubinaemia, reducing the risk of kernicterus.
- However, bile is hepatotoxic, leading to progressive liver damage.
- Left untreated, it progresses to early-onset liver cirrhosis and portal hypertension.

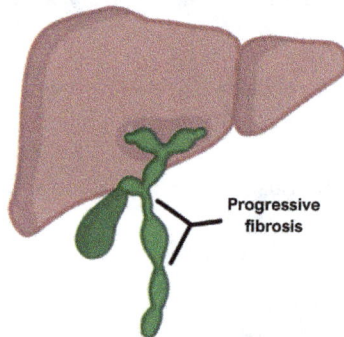

Progressive fibrosis

Symptoms

- Mild jaundice in the first few weeks of life
- Cholestasis – pale stools, dark urine
- Normal birthweight which is then followed by poor levels of growth and appetite
- If untreated, signs of liver cirrhosis (hepatosplenomegaly due to portal hypertension)

Key tests

- Blood test shows high ALP, ALT, and high levels of conjugated bilirubin
- Ultrasound shows biliary tract distension with a contracted or absent gallbladder
- ECRP fails to outline a normal biliary tree

Management

- 1st line is the Kasai procedure – this is a hepatoportoenterostomy (loop of jejunum anastomosed to cut surface of porta hepatis)
- If unsuccessful, a liver transplant maybe required

Renal Conditions

- **Potter's sequence**

This is a complication which occurs due to severe oligohydramnios in the uterus which affects foetal development.

- It usually occurs due to problems with the foetus' kidneys, which reduce urine production, reducing the amount of amniotic fluid in the uterus.
- The lack of cushioning fluid results in foetal compression giving deformities.
- As amniotic fluid is essential for foetal lung development, reduced urine production leads to underdeveloped lungs, leading to respiratory failure after birth.

Symptoms

- Lung deformities – pulmonary hypoplasia giving respiratory failure
- Facial deformities – low-set ears, parrot beak nose, prominent epicanthic folds
- Organ deformities – anal atresia, absence of rectum/colon, diaphragmatic hernia
- Limb deformities – clubbed feet

Management

- Very difficult to treat. Baby is usually stillborn or dies soon due to respiratory failure

- **Multicystic dysplastic kidney**

This is a congenital malformation resulting in a non-functioning kidney with multiple fluid-filled cysts.

- This kidney lacks renal tissue and has no connection to the bladder.
- It occurs due to failed interaction between the ureteric bud (forms ureter, pelvis, calyces, collecting ducts) and nephrogenic mesenchyme (forms kidney tissue).

Symptoms

- The affected kidney is non-functional
- Potter's syndrome (severe oligohydramnios and poor foetal development) will result if both kidneys are affected

Management

- Around 50% of affected kidneys involute by the age of 2
- If the kidney remains large or causes complications (e.g. hypertension), a nephrectomy may be needed

- **Vesicoureteral reflux**

This is characterised by the backflow of urine from the bladder into the ureter.
- The backflow of urine predisposes children to recurrent urinary tract infections which can eventually lead to renal scarring and chronic kidney disease.

o **Primary VUR**

This is the most common type of VUR, which occurs due to a congenital defect in the vesicoureteral junction.
- This defect causes the ureters to enter the bladder at a perpendicular angle.
- This reduces the length of the ureter in the wall of the bladder, affecting the function of the vesicoureteral junction.
- Urine can flow backwards from the bladder into the ureter causing complications.
- Primary VUR usually resolves with age.

o **Secondary VUR**

In secondary VUR, the cause of urine backflow is not due to a defect in the vesicoureteral junction but instead secondary to another pathology.
- Causes include urethral obstruction, urinary tract infections causing inflammation of the urinary tract or a neuropathic bladder.

Symptoms

- Recurrent UTIs at a young age
- Abdominal pain, dysuria and frequency

Key tests

- Voiding cystourethrogram shows urine backflow into ureters
- This involves catheterisation of the bladder and filling it with a contrast agent (dye) that shows up on X-rays
- The patient then urinates while X-ray images are taken to observe the flow of urine

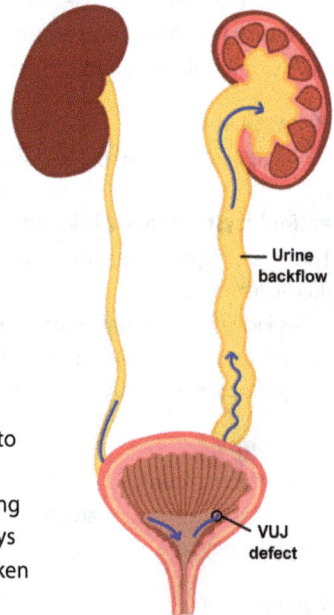

Urine backflow

VUJ defect

Management

- Encourage fluid intake, regular voiding, complete bladder emptying
- For recurrent infections, patients can be offered antibiotic prophylaxis
- If persistent, consider surgical approaches to repair the VUJ

It is important to check for underlying causes in children with recurrent UTIs.
- A DMSA scan, also known as a dimercaptosuccinic acid scan, is a nuclear medicine test used to assess kidney function and structure.
- It involves injecting a small amount of radioactive tracer (isotope) into a vein, which is then absorbed by the kidneys.
- The scan captures images of the kidneys, helping doctors identify any problems, such as scarring or reduced function.

For children < 6 months, organize an ultrasound within 6 weeks for 1st UTI.
- If recurrent UTIs, then perform an US during infection and a DMSA after.
- If child is > 6 months, no investigation is required for the 1st UTI.
- If recurrent UTIs, request an US within 6 weeks and then DMSA.

- **Wilm's tumour (nephroblastoma)**

This is a malignant kidney tumour of the young renal tubules and kidney cells.
- It is the most common abdominal malignancy in children, usually presenting around the age of 3. In children < 1, it is called a metanephric blastema.

Causes
- Most cases are sporadic, but can also be associated with hereditary disorders:
- WAGR syndrome – Wilms tumour, aniridia (absence of iris), genito-urinary anomalies and range of developmental delays.
- Beckwith-Wiedemann syndrome – this causes a Wilms tumour as well as organomegaly due to mutations in IGF-2.
- Denys-Drash syndrome – this gives a Wilms tumour as well as glomerulonephritis and male pseudohermaphrotidism.

Symptoms
- Triad of painless haematuria, loin mass and lumbar pain
- Weight loss, failure to thrive
- Enlarged abdominal mass (due to enlarged kidneys)

Management
- Nephrectomy to remove the affected kidney
- Chemotherapy/radiotherapy may be required

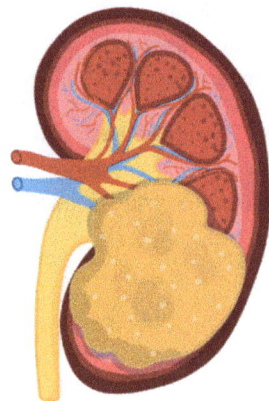

- **Enuresis**

This refers to the involuntary discharge of urine in a child older than the age of 5 years.
- Whilst it is common, less than 10% of bedwetting cases have a pathological medical cause, and most of the time children grow out of this pattern of behaviour with training.
- Primary enuresis is diagnosed where the child never achieved continence.
- Secondary enuresis is used in cases where the child had achieved continence for at least 6 months.

○ **Primary enuresis**

This is the involuntary of discharge of urine in a child who never achieved continence.
- It can be divided into two types, depending on whether there are daytime symptoms.

▪ **Primary nocturnal enuresis**

This is commonly referred to as bedwetting and describes when the child is dry during the day but involuntarily passes urine during sleep.
- This is most likely to be due to behavioural issues, such as the child not using the toilet before bed. However, it can also be due to biological causes.

Causes
- Behavioural – drinking water before bed, not emptying bladder before bed
- Sleep arousal difficulties – inability to wake to noise or the sensation of a full bladder
- Bladder dysfunction – small capacity or overactive bladder

Management
- Reward systems (star charts) given for good behaviour such as using the toilet before bed to train good habits
- 1st line is enuresis alarm – this senses moisture in the nappy and will wake the child up if moisture detected
- If unresolving, then can try desmopressin which reduces urine production
- If persistent after 2 treatment courses, refer to enuresis clinic for specialist input

▪ **Primary enuresis with daytime symptoms**

This is the involuntary of discharge of urine in a child during the night and daytime.
- It is usually due to lower urinary tract disorders which require further investigation.

Causes
- Overactive bladder, structural abnormalities
- Neurological disorders (e.g. neurogenic bladder due to spinal dysraphism)

Symptoms
- Bedwetting at night alongside daytime wetting, urgency, frequency, dysuria
- Neuropathic bladder is associated with neurological symptoms
- If ectopic ureter, associated with constant dribbling, child will be always damp
- Incontinence increases risk of secondary UTI

Key tests
- Urinalysis to rule out UTI
- May require imaging to assess for structural causes

Management
- Refer to specialist for further investigation

o **Secondary enuresis**
This is the involuntary passing of urine in children older than 5 years of age who had previously achieved continence for 6 months.
- This is more likely to be due to an acute problem, such as a UTI or a change in the family situation.

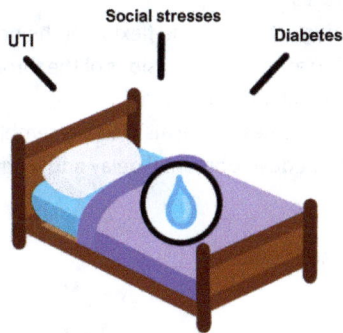

Causes
- Medical – diabetes, UTI, constipation, CKD, seizures
- Behavioural – family problems, psychological problems

Management
- Manage underlying cause

Epilepsy

Epilepsy in children is a neurological condition characterised by recurring seizures.
- Children can develop seizures after an insult to the brain, such as inflammation, space-occupying lesions and infections.
- However, seizures can also be secondary to specific syndromes.
- The main investigations for seizures include an MRI (structural causes) and EEG.

- **Benign sleep myoclonus**

These are myoclonic jerks that occur during sleep in young children and stop when the child is woken up.
- They are not real seizures, are benign and self-limiting.
- No treatment is required other than reassurance.

- **Epileptic (infantile) spasms (West's syndrome)**

This is a rare and severe form of epilepsy which is seen in infants < 2 years old.
- It is typically associated with an underlying neurological abnormality.
- It is believed to result from a dysfunction in the regulation of GABA (gamma-aminobutyric acid) transmission.

Symptoms
- Triad of muscle spasm attacks
- Initially starts with "lightning attacks", rapid flexion of the head, trunk and limbs
- This is followed by "nodding attacks", convulsions of the throat and neck flexor muscles where the chin jerks down and head draws in
- "Salaam/jack-knife attacks" are flexor spasms which resemble the salaam greeting
- Patients typically also exhibit developmental delay and learning difficulties

Key tests
- EEG – hypsarrthymia, a chaotic electrical activity with no pattern

Management
- Management options include hormonal therapy such as steroids or ACTH
- Vigabatrin inhibits GABA breakdown to increase inhibitory transmission

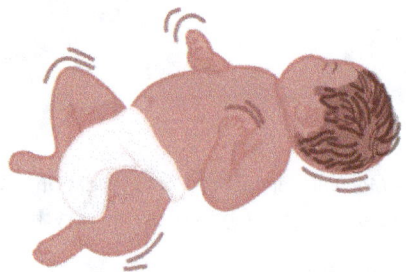

- **Lennox-Gastaut syndrome (LGS)**

This is a rare condition which causes epilepsy in children around the age of 3–5 and persists into childhood.
- Around 20% of children with West's syndrome will go on to develop LGS.

Symptoms

- Seizures (most commonly tonic seizures) which occur during non-REM sleep
- Seizures can occur daily and are difficult to treat with anticonvulsive medication
- There may be a clinical history of West's syndrome
- Eye problems – refractive errors, strabismus

Key tests

- EEG – characteristic slow wave spike

Management

- Anti-epileptics e.g. sodium valproate
- Ketogenic diet also helps to decrease the frequency of seizures

- **Childhood absence epilepsy**

This is an idiopathic epilepsy disorder that causes absence seizures in otherwise healthy children.
- The seizures are brief but can occur numerous times per day.
- Minor automatisms may be present, but the occurrence of major motor symptoms rules out the diagnosis.

Symptoms

- Multiple short (4–20 s) absence seizures with quick recovery
- Children usually develop normally (most will become seizure free in adolescence)
- No major motor symptoms

Key tests

- MRI is typically normal
- EEG – characteristic 3 Hz, generalised symmetrical spikes

Management

- Anti-epileptics e.g. sodium valproate or ethosuximide

- **Benign Rolandic epilepsy**

This is the most common epilepsy syndrome in children.
- It starts between the ages of 3–13 and stopping at 14–18 years.
- Seizure activity starts close to the central sulcus around the Rolandic fissure.
- Children usually have normal intelligence and development.

Symptoms

- Single focal seizures giving unilateral face
  paraesthesia when waking up

Key tests

- EEG – characteristic spikes in the centro-
  temporal area

Management

- No treatment is required if the symptoms are
  mild
- If more severe, then 1st line is usually carbamazepine
  for focal seizures

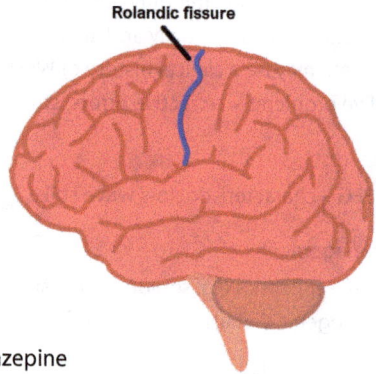
Rolandic fissure

- **Febrile convulsions**

These are seizures associated with a fever over 38°C in an otherwise healthy child.
- They usually occur before age 5 and are less common in older children.
- Importantly, they result from the acute infection and are not linked to an underlying
  neurological disorder.

Symptoms

- Brief tonic-clonic seizures
- Often triggered by a viral infection, so may have signs of concurrent illness

Febrile seizures are typically classified by duration.
- Simple – these last < 15 minutes, resemble generalised seizures, and do not recur
  within 24 hours
- Complex – these last 15–30 minutes and may appear focal. They may recur within
  24 hours and can lead to incomplete recovery (e.g. Todd's palsy)
- Status epilepticus – this lasts > 30 minutes

Key tests

- Clinical diagnosis based on history, MRI or EEG are not usually required

Management

- If it is the first seizure or shows features of a complex seizure, will need admission
- For recurrent seizures, train parents to use rectal diazepam or buccal midazolam
- Acute seizure management according to guidelines

- **Reflex anoxic seizures**

This refers to seizures that occur in otherwise healthy children in response to painful or emotional stimuli.
- They are caused by neurally-mediated transient asystole in children with very sensitive vagal cardiac reflexes and are not epileptic seizures.

Symptoms

- Child turns pale and falls to floor, followed by rapid recovery

Key tests

- Clinical diagnosis

Management

- No treatment is usually required, and it carries a good prognosis

- **Juvenile myoclonic epilepsy (Janz syndrome)**

This is a common type of generalised epilepsy in adolescents aged 12–18.
- It is more frequently seen in girls than boys.
- Seizures typically occur in the early morning and are triggered by sleep deprivation.

Symptoms

- Brief episodes of involuntary muscle jerks, usually in the morning or before sleep
- Myoclonic jerks are more common in the arms than legs
- The jerks can cause the patient to drop objects
- Generalised tonic-clonic seizures may develop after a few months of myoclonic jerks

Key tests

- EEG – characteristic 4–6 Hz polyspike and slow wave discharges

Management

- Avoid sleep deprivation
- Treat with anti-epileptics e.g. sodium valproate

Motor Conditions

- **Muscular dystrophies**

This refers to a group of degenerative disorders that cause progressive skeletal muscle weakness and breakdown.

- There are over 30 distinct types, though a few subtypes are more common.
- Each subtype has a unique pattern of inheritance.

○ **Duchenne muscular dystrophy (DMD)**

This form of muscular dystrophy is caused by an X-linked recessive mutation in the dystrophin gene. The mutation is typically a severe nonsense or frameshift mutation.

- Dystrophin connects the muscle fibre cytoskeleton to the extracellular matrix via a membrane protein complex, helping to stabilise the muscle cell membrane.
- Without dystrophin, muscle cell membranes become unstable.
- Damaged muscle cells release creatine kinase and calcium influx causes cell death.
- Over time, muscle fibres atrophy and are replaced by fat and fibrotic tissue.

Symptoms

- Poor balance and a progressive loss of walking ability
- Proximal muscle weakness, typically starting between ages 4–5
- Gowers' sign – using the arms to rise from a squatting position
- Calf pseudohypertrophy
- May be associated with intellectual impairment
- Death usually occurs due to cardiac or respiratory failure, or dilated cardiomyopathy

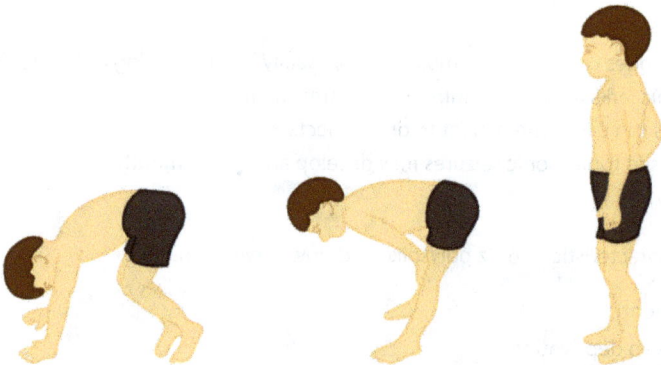

Gowers' sign

○ **Becker muscular dystrophy**

This condition is similar to Duchenne muscular dystrophy but is caused by a missense mutation in the dystrophin gene.

- The mutation allows partial function of dystrophin, enabling one end of the protein to anchor the cytoskeleton, providing greater muscle stability than in Duchenne's.
- As a result, it causes a milder form of the disease with a later onset.

Symptoms

- Similar to Duchenne, but symptoms typically appear around 5 years later
- Progressive proximal muscle weakness
- Less likely to involve cognitive impairment or learning disabilities

○ **Myotonic dystrophy**

This refers to a type of muscular dystrophy where muscles contract but are unable to relax properly, causing myotonia.

- It is an autosomal dominant condition caused by mutations in the DMPK gene (type 1) or CNBP gene (type 2).
- In type 1, a CTG trinucleotide repeat expansion (over 50 repeats) leads to disease manifestation.
- Symptoms can present at any time from childhood to early adulthood.

Symptoms

- Progressive muscle weakness and wasting
- Myotonia – delayed muscle relaxation after contraction
- Associated features include intellectual disability and cataracts
- Diabetes mellitus, dysarthria
- Facial features – long, thin face with hollow temples, drooping eyelids and frontal balding in males

Key tests

- Blood tests show elevated creatine kinase due to muscle breakdown
- Genetic testing and muscle biopsy confirm the diagnosis

Management

- Multidisciplinary care focuses on maximising quality of life as there is no cure
- Steroids may slow muscle degeneration; anticonvulsants help manage seizures
- Manage associated complications such as diabetes

- **Cerebral palsy (CP)**

This refers to a group of permanent motor disorders that arise in early childhood due to damage to the developing motor pathways in the central nervous system.
- Although primarily affecting movement and posture, it is often associated with additional symptoms due to involvement of other neurological structures.

It is classified depending on the nature of the motor disorder:
- Spastic – due to UMN damage, causes muscle stiffness, hypertonia, hyperreflexia
- Dyskinetic – due to basal ganglia damage, leading to involuntary movements
- Ataxic – due to cerebellar damage, resulting in poor coordination and balance
- Mixed – where the patient will have symptoms of more than one subtype

Causes

- Maternal infection – associated with CMV and rubella
- Foetal infection – neonatal meningitis
- Birth ischaemia – asphyxia during birth, trauma

Symptoms

- Delayed motor milestones – late development of rolling, crawling, and walking
- Gait abnormalities – spastic or ataxic gait may be seen
- Persistence of primitive reflexes
- May also have associated learning difficulties, seizures, or sensory impairments

Key tests

- It is predominantly a clinical diagnosis, based on history and examination
- MRI can help identify the underlying cause or extent of brain involvement

Management

- Multidisciplinary team (MDT) approach as there is no cure
- Focus is on maximising independence through occupational therapy, physiotherapy, speech therapy
- Anticonvulsants used for seizures
- Benzodiazepines and baclofen can be used for spasticity

Infectious Diseases

Neonates are at high risk of infection, as their immune systems are underdeveloped.

- In babies, it can be difficult to localise the source of infection as it is impossible to take a clinical history from the patient and the symptoms can be very ambiguous.
- We can divide neonatal sepsis into early and late onset infections.

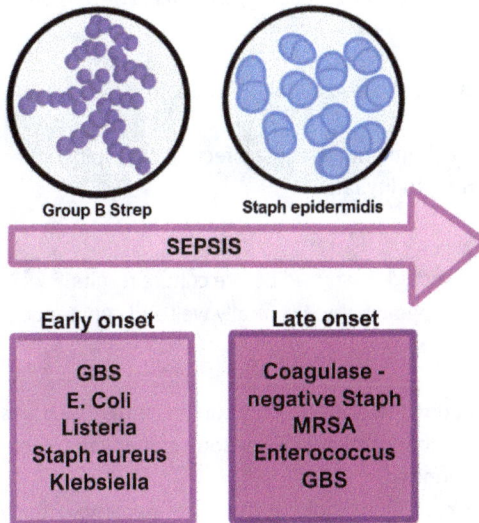

| Group B Strep | Staph epidermidis |

SEPSIS

Early onset	Late onset
GBS E. Coli Listeria Staph aureus Klebsiella	Coagulase - negative Staph MRSA Enterococcus GBS

- **Early onset infection**

This refers to an infection that occurs within the first 72 hours after birth.

- Common pathogens are Group B Streptococcus, followed by E. coli and Listeria.
- Infections may originate from various sources, but the most frequent source is an ascending infection from the birth canal.
- Bacteria ascend from the maternal genital tract and invade the amniotic fluid.
- The foetus becomes infected as the foetal lungs come into direct contact with the contaminated amniotic fluid.
- This typically results in pneumonia and sepsis.

Risk factors

- Prematurity
- Premature rupture of membranes, chorioamnionitis
- Intravenous antibiotics given to the mother within 24 hours of delivery
- Infection in a sibling in cases of multiple pregnancies

Symptoms

- Respiratory distress – cyanosis, grunting, tachypnoea
- Shock, floppiness
- Seizures
- Non-blanching rash
- Fever
- Gastrointestinal symptoms – poor feeding, abdominal distension, vomiting

Key tests

- Septic screen including full blood count, inflammatory markers, blood cultures, blood gas, and urine sample
- Lumbar puncture is recommended, as the infection can rapidly spread to the meninges which carries a high mortality rate

Management

- Empirical antibiotics should be started before culture results
- Antibiotics can be stopped if baby is clinically well and cultures come back negative

- **Late onset infection**

This refers to an infection in neonates that occurs more than 72 hours after birth.
- Unlike early onset infections, the primary source is environmental, either from the hospital or the community.
- The most common pathogens include coagulase-negative Staphylococcus, such as Staphylococcus epidermidis.
- Other common organisms include Staphylococcus aureus and Escherichia coli.

Risk factors

- Prematurity
- Underlying comorbidities – cardiac or respiratory disease
- Admission to a neonatal intensive care unit (NICU)

Symptoms

- Similar to early onset infection

Key tests

- Septic screen and lumbar puncture

Management

- First-line treatment involves empirical antibiotics, e.g. flucloxacillin and gentamicin
- If no clinical improvement, microbiology discussion to guide antibiotics

Specific Infections

- **Scarlet fever**

This is a bacterial infection, typically affecting children, that causes a distinctive red rash, sore throat and fever.

- It occurs due to a systemic reaction to the toxin produced by Group A haemolytic streptococci (usually Streptococcus pyogenes).
- The infection typically affects children aged 3–5 years and is a notifiable disease.
- It spreads through the inhalation of respiratory droplets or direct contact with infected secretions.
- Only a small number of patients with strep throat or skin infections (such as impetigo) develop scarlet fever.

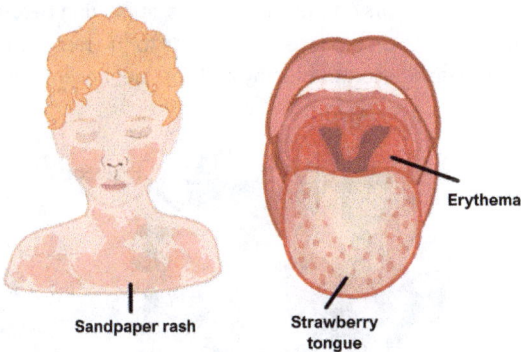

Sandpaper rash

Strawberry tongue

Erythema

Symptoms

- General – fever, malaise, headache, sore throat, swollen lymph nodes
- Strawberry tongue – initially coated white, then red papillae emerge
- Rash – punctate erythema with a sandpaper-like texture. It starts on the torso and spreads to the palms and soles, and is more pronounced in the skin folds
- Desquamation (peeling) occurs later, especially around the fingers and toes
- Complications include otitis media, rheumatic fever and post-streptococcal glomerulo-nephritis

Key tests

- Can be diagnosed clinically. Throat swab can be used to confirm diagnosis

Management

- 1st line is oral phenoxymethylpenicillin for 10 days
- Children should be excluded from school for 24 hours after starting antibiotics

- **Measles**

This is a highly infectious illness caused by the measles RNA paramyxovirus.

- The virus initially infects epithelial cells in the trachea and bronchi, then spreads to nearby lymph nodes.
- It enters the bloodstream and disseminates to organs such as the lungs, intestines, and brain.
- Transmission occurs via respiratory droplets and individuals are infectious from the prodromal phase until four days after the rash appears.
- Although now rare due to the MMR vaccine, outbreaks still occur.
- It is a notifiable disease and must be reported to public health authorities.

Symptoms

- Prodrome of high fever, runny nose, red eyes (conjunctivitis)
- Koplik spots – small white spots on the inner cheeks, appearing before the rash
- Maculopapular rash – starts on the face and spreads to the rest of the body (typically around days 3–5). The rash becomes blotchy and confluent over time

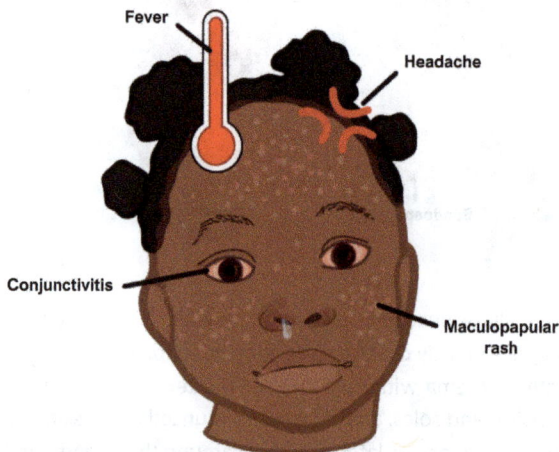

Complications

- Ears – otitis media (most common complication)
- Brain – encephalitis (1–2 weeks after infection)
- Chest – pneumonia (most common cause of death) and myocarditis
- Abdomen – diarrhoea and possible risk of appendicitis
- CNS – subacute sclerosing panencephalitis is a slow progressive brain infection caused by the measles virus. It leads to demyelination in adulthood, causing upper motor neuron signs similar to multiple sclerosis

Key tests
- Clinical diagnosis is often sufficient; if unclear, confirm with serology (IgM measles specific antibodies), the sensitivity is highest 3 to 14 days after rash onset

Management
- Supportive care with rest, fluids, and pain relief
- Admit if pregnant or immunocompromised
- If an unvaccinated child is exposed to measles, offer MMR vaccine within 72 hours
- Management of complications

- **Hand, foot, and mouth disease**
This is a viral infection seen in children, caused by intestinal picornaviruses.
- It us usually caused by viruses Coxsackie A16 and Enterovirus 71.
- It is highly contagious and tends to spread in school outbreaks.
- Transmission occurs via nasopharyngeal secretions and close personal contact.

Symptoms
- General – fever, nausea, vomiting, general discomfort
- Painful ulcers, blisters, or lesions around the mouth and nose
- Flat, discoloured spots followed by vesicular sores which are seen on the palms, soles, buttocks and lips
- Rash is rarely itchy in children but may be itchy in adults

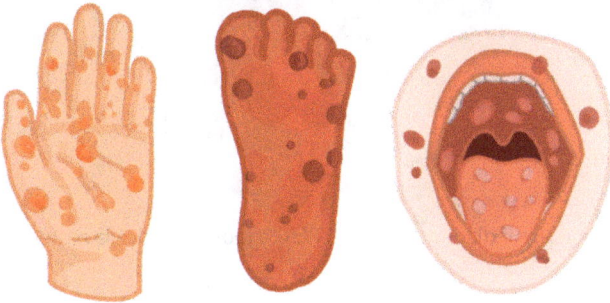

Key tests
- Clinical diagnosis

Management
- Supportive management with hydration and analgesia, self-resolves in about a week
- Children do not need to be excluded from school

- **Chickenpox**

This is a primary infection usually seen in children due to the varicella zoster virus.

- It is spread via the airways and gives a rash usually 4 days post infection.
- The most infectious period is 1–2 days before you get the rash and continues till all lesions are dry and crusted over.

Symptoms

- Prodrome of high temperature
- Pruritic vesicular rash on the head and torso before spreading to limbs
- Can be followed by a secondary bacterial infection of the skin lesions
- Complications include pneumonia, encephalitis and disseminated haemorrhagic chickenpox, seen in immunocompromised patients

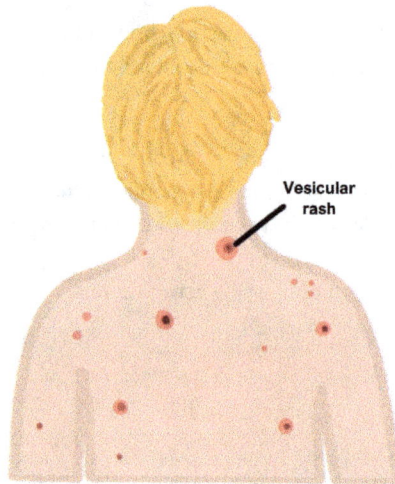

Vesicular rash

Key tests

- Diagnosed clinically. If diagnostic doubt, PCR to look for varicella zoster DNA

Management

- Supportive treatment – antipyretics, applying calamine lotion for vesicles
- Exclude from school until all lesions are dry and crusted over
- If patient is aged > 14 and presents within 24 hours of rash onset, can give acyclovir (e.g. 800 mg 5 times a day for 7 days)
- If immunocompromised, pregnant, or neonatal and exposed to chickenpox, discuss with a specialist as they may need varicella zoster Ig if varicella antibody negative (implying no immunity to the virus)

- **Pityriasis rosea**

This is a skin rash typically seen in young people between the ages of 10–30.
- It is thought to be associated with human herpesvirus 7 but is not considered to be highly contagious.

Symptoms

- Symptoms may follow a recent upper respiratory tract infection
- Prodrome of headache, joint pain, fever, and tiredness
- Herald patch – red, scaly area resembling a fungal infection, on the trunk or neck
- This is followed by smaller red, oval patches on the body and arm. These align along skin cleavage lines, giving a "fir-tree" or "Christmas tree" appearance

Key tests

- It is diagnosed clinically

Management

- Reassurance as it is a self-limiting condition

- **Roseola infantum (sixth disease)**

This is a viral illness caused by human herpesvirus 6 (most common) or 7.
- It commonly affects children under 3, with peak incidence around the age of 1.
- The classic pattern is a high fever followed by a rash, but interestingly, the child usually appears well by the time the rash emerges.

Symptoms

- Prodrome of fever lasting 3–6 days; many children appear well despite fever
- Increased risk of febrile seizures
- Maculopapular rash appears as the fever subsides
- Pink, raised lesions typically start on the torso and spread to the limbs
- May also cause diarrhoea and cough
- Nagayama spots – red papules on the soft palate and uvula

Key tests

- It is diagnosed clinically

Management

- Reassurance as it is a self-limiting condition which resolves spontaneously

Hypermobility Conditions

These are conditions that result in excessive movement of the joints with an increased risk of subluxation or dislocation.
- Mild hypermobility is common, especially in girls and is often a normal variation.
- Many individuals with hypermobility are asymptomatic and benefit from the increased range of motion.
- However, some may experience recurrent joint and muscle pain, often triggered by physical activity.
- Management includes wearing supportive footwear and using orthotics to reduce discomfort and improve joint stability.

However, in some cases, hypermobility can be part of an underlying condition that causes pathological laxity and leads to further complications.

● **Marfan's syndrome**
This is an autosomal dominant connective tissue disorder caused by a mutation in the FBN1 gene.
- The FBN1 gene encodes fibrillin-1, a glycoprotein that is a key component of the extra-cellular matrix.
- Fibrillin-1 is essential for connective tissue structure and also plays a role in regulating growth factor signalling.

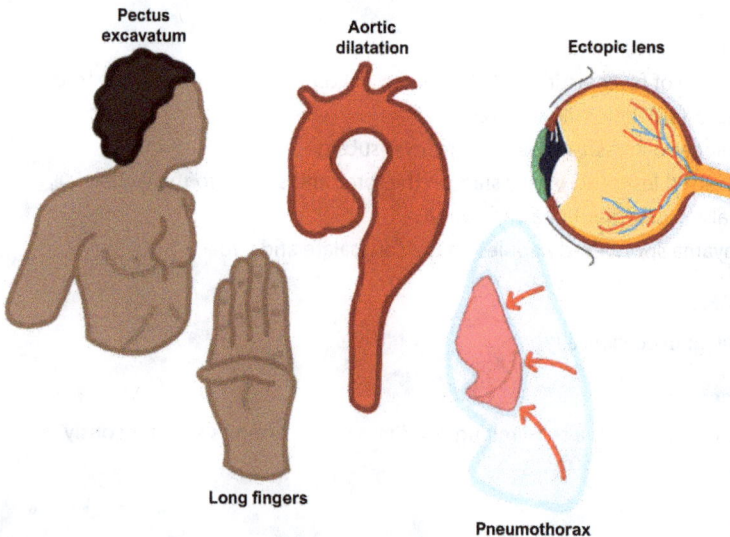

Pectus excavatum

Aortic dilatation

Ectopic lens

Long fingers

Pneumothorax

Symptoms

- Skeleton – tall stature, increased arm span, scoliosis, pectus excavatum
- Limbs – hypermobile joints, flat feet (pes planus), arachnodactyly (long, slender fingers and toes)
- Respiratory – increased risk of spontaneous pneumothorax
- Cardiac – aortic sinus dilation (increasing the risk of aortic regurgitation and aneurysms), mitral valve prolapse
- Eyes – lens subluxation, blue sclera, myopia
- CNS – weakening of the connective tissue surrounding the spinal cord

Management

- There is no cure, management uses an MDT approach to monitor complications such as aortic root dilation and ocular issues

- **Ehler-Danlos syndrome**

This is an autosomal dominant condition that affects collagen synthesis.
- Collagen is a key component of connective tissue, providing strength and stability.
- Mutations in various genes can cause the condition, which result in increased elasticity of connective tissue in the skin, joints, blood vessels, and heart valves.

Symptoms

- Musculoskeletal – hypermobile joints prone to dislocation, increased risk of early-onset osteoarthritis
- Skin – soft, stretchy, and fragile skin that bruises easily
- Cardiovascular – mitral valve prolapse, arterial aneurysms and dissections
- Raynaud's phenomenon
- Increased risk of spontaneous pneumothorax
- Flat feet (pes planus)

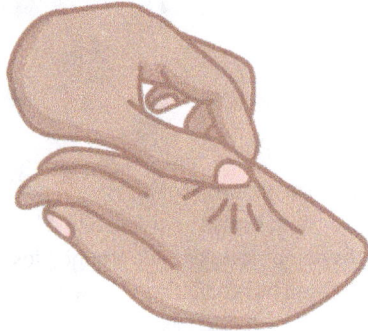

Stretchy, elastic skin

Management

- No cure; treatment is supportive and aimed at monitoring and managing complications, especially cardiovascular and joint-related issues

Hip Conditions

- **Developmental dysplasia of the hip (DDH)**

This is a group of conditions affecting the proximal femur and acetabulum in babies.

- The joint between the femur and acetabulum is underdeveloped, leading to deformity ranging from mild dysplasia to subluxation or full dislocation of the hip.
- It is more common in females and typically affects the left hip.
- Major risk factors include breech presentation, a positive family history and oligo-hydramnios.
- All breech babies born at or after 36 weeks' gestation should have a bilateral hip ultra-sound at 6 weeks to screen for developmental dysplasia of the hip.

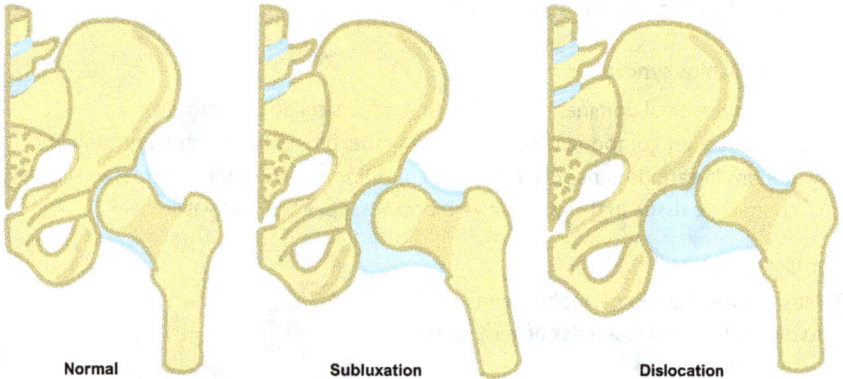

Normal   Subluxation   Dislocation

Symptoms

- Limp or abnormal gait
- Ability to sublax or dislocate the hip
- Asymmetrical skinfolds around hips
- Limited hip abduction
- Shortening of the affected leg
- If untreated, may lead to early-onset arthritis

Key tests

- Two screening tests are performed at birth as part of the NIPE examination
- Barlow test attempts to dislocate an articulated femoral head posteriorly
- Ortolani test attempts to relocate a dislocated femoral head into the acetabulum upon abduction
- If either test is positive, perform an ultrasound of the hip (diagnostic test), or an X-ray if the child is older than 4.5 months

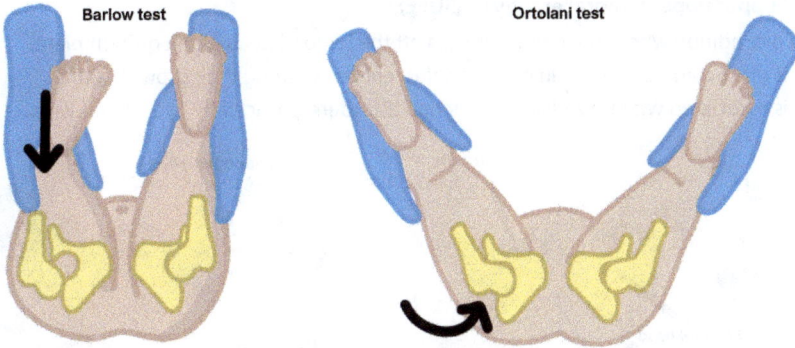

Barlow test

Ortolani test

Management
- Mild dysplasia may resolve spontaneously
- Moderate to severe cases are treated with a Pavlik harness, which positions the hip in flexion and abduction
- Surgery is required for older children or when conservative treatment fails

- **Transient synovitis**

Known as "irritable hip", this condition involves temporary inflammation of the synovium (inner lining) of the hip joint capsule.
- It is the most common cause of hip pain in children, especially those under 10 years.
- It often follows a recent viral infection, and while a low-grade fever may be present, the exact cause is unknown.

Symptoms
- Acute onset of hip pain
- Limping, with or without pain
- May have a mild fever
- In younger children, may present as unexplained crying when having nappy changed
- Reduced range of motion, particularly internal rotation of the hip

Key tests
- It is a diagnosis of exclusion, made after ruling out more serious conditions such as septic arthritis, which may require a joint aspirate

Management
- Rest and non-steroidal anti-inflammatory medication
- The condition is usually self-limiting and resolves within a few days

- **Slipper upper femoral epiphysis (SUFE)**

A hip condition where the epiphysis slips off the femoral head at the growth plate.
- It is most commonly seen in obese adolescent boys during their growth spurt.
- It is associated with underlying endocrine disorders, particularly hypothyroidism.

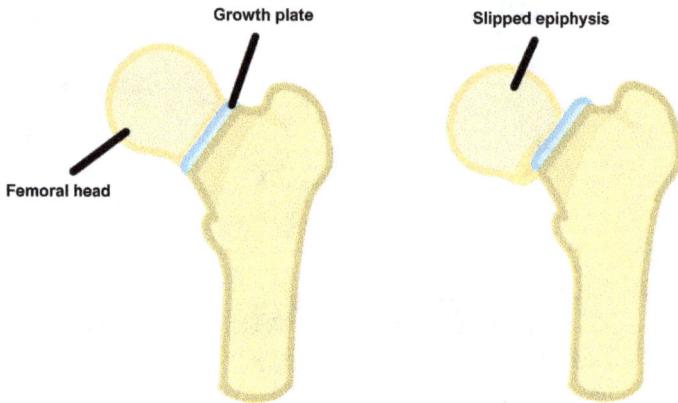

Growth plate   Slipped epiphysis

Femoral head

Symptoms
- Can present acutely following trauma or develop gradually over time
- Hip pain, though it may also present as isolated groin or knee pain
- Reduced internal rotation of the hip, especially when flexed
- Limping and discomfort with movement
- If untreated, there is a risk of avascular necrosis of the femoral head

Key tests
- X-ray (anteroposterior and frog-leg lateral views) shows displacement of the epiphysis relative to the femoral neck

Management
- Most cases are managed surgically, with an open reduction and fixation using a screw placed through the centre of the epiphysis to stabalise the joint

- **Legg-Calve-Perthes' disease**

This condition is characterised by disruption of the blood supply to the femoral head.
- It is typically seen in young boys aged between 4 and 8 years old.
- The lack of blood flow leads to avascular necrosis of the capital femoral epiphysis.
- Over time, the bone undergoes revascularisation and necrotic tissue is resorbed.
- However, this process results in the overall loss of bone mass and weakening of the femoral head, which may cause long-term complications.

Symptoms

- Hip pain (which can be bilateral)
- Pain may be referred to the knee and is often initially mistaken for growing pains
- Joint stiffness with reduced range of movement
- Difficulty weight bearing, leading to a limp
- Potential later complications include osteoarthritis and early fusion of the growth plates, affecting limb growth

Key tests

- Hip X-ray – early findings include joint space widening and increased density in the femoral head, later on can show flattening and irregularity of the femoral head
- Bone scan or MRI are used when symptoms persist despite a normal X-ray

Management

- The goal is to minimise stress on the hip while the condition progresses
- Younger children are more likely to be managed conservatively with observation
- Supportive management includes traction, bracing to maintain range of motion, and physiotherapy
- Surgery may be required in cases where joint damage is significant and irreversible

• Growing pains

This is the colloquial term for nocturnal idiopathic pain, which refers to a common and benign cause of limb pain in children aged 3–12 years.
- The exact cause is not well understood, but it typically affects younger children before their adolescent growth spurt.
- It presents as episodes of pain in the lower limbs that often wake the child from sleep and usually ease with massage or comfort.

Symptoms

- Symmetrical pain in the lower limbs, not limited to joints
- Pain never present on waking in the morning
- Pain does not limit daily physical activities (no limping)
- Physical examination should be normal (some children can have hypermobility)

Key tests

- A diagnosis of exclusion after ruling out other more serious causes

Management

- Reassurance as the condition is harmless and self-resolving

Knee Conditions

- **Chondromalacia patellae (CMP)**

This condition is characterised by inflammation and softening of the articular cartilage on the underside of the patella and is more commonly seen in adolescent girls.
- The cartilage gradually deteriorates, becoming rough and uneven.
- This increases friction during movement, leading to pain and discomfort.
- It can be triggered by an acute knee injury or by long-term friction between the patella and the femoral groove.

Symptoms

- Pain at the front of the knee, particularly during sports like football, rowing and tennis
- Discomfort worsens after prolonged sitting

Key tests

- Usually a clinical diagnosis
- MRI can be used in cases of diagnostic uncertainty to visualise cartilage damage

Management

- RICE (rest, ice compression, elevation), anti-inflammatory medication
- Physiotherapy to strengthen surrounding muscles and improve patellar tracking

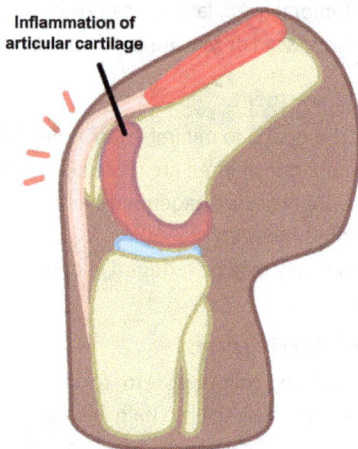

Inflammation of articular cartilage

- **Osgood-Schlatter disease**

This condition, known as tibial apophysitis, refers to inflammation at the patellar tendon insertion on the tibial tuberosity, due to repeated stress on the growth plate.
- It causes a painful swelling just below the knee, which worsens with activity.
- It is most commonly seen in active teenage boys, and associated with overuse and participation in high-impact sports involving frequent jumping or sprinting.

Symptoms

- Pain over the lower front of the knee that improves with rest
- Knee pain worsens with activity, particularly high-impact sports
- Pain is reproduced when the knee is extended against resistance
- Localised tenderness and swelling over the tibial tuberosity

Key tests
- It is diagnosed clinically, can consider MRI if diagnostic doubt

Management
- RICE, anti-inflammatory medication and physiotherapy
- Surgery may be required in severe or persistent cases

- **Osteochondritis dissecans**

This condition involves the formation of cracks in the articular cartilage and the underlying subchondral bone, commonly affecting the knee in active teenagers.
- Whilst the exact cause is unknown, it involves avascular necrosis of the subchondral bone due to a temporary loss of blood supply.
- The affected bone is gradually reabsorbed, weakening the cartilage above and increasing the risk of fragmentation.
- Unlike osteoarthritis, which affects the cartilage surface, this condition originates in the bone beneath the cartilage and secondarily affects the overlying cartilage.

Symptoms
- Pain following exercise, often with a crackling or grinding sound on movement
- Intermittent swelling and joint locking
- If untreated, can cause a joint effusion

Avascular necrosis

Key tests
- X-ray or MRI to detect subchondral bone necrosis

Management
- Physiotherapy to reduce stress on the joint
- Surgical intervention may be necessary in more severe or persistent cases

- **Patellar dislocation**

This refers to the displacement of the patella from its groove in the femur.
- It typically occurs when the knee is straight and the lower leg twists outward, often during sports such as football.
- The patella usually sublaxates laterally due to the stronger pull of the vastus lateralis muscle compared to the vastus medialis.
- A partial dislocation is known as a subluxation, which is more common than a full dislocation but can be equally disabling.

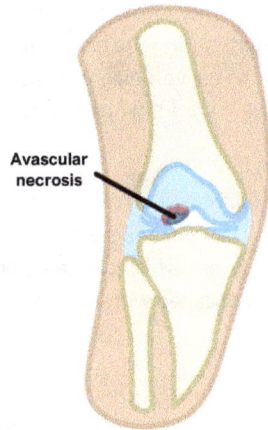

Symptoms

- Pain felt deep inside the kneecap
- Visible lateral displacement or subluxation of the patella
- Sensation of instability (the knee "giving way")

Management

- Physiotherapy to strengthen supporting muscles and improve patellar tracking
- Surgery may be required in recurrent cases or to correct misalignment of the quadriceps' pull on the patella

- **Juvenile idiopathic arthritis (JIA)**

This is a condition characterised by arthritis in children under the age of 16, which lasts for more than six weeks.
- There are seven recognised JIA subtypes, but oligoarticular JIA is the most common.
- If untreated, it can result in joint deformities, growth restriction and delayed puberty.

○ **Oligoarticular JIA**

This is the most common subtype of juvenile idiopathic arthritis, affecting four or fewer joints during the first six months of the disease.
- To receive a diagnosis, patients should be < 16 years old, have persistent joint swelling (> 6 weeks) without evidence of infection or any other cause.

Symptoms

- Stiffness, worse in the morning, which worsens after periods of inactivity
- Joint pain and swelling, usually in medium-sized joints such as the knees, ankles, and elbows, which can cause limping
- Associated with anterior uveitis, so regular ophthalmology screening is important

Key tests

- Inflammatory markers (CRP, ESR) may be raised but are often normal in early stages
- ANA may be positive; rheumatoid factor can be positive or negative

Management

- Referral to paediatric rheumatology for specialist care
- NSAIDs for symptom relief during flares
- Intra-articular steroid injections can be used in oligoarticular disease
- Immunosuppressants such as methotrexate may be needed in refractory cases

Bone Tumours

Tumours arise from an abnormal proliferation of cells and may be benign or malignant.
- One of the most common presenting symptoms is bone pain.
- However, bone pain can often be poorly localised and associated with a wide range of other conditions.
- For this reason, it is important to identify red flag symptoms that may indicate an underlying bone malignancy.

Red flag symptoms
- Bone pain that worsens at night or wakes the patient from sleep
- Inability to bear weight
- Pain that does not improve with medication
- Pathological fractures
- Systemic features such as anaemia or weight loss

Guidelines
- Unexplained bone pain or swelling in children and young people requires an urgent X-ray within 48 hours
- If imaging suggests sarcoma, then a 2 week-wait referral for adults and 48-hour referral for children is required

- **Osteosarcoma**

This is a malignant tumour resulting from the proliferation of primitive cells that differentiate into osteoblasts.
- It is the most common primary malignant bone cancer.
- It typically affects children and adolescents, usually involving the metaphysis of long bones in the legs.
- It is associated with mutations in the retinoblastoma gene and may occur in individuals with a history of retinoblastoma.

As the tumour cells are osteoblast-derived, they produce immature bone, creating a sclerotic (dense) pattern on imaging.
- Early on, the tumour lays down new bone, producing a white appearance on X-ray.
- As the tumour expands, it lifts the periosteum off the bone.

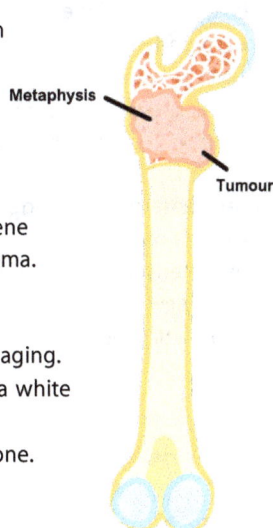

Metaphysis

Tumour

In response, the periosteum attempts to lay down new bone, a phenomenon known as a periosteal reaction.
- This forms a radiographic feature called the Codman triangle.

In fast-growing tumours, the periosteum cannot respond quickly enough.
- Instead, Sharpey's fibres stretch outward, creating a radiating or sunburst appearance on imaging, a classic sign of aggressive disease.

Symptoms
- Red flag symptoms such as bone pain that worsens at night
- May have constitutional symptoms – weight loss, anaemia, lethargy

Key tests
- X-ray showing a sclerotic lesion with possible Codman triangle or sunburst pattern
- CT or MRI for detailed assessment and staging
- Bone biopsy to confirm diagnosis

Management
- Surgical resection +/- chemotherapy and radiotherapy

- **Ewing sarcoma**

This is a malignant tumour arising from the proliferation of primitive neuroectodermal cells, typically seen in children and adolescents.
- In contrast to an osteosarcoma, Ewing sarcoma commonly affects the diaphysis (middle) of long bones and the pelvis.
- It is caused by a chromosomal translocation between chromosomes 11 and 22, involving the EWSR1 gene.
- It is an aggressive tumour that metastasises early, and many patients have established metastatic disease at the time of diagnosis.

Unlike osteosarcoma, Ewing sarcoma produces lytic lesions that destroy bone, appearing more lucent on X-ray.
- A characteristic finding on imaging is the onion-skin appearance due to concentric layers of new bone laid down by the periosteum.
- Multiple lytic lesions may create a moth-eaten appearance.
- A periosteal reaction can also produce a Codman triangle, similar to osteosarcoma.

Symptoms

- Red flag signs such as bone pain that worsens at night or causes waking from sleep

Key tests

- X-ray shows a lytic lesion with onion-skin or moth-eaten appearance
- CT or MRI for staging and further assessment
- Bone biopsy is diagnostic and shows a small round blue cell tumour, typically staining positive for CD99

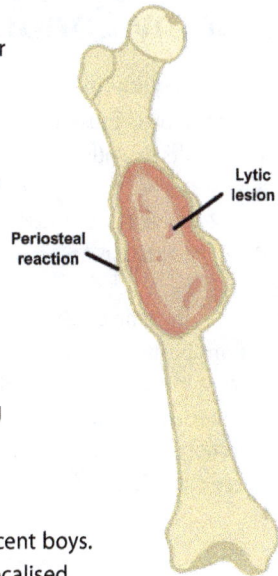

Lytic lesion

Periosteal reaction

Management

- Surgery +/- chemotherapy and radiotherapy depending on the location and extent of disease

- **Osteoid osteoma**

This is a benign bone tumour that typically affects adolescent boys.
- It usually involves the spine, femur, or tibia and causes localised bone pain.
- Osteomas in general are benign tumours made of bone and are the most common benign neoplasms of the nose and paranasal sinuses.

Symptoms

- Bone pain that is worse at night and improves with NSAIDs
- Localised tenderness and swelling over the affected area

Key tests

- X-ray shows a well-demarcated radiolucent (dark) nidus of osteoid tissue, often surrounded by sclerotic bone

Management

- Surgical removal or radiofrequency ablation of the nidus (core of the osteoma)
- Amputation is not typically required for benign lesions like an osteoid osteoma

Trisomy Conditions

- **Down's syndrome**

This condition is caused by the presence of an extra copy of chromosome 21.

- This results in a number of physical and developmental complications.
- It is caused by non-disjunction during meiosis which produces a sex cell (sperm or egg) with 2 copies of chromosome 21 rather than 1.
- When fertilisation occurs, this results in 3 overall copies of chromosome 21.

However, in some cases it can also be due to a Robertsonian translocation.

- A translocation is a type of structural chromosomal abnormality where part of one chromosome breaks off and attaches to another chromosome.
- A Robertsonian translocation is a specific type of translocation involving acrocentric chromosomes (chromosomes with the centromere near one end).
- These chromosomes (13, 14, 15, 21, and 22) have a short arm and a long arm.

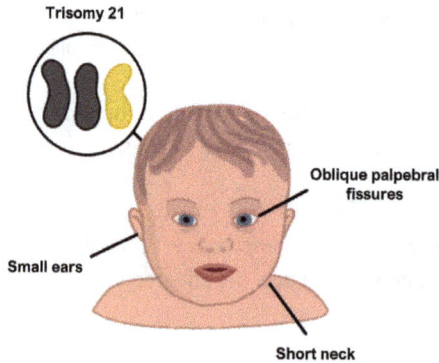

In a Robertsonian translocation, the long arms of two acrocentric chromosomes fuse, and the short arms are usually lost.

- If the long arm of chromosome 21 fuses with the long arm of another acrocentric chromosome (like 14 or 15), and the individual inherits this fused chromosome along with a normal chromosome 21, they will have three copies of the long arm of chromosome 21 (trisomy 21), resulting in Down's syndrome.

The likelihood of Down's syndrome increases significantly with maternal age.

Maternal age (years)	20	30	40	45
Risk	1 in 1500	1 in 800	1 in 100	1 in 50

Symptoms

- Intellectual – learning disability, features of autism, delayed developmental milestones, early-onset Alzheimer's disease
- Facial – flat facial profile, small ears, large protruding tongue, oblique palpebral fissures, Brushfield spots in the iris
- Respiratory – recurrent respiratory tract infections
- Cardiac – endocardial cushion defect (most common), ventricular septal defect, secundum atrial septal defect, patent ductus arteriosus, tetralogy of Fallot
- Gastrointestinal – duodenal atresia, Hirschsprung's disease
- Limbs – single palmar crease, wide sandal gap between first and second toes, hypotonia, short stature
- Endocrine – hypothyroidism
- Reproductive – subfertility in both males and females

Key tests

- Diagnosis is via chromosomal analysis (karyotyping)

Management

- No cure, requires lifelong MDT support and management of complications

- **Patau syndrome**

This is caused by the presence of an extra copy of chromosome 13 (trisomy 13).

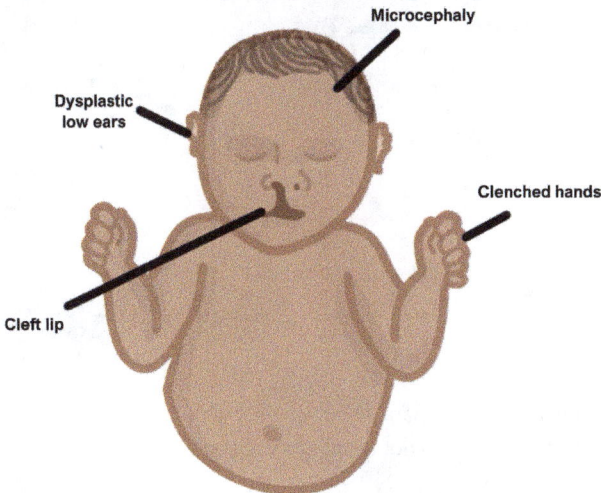

Symptoms

- Head and neck – scalp lesions, cleft lip or palate, microcephaly
- Eyes – microphthalmia, cataracts, retinal detachment
- Limbs – polydactyly, clenched hands
- Congenital heart defects – dextrocardia
- Urogenital – abnormal external genitals, renal abnormalities

Management

- No cure available. Most (90%) children die within the first year of life

- **Edwards' syndrome**

This condition is caused by the presence of an extra copy of chromosome 18.

Symptoms

- Head and neck – prominent occiput, low-set ears, micrognathia
- Chest – short sternum, oesophageal atresia
- Limbs – flexed and overlapping fingers, rocker-bottom feet
- Heart defects – ventricular septal defect, atrial septal defect, patent ductus arteriosus

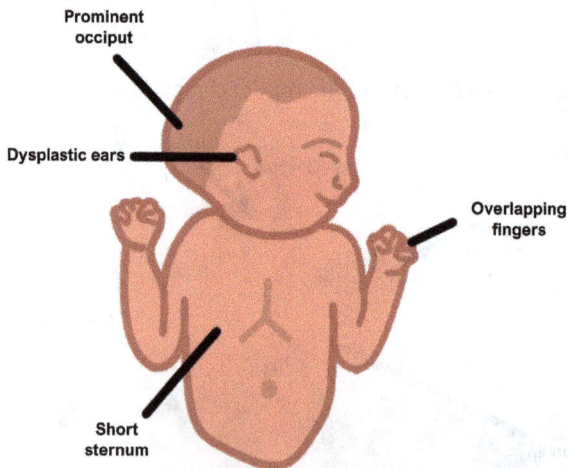

Management

- There is no cure available, manage complications with an MDT approach
- Most pregnancies affected do not result in a live birth, and 90% of children die within the first year of life

Sex Chromosome Conditions

- **Klinefelter's syndrome**

This condition results from the presence of an additional sex chromosome, giving a karyotype of 47, XXY.
- Individuals are genetically male due to the presence of the Y chromosome.
- However, they may have a range of physical and reproductive abnormalities.
- It is caused by nondisjunction of chromosomes during meiosis in either parent, resulting in an extra X chromosome in the zygote.

Symptoms

- Body – tall stature
- Feminisation – gynaecomastia (increased risk of breast cancer), reduced body hair, decreased muscle mass
- Genitals – small, underdeveloped testicles, reduced libido
- Endocrine – lack of secondary sexual characteristics and infertility

Key tests

- Blood tests typically show elevated FSH and LH, with low testosterone
- Chromosomal analysis (karyotyping)

Management

- Testosterone replacement therapy to support development of male characteristics
- Infertility treatment such as ICSI or IVF may help with reproduction
- Breast tissue may be surgically removed due to increased breast cancer risk

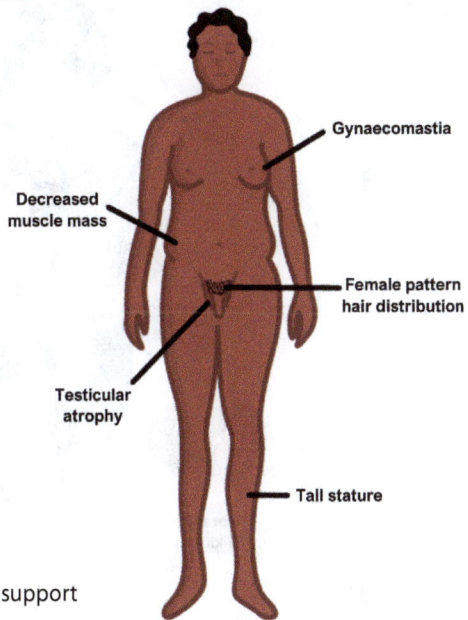

- **Turner's syndrome**

This condition results from the absence of one sex chromosome, giving the karyotype 45, XO.
- Without a Y chromosome, individuals are female and have female sexual organs.
- It occurs due to the complete loss of one X chromosome, or deletion of the short arm of one X chromosome.

Symptoms

- Antenatal – early miscarriage, foetal hydrops, cystic hygroma
- Body – short stature, multiple pigmented naevi
- Head and neck – webbed neck, high-arched palate
- Chest – widely spaced nipples, broad shield-shaped chest
- Limbs – spoon-shaped nails, lymphoedema of hands and feet
- Heart – bicuspid aortic valve, coarctation of the aorta
- Ovaries – ovarian dysgenesis leading to primary amenorrhoea

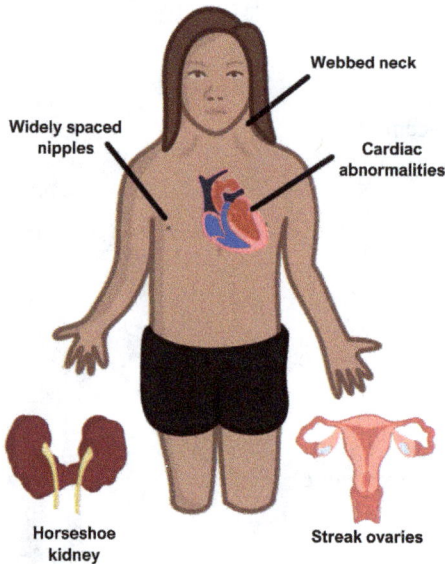

Widely spaced nipples

Webbed neck

Cardiac abnormalities

Horseshoe kidney

Streak ovaries

Complications

- Endocrine – primary amenorrhoea, hypothyroidism
- Autoimmune – increased risk of conditions such as Crohn's disease
- Infertility due to underdeveloped ovaries

Key tests

- Karyotyping is diagnostic, this can be performed antenatally (via amniocentesis or chorionic villus sampling) or postnatally

Management

- No cure available; treatment focuses on symptom management
- Growth hormone therapy is often used to promote height development
- Oestrogen replacement for the development of secondary sexual characteristics

- **Swyer syndrome**

This is a rare condition caused by a mutation in the SRY gene on the Y chromosome.

- The SRY gene is essential for the masculinisation of the embryo. Without its function, the undifferentiated gonads fail to develop into testicles, even in an XY foetus.
- As a result, individuals with Swyer syndrome have an XY karyotype but develop as phenotypic females, with a uterus, fallopian tubes, and vagina.
- They are born with a female appearance but have non-functional streak gonads.
- During puberty, the lack of functional gonads means insufficient oestrogen is produced, leading to absent breast development and primary amenorrhoea.

Management

- Oestrogen and progestogen hormone replacement therapy is required to induce and maintain secondary sexual characteristics and menstrual cycles

- **Noonan syndrome**

This is a genetic condition often referred to as the male version of Turner's syndrome.

- However, unlike Turner's syndrome, the mutation is not on the sex chromosomes but is autosomal dominant, usually due to a mutation in the PTPN11 gene on Chr 12.

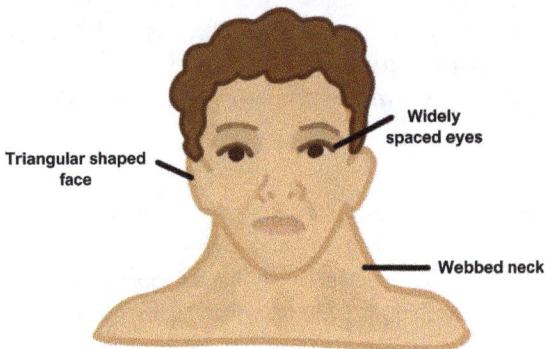

Triangular shaped face

Widely spaced eyes

Webbed neck

Symptoms

- Face – low-set ears, triangular-shaped face, large head with excess nuchal skin
- Eyes – hypertelorism (widely spaced eyes)
- Skin – lymphoedema
- Body – webbed neck, short stature, widely spaced nipples
- Heart – pulmonary valve stenosis (most common cardiac defect)

Management

- Multidisciplinary approach to manage complications

Specific Gene Conditions

- **Fragile X syndrome**

This condition is caused by a trinucleotide (CGG) repeat expansion in the FMR1 gene.

- The FMR1 gene encodes the FMRP protein, which is most concentrated in the brain and testes and plays a role in transporting mRNA to the nucleus and synapses for neural development.

Inheritance

- X-linked dominant, more commonly affecting males
- Females are less affected due to random X-chromosome inactivation
- The condition shows variable expressivity, meaning that people with the same mutation may experience the condition differently, with varying degrees of severity
- The condition also shows genetic anticipation, a phenomenon where the age of onset and/or severity of symptoms of a genetic disorder become more pronounced in successive generations of a family

In unaffected individuals, the FMR1 gene has 5–44 CGG repeats

- 45–54 repeats is a grey zone
- 55–200 repeats is known as a premutation. Women with a premutation have an increased risk of having a child with the full mutation
- People with > 200 repeats have the full mutation, which results in the syndrome

Symptoms

- Intellectual – learning difficulties, autism spectrum disorder
- Facial – long face, large protruding ears, high-arched palate
- Behavioural – social anxiety, hypersensitivity, hand flapping, biting, poor eye contact
- Other features – macroorchidism, hypotonia, mitral valve prolapse

Key tests

- Diagnosis is by PCR and Southern blot to detect the CGG repeat expansion
- It can be made antenatally via chorionic villus sampling (CVS) or amniocentesis

Management

- No cure is available. Mainstay of management is multidisciplinary support including behavioural therapy, speech and language therapy, and educational interventions

- **Prader-Willi syndrome (PWS)**

This is a genetic condition caused by the loss of function of genes in the PWS region of chromosome 15 (15q11–13).
- The condition is a prime example of genetic imprinting, where gene expression depends on parental origin of the chromosomes.
- The absence of a functioning paternal copy of the gene in the PWS region leads to Prader-Willi syndrome.
- The absence of a functioning maternal copy results in Angelman syndrome.

There are two main mechanisms by which the condition can arise:
- Deletion of the PWS region on the paternal chromosome (most common).
- Uniparental disomy – this is where the child inherits two maternal copies of chromosome 15 and no paternal copy, due to errors in meiosis.
- The maternal chromosomes retain their imprint, meaning that the PWS region on these chromosomes remains inactive.
- As a result, no PWS genes are expressed and the child develops the syndrome.

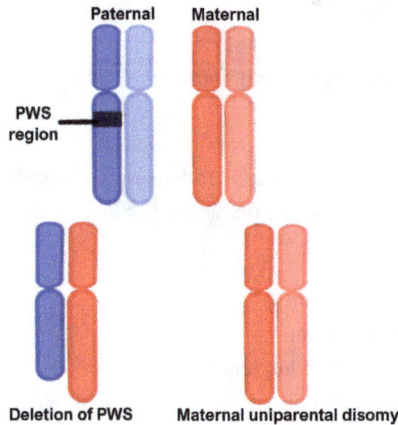

Symptoms
- CNS – developmental delay, learning difficulties, behavioural issues in adolescence
- Appetite – hyperphagia, leading to obesity and type 2 diabetes
- Short stature with hypotonia
- Distinctive facial features
- Hypogonadism and infertility

Management
- No cure; treatment focuses on managing symptoms
- Restricting access to food is essential to prevent severe obesity

- **Pierre-Robin syndrome**

This is a genetic condition caused by a mutation near the SOX9 gene.
- It leads to distinctive facial abnormalities.
- It presents with features similar to Treacher-Collins syndrome, but Pierre-Robin usually occurs due to de novo mutations, making a family history less common.

Symptoms
- Micrognathia (small lower jaw and receding chin)
- Posterior displacement of the tongue, can cause upper airway obstruction
- Cleft palate
- May also lead to hearing loss and speech difficulties

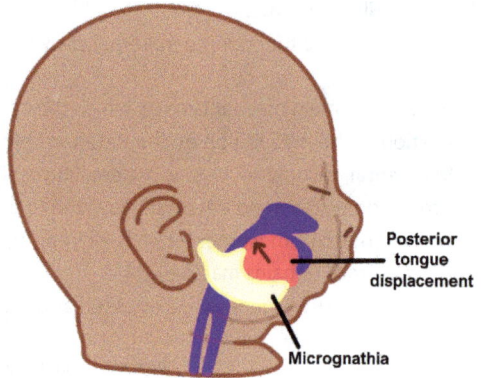

Posterior tongue displacement

Micrognathia

Management
- Supportive care with interventions to assist breathing and feeding
- Corrective procedures as needed for deformities

- **Williams syndrome**

This is a genetic condition caused by a microdeletion on chromosome 7.
- It can be inherited in an autosomal dominant fashion, though most cases are usually due to de novo mutations.

Symptoms
- General – failure to thrive, low muscle tone
- Elfin-like facies (features resembling an elf)
- Neurological – learning difficulties, motor issues such as hyperreflexia
- Behaviour – highly social and friendly personality, often with ADHD traits
- Heart – supravalvular aortic stenosis

Key tests
- FISH studies show deletion on chromosome 7

Management
- MDT managed of complications

- **DiGeorge syndrome (Velocardiofacial syndrome)**

This condition is caused by a deletion a segment of chromosome 22 (22q11.2).

- It results in a combination of facial abnormalities, congenital heart defects and developmental delays.
- Most cases are due to sporadic mutations, though it can be inherited in an autosomal dominant manner.

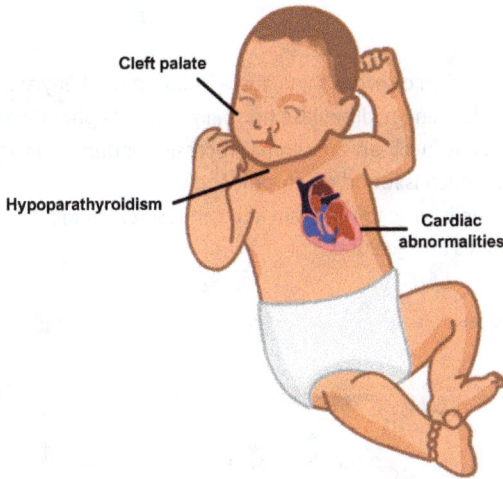

Cleft palate

Hypoparathyroidism

Cardiac abnormalities

Symptoms

- Can be remembered using the mnemonic CATCH-22:
- Cardiac – tetralogy of Fallot, aortic arch anomalies, truncus arteriosus
- Face – small palpebral fissures, epicanthic folds, smooth philtrum, low nasal bridge
- Thymus abnormality leads to immunodeficiency
- Cleft palate
- Hypoparathyroidism causes hypocalcaemia, which may lead to seizures

Management

- No cure; managing individual complications through multidisciplinary approach

- **Rett syndrome**

This is a rare genetic disorder that presents with features similar to autism, along with additional neurological impairments.

- It is most commonly diagnosed in females between 6 and 18 months of age.
- It is due to a genetic mutation in the MECP2 gene, which encodes a protein called MeCP2, which is crucial for normal brain development and function.

Symptoms

- Autistic – poor communication, language problems, repetitive hand movements
- General – slowed growth, small head circumference (acquired microcephaly)
- Neurological – seizures, sleep disturbances

Management

- No cure; treatment is supportive and focused on managing symptoms

- **Phenylketonuria**

An amino acid metabolism disorder that causes build-up of phenylalanine in the blood.
- The enzyme phenylalanine hydroxylase normally converts phenylalanine to tyrosine.
- This condition is caused by an autosomal recessive mutation in the phenylalanine hydroxylase gene, which is found on chromosome 12.
- Excess phenylalanine is toxic to the brain and can result in neurological problems such as learning difficulties and seizures.

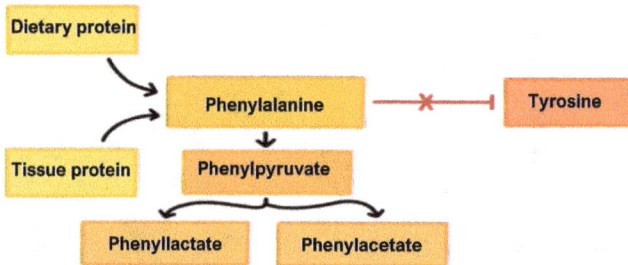

Symptoms

- Developmental delay
- CNS – learning difficulties, seizures
- Facial – fair hair and blue eyes
- Physical – heart defects, small head, low birth weight, lighter skin complexion
- Distinctive "musty" odour in urine and sweat (due to phenylacetate)

Key tests

- Guthrie screening test (heel-prick test) performed between days 5–9 of life
- Confirmed by blood tests showing elevated phenylalanine levels

Management

- Lifelong dietary restriction of phenylalanine, especially important during pregnancy for affected mothers
- Use of amino acid supplements to ensure adequate nutrition

Sexual Development

The foetal gonads begin as bipotential and undifferentiated.
- In males, the presence of the SRY gene on the Y chromosome triggers gonadal differentiation into testicles.
- The testes produce testosterone and its more potent derivative, dihydrotestosterone (DHT), which drives the development of male internal and external genitalia.
- In the absence of SRY, the gonads will develop into ovaries and female genitalia.

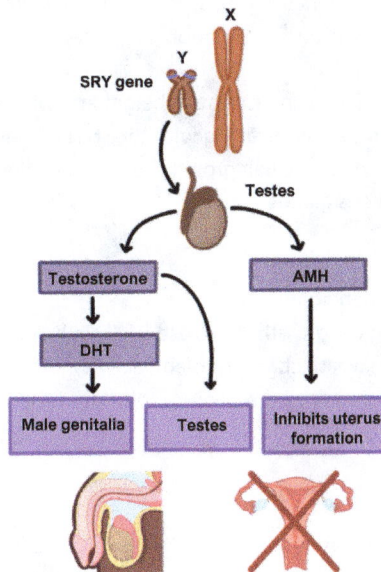

During puberty, the hypothalamus begins to secrete gonadotropin-releasing hormone (GnRH) in a pulsatile manner.
- This stimulates the anterior pituitary to release luteinising hormone (LH) and follicle-stimulating hormone (FSH), which act on the gonads.
- In males, LH stimulates Leydig cells to produce testosterone, while FSH promotes spermatogenesis via Sertoli cells.
- In females, LH triggers ovulation and stimulates theca cell androgen production, and FSH stimulates follicular growth and oestrogen production by the granulosa cells.

Puberty

Puberty is initiated by activation of the hypothalamic-pituitary-gonadal (HPG) axis, leading to increased sex hormone production.
- This drives the development of both primary and secondary sexual characteristics.

Primary sexual characteristics refers to the genitals, which are directly involved in sexual reproduction.

Secondary sexual characteristics refers to sex-specific traits not directly involved in sexual reproduction (e.g. breast development, body hair).
- While both sexes experience similar features, the sequence of changes differs.

Females
- First sign is breast development (may be asymmetrical initially)
- This is followed by growth and maturation of the external genitalia and internal reproductive organs
- The growth spurt follows, with an increase in height and widening of the pelvis
- Menarche (first period) occurs after, along with the start of regular menstrual cycles
- Additional changes include pubic hair growth, voice deepening and increased activity of the sweat and sebaceous glands

Males
- The first sign is testicular enlargement
- This is followed by a marked growth spurt, especially in height
- Increased muscle mass, sweat/sebaceous gland activity and lowering of the voice
- Other features include growth of the penis, pubic hair development, and facial/body hair growth

- **Precocious puberty**

This is defined as the development of secondary sexual characteristics at an abnormally early age.
- In females, this is before age 8; in males, before the age of 9.
- In girls, it is usually due to premature activation of normal puberty.
- In boys, it is more often due to an underlying pathological cause.

Precocious puberty can be classified into two types:

o **Central (gonadotropin-dependent)**

This is caused by disturbances in the central nervous system leading to early activation of the HPA axis.
- Elevated GnRH stimulates the production of LH and FSH, resulting in increased sex hormones and early development of secondary sexual characteristics.

Causes
- Genetic (familial)
- Hypothyroidism
- CNS abnormalities – tumours, hydrocephalus, surgery/brain injury

Symptoms
- Early appearance of puberty features in normal developmental order (consonant)

Key tests
- Blood tests show high LH and FSH (with LH > FSH) and high testosterone/oestrogen

Management
- GnRH analogues can be used to delay puberty
- It is important to address any underlying cause

○ **Peripheral (gonadotropin-independent)**
This is when sex hormone levels are elevated independently of GnRH stimulation.
- The cause lies downstream of the pituitary gland in the HPA axis.

Causes
- Adrenal gland – tumour, congenital adrenal hyperplasia
- Gonads – granulosa cell tumour (ovaries), Leydig cell tumour (testes)
- Exogenous sex steroids

Symptoms
- Early development of puberty features, often in an abnormal sequence (dissonant)

Key tests
- Blood tests show low levels of LH and FSH (due to negative feedback) but high levels of testosterone and oestrogen

Management
- Identify and treat any underlying cause
- Androgen or oestrogen inhibitors may be used to delay further development

- **Delayed puberty**

This refers to the development of secondary sexual characteristics occurring later than expected during adolescence.

- It is defined as the absence of secondary sexual characteristics by age 14 in females and age 15 in males.
- Unlike precocious puberty, delayed puberty in males is more often a normal variant, while in females it is more likely to be due to an underlying biological cause.

Delayed puberty can be categorised into 3 types.

○ **Constitutional delay of growth and puberty**

This is the most common type of delayed puberty which refers to a variation in the normal timing of puberty, without an underlying pathological process.

- It is usually more common in boys than girls.
- Delays may be due to inherited genetic factors, but can also be influenced by external factors such as excessive dieting or physical training.

Symptoms

- Delayed development of secondary sexual characteristics
- Moderate delay in growth (but eventually target height is reached at an older age)

Key tests

- Check full hormonal profile (LH, testosterone, prolactin)

Management

- No treatment is usually required
- If the child is significantly distressed, then can consider giving hormones to speed up the puberty process

○ **Hypergonadotropic hypogonadism**

This type is characterised by high levels of gonadotrophins FSH and LH with under-development of the gonads.

- In this type, direct ovarian or testicular failure leads to poor production of testosterone and oestrogen, resulting in reduced growth of the gonads and delay of secondary sexual characteristics.
- However, low sex steroids mean there is less negative feedback on the pituitary gland leading to high levels of FSH and LH.

Causes

- Steroid hormone enzyme deficiencies – 5-a-reductase deficiency
- Acquired testes/ovarian damage – surgery, chemo/radiotherapy, trauma
- Chromosomal abnormalities – Klinefelter syndrome, Turner syndrome

Key tests

- Blood tests show high levels of FSH/LH with low levels of testosterone/oestrogen

Management

- Treat the underlying cause. May require exogenous sex hormone replacement

○ **Hypogonadotropic hypogonadism**

This type is due to dysfunction of the hypothalamus or pituitary gland which results in low levels of FSH and LH.

- This leads to poor downstream stimulation of the gonads.
- This causes reduced production of oestrogen and testosterone, resulting in poor gonad development and a delay in secondary sexual characteristics.

Causes

- Systemic diseases – cystic fibrosis, anorexia, Crohn's disease
- CNS disorders – intracranial tumours (craniopharyngiomas), pituitary insufficiency
- Hypothyroidism

Key tests

- Blood tests show low GnRH, FSH/LH, oestrogen, and testosterone

Management

- Sex hormone replacement therapy

A condition that causes hypogonadotropic hypogonadism is **Kallman's syndrome**
- This is an X-linked recessive condition.
- There is a failure of GnRH secreting neurons which originate in the olfactory epithelium to migrate to the hypothalamus, resulting in poor GnRH secretion.
- It gives delayed puberty and anosmia (lack of smell).
- It is also associated with facial deformities such as cleft lip/palate.
- CNS problems include hearing loss and abnormal eye movements.
- It is also associated with renal agenesis and abnormal finger/toe bones.
- Patients are typically quite tall.

Androgen Disorders

There are a host of conditions that interfere with androgen signalling, which can lead to disorders of sexual development.

● **Congenital adrenal hyperplasia (CAH)**

This is an autosomal recessive disorder that causes excessive sex steroid production and hyperplasia of the adrenal glands.
- It results from mutations in enzymes involved in aldosterone and cortisol synthesis.
- Enzyme deficiency causes precursors to be shunted toward sex steroid production.
- This increases androgen levels leading to masculinization of the phenotype.
- Cortisol deficiency also leads to elevated ACTH levels due to lack of negative feedback, causing bilateral adrenal hyperplasia.

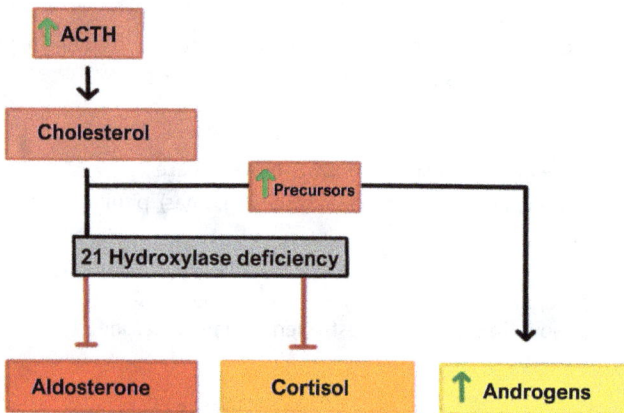

The clinical presentation of CAH depends on the specific enzyme deficiency.

○ **21-hydroxylase deficiency**

This is the most common form which leads to salt wasting due to low cortisol and aldosterone, with high androgen levels.
- In females, it causes masculinisation of the female genitalia.
- In males, it can cause precocious puberty.

Lack of cortisol and aldosterone may result in a salt wasting crisis during the first few weeks of life.
- This presents with hypotension, circulatory collapse, vomiting, and diarrhoea.
- This is more commonly seen in males with 21-hydroxylase deficiency.

○ **11β-hydroxylase deficiency**

This subtype is less common.

- It causes virilisation of female genitalia and precocious puberty.
- These is less salt wasting, and it causes hypertension and hypokalaemia.

○ **17-hydroxylase deficiency**

This is a milder, non-virilising form seen in females.

- It presents later and may cause menstrual irregularities or infertility.

Key tests

- Bloods show electrolyte derangement (Na, K) and high 17a-hydroxyprogesterone
- Genetic testing is used to confirm the diagnosis

Management

- Hormone replacement therapy with cortisol and aldosterone
- In some XX individuals, surgical correction of the external genitalia may be considered to reverse virilisation

● **Androgen insensitivity syndrome (AIS)**

This is an X-linked recessive disorder caused by a mutation in the gene which encodes the androgen receptor, also known as Morris syndrome.

- This reduces the body's ability to respond to androgens, such as testosterone.
- Since female development is the default pathway and androgens are required to masculinise, the lack of androgen effect leads to externally female genitalia.
- However, XY individuals have an active SRY gene so they develop testes.
- The inability to respond to testosterone results in failed external virilisation, giving a female phenotype despite the presence of testes.

AIS exists on a spectrum and can be classified according to the degree of insensitivity.

○ **Complete androgen insensitivity**

Here, the body is completely unresponsive to testosterone.

- It results in female external genitalia and secondary sexual characteristics, but male internal gonads (testes).
- Individuals are usually raised as females and may not be diagnosed until puberty.

Symptoms

- Primary amenorrhoea (due to absence of a uterus)
- Inguinal/groin masses from undescended testes
- Affected females may appear more masculine in build than typical XX females

○ **Partial androgen insensitivity**

The body is partially responsive to testosterone.
- Individuals may be raised as male or female depending on the degree of virilization.

Symptoms

- Genitalia may be ambiguous, or appear typically male or female
- May have undervirilised male features and show breast development at puberty
- Subfertility

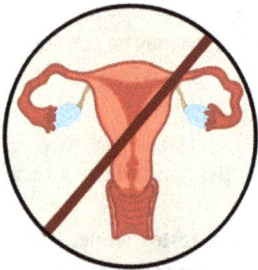

Absent female   Feminine appearance   Undescended testes
reproductive organs

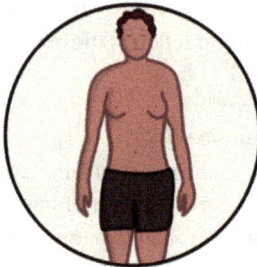

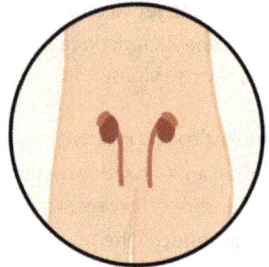

Key tests

- Karyotype (e.g. buccal smear or chromosomal analysis) shows 46, XY
- Blood tests show elevated testosterone, oestrogen and LH levels due to impaired negative feedback

Management

- For complete androgen insensitivity, individuals are typically raised as females
- Counselling is essential for psychological support
- Bilateral orchidectomy to remove undescended testes reducing malignancy risk
- Hormone therapy with oestrogen to support feminisation and bone health

- **5-alpha reductase deficiency**

This is an autosomal recessive condition caused by a mutation in the SRD5A2 gene.

- 5-alpha reductase is the enzyme that converts testosterone into its more potent form, dihydrotestosterone (DHT).
- DHT is essential for the virilisation of external male genitalia in XY foetuses.
- Enzyme deficiency reduces DHT levels, leading to underdeveloped male genitalia.
- However, at puberty, a surge in testosterone levels overcomes the deficiency and causes masculinisation and sexual maturation.

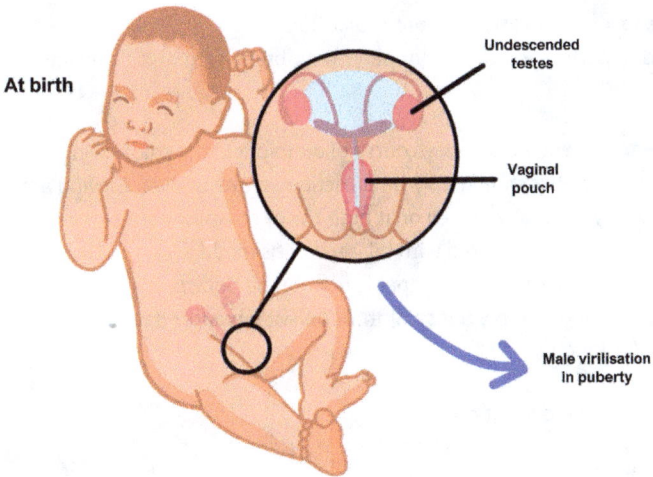

Symptoms

- Ambiguous genitalia at birth, commonly with hypospadias
- Affected children may be raised as females
- At puberty, masculinisation occurs, including rapid hair growth, deepening of the voice, growth in height and enlargement of genitalia

Key tests

- Karyotype reveals XY chromosomes
- Hormone profile shows normal testosterone levels, but low DHT with a high testosterone: DHT ratio

Management

- Hormone replacement therapy based on the gender identity adopted
- Genital surgery may be considered depending on individual preference

ENT Conditions

- **Otitis media**

This refers to an infection of the middle ear, most commonly seen in children due to Eustachian tube dysfunction.
- It often follows an upper respiratory tract infection and presents with concurrent fever and history of coughing.

Symptoms

- Earache, fever, irritability, sometimes diarrhoea
- Can lead to perforation of the tympanic membrane with associated ear discharge

Management

- First-line treatment is a 5–7-day course of antibiotics (e.g. amoxicillin)
- However, antibiotics should only be prescribed if one of the following applies:
- The child is systemically unwell or at high risk of complications
- The child is under 2 years old with bilateral otitis media
- There is otorrhoea following tympanic membrane perforation
- If none of the above apply but symptoms persist beyond 3 days, a back-up prescription may be considered

For children with recurrent otitis media, tympanostomy tubes (grommets) may be inserted to reduce the risk of glue ear and improve drainage.

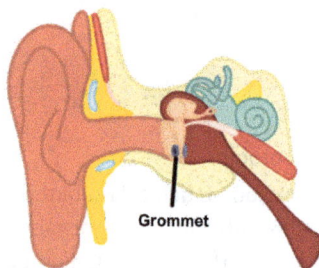

Grommet

- **Otitis media with effusion (glue ear)**

This is a condition where fluid accumulates in the middle ear and mastoid air cells due to negative pressure caused by Eustachian tube dysfunction.
- It is often a complication of acute otitis media, following a viral or bacterial infection.
- The fluid interferes with sound transmission, leading to conductive hearing loss.

Symptoms

- Often asymptomatic except for reduced hearing
- If left untreated, it can cause secondary problems such as speech delay, learning difficulties, or balance problems

Key tests
- Otoscopy shows a retracted tympanic membrane, sometimes with visible fluid levels
- Audiometry may reveal conductive hearing loss

Management
- Initial management may involve observation, as many cases resolve spontaneously
- Antibiotics are not routinely required unless there is evidence of infection
- If persistent or causing significant hearing impairment, tympanostomy tubes (grommets) may be considered
- Adenoidectomy may be offered in some cases to improve Eustachian tube function

• Adenoidal hyperplasia
This refers to the enlargement of the adenoid (pharyngeal) tonsils, which can partially obstruct the nasal airway.
- Adenoidal tissue normally increases in size until around 8 years of age, after which it gradually regresses.
- In children aged 2–8 years, the adenoids can grow faster than the surrounding airway structures, narrowing the lumen and reducing airflow.
- This predisposes children to respiratory tract infections and related complications.

Symptoms
- Can be asymptomatic
- Airway obstruction – mouth breathing, nasal voice, snoring
- Increased infection risk – recurrent otitis media, sore throats, and persistent cough

Key tests
- Nasal endoscopy allows direct visualisation of the adenoids

Management
- Adenoidectomy may be indicated in cases of obstructive sleep apnoea or recurrent otitis media with effusion

• Choanal atresia
Choanal atresia is a congenital condition in which the back of the nasal passage (choana) is blocked due to abnormal development of bony or soft tissue structures.
- This can obstruct normal airflow.
- It typically presents at birth and may be associated with other congenital anomalies, including learning disabilities and colobomas.

Symptoms

- Unilateral – often asymptomatic, may present later with nasal discharge/obstruction
- Bilateral – presents shortly after birth with respiratory distress, particularly cyanosis, as neonates are obligate nose breathers
- Cyanosis may worsen during feeding and improve when crying (as mouth is open)

Key tests

- Usually diagnosed clinically
- CT scan can be used to confirm the diagnosis and defines the extent of obstruction

Management

- Surgical intervention (fenestration procedures) to create or maintain a patent airway

- **Cleft lip and palate**

This is the most common congenital facial anomaly.
- Cleft lip results from failure of the frontonasal and maxillary processes to fuse properly during embryonical development.
- Cleft palate occurs when the palatine processes and nasal septum fail to fuse.
- It is associated with maternal use of anti-epileptic medications in pregnancy as well as genetic disorders.

Symptoms

- Facial deformity
- Feeding difficulties due to poor suction
- Speech and language development problems
- Delayed eruption and development of teeth
- Increased risk of otitis media with cleft palate

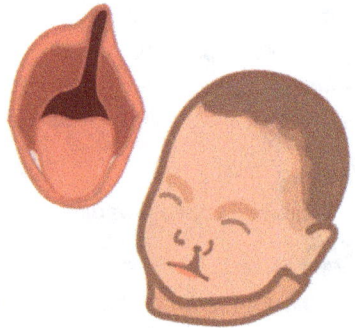

Key tests

- Antenatal detection via ultrasound, usually at the 20-week anomaly scan
- Postnatal detection during clinical assessment with the NIPE

Management

- Surgical correction at age-appropriate intervals
- Cleft lip is typically repaired at 10 weeks (within the first 2–3 months)
- Cleft palate is typically repaired between 6–12 months of age

Paediatric Ophthalmology

- **Squint (strabismus)**

This is a condition where the eyes are misaligned and do not focus on the same point when viewing an object.
- It can be constant or intermittent and typically affects one eye.
- If untreated in childhood, it can lead to amblyopia and impaired depth perception.

○ **Concomitant**

This is where deviation remains the same in all directions of gaze.
- It is caused by an imbalance in the strength of extraocular muscles.
- It can be convergent (esotropia – more common) or divergent (exotropia).

○ **Incomitant**

This is a squint where the degree of deviation varies with direction of gaze.

○ **Paralytic**

This is a rare subtype, due to paralysis of one or more extraocular muscle.

Complications

- The most significant complication is amblyopia (lazy eye)
- In amblyopia, the brain suppresses input from the misaligned eye, disrupting visual development
- This leads to reduced vision in the affected eye despite a normal appearance
- It is the most common cause of unilateral vision loss in children and young adults

Key tests

- Corneal light reflex test – shine a light from ~30 cm away to check for symmetrical reflection in both eyes
- Cover test – ask the child to fixate on an object; cover one eye and observe the uncovered eye for movement to detect misalignment

Management

- Children should be referred to ophthalmology
- Correct refractive errors with glasses
- Use occlusion therapy (patching the stronger eye) to stimulate the weaker eye and prevent amblyopia

- **Congenital cataract**

This refers to clouding of the lens present at birth, leading to reduced vision.
- The severity varies widely, from minimal impact to profound visual impairment.
- Prompt treatment is crucial, as delayed management can result in amblyopia.

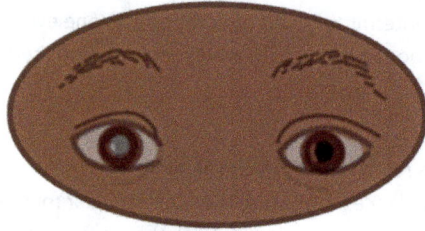

Right eye cataract

Causes

- Infections in utero – rubella, CMV, toxoplasmosis
- Genetic conditions – Down syndrome, Marfan syndrome, Alport syndrome
- Can also be idiopathic

Symptoms

- Visual difficulties, though this is hard to detect in newborns

Key tests

- Ophthalmoscopy shows loss of red reflex in the affected eye

Management

- Surgical removal of the cataract to avoid amblyopia

- **Retinoblastoma**

This is a malignant proliferation of immature cells of the retina, which is the most common primary malignant tumour of the eyes, seen in young children.
- It does not have a high mortality rate, but children may suffer irreversible loss of vision in the affected eye.
- Up to 40–45% of affected children have an inherited predisposition of the condition.
- This is due to an autosomal dominant mutation in the tumour suppressor gene Rb on chromosome 13, which is passed down from their parents.
- Whilst both alleles need to be mutated to cause the condition, if children inherit one faulty allele, then only one other mutation is required to give rise to retinoblastoma.
- This is known as the "two-hit model".

Symptoms

- Difficulties in vision, although this can be difficult to assess in newborns
- Leukocoria (white pupil)
- Squint

Key tests

- Ophthalmoscopy shows loss of red reflex
- CT/MRI shows an intraocular mass with calcifications and retinal detachment

Management

- Depends on size/location – chemotherapy, radiotherapy, laser and cryotherapy
- Surgical removal of the eye (enucleation) if large tumour or other treatments failed

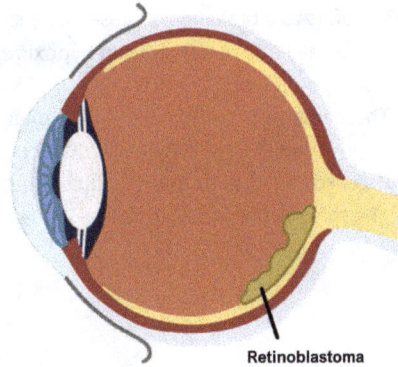

Retinoblastoma

- **Ophthalmia neonatorum/neonatal conjunctivitis**

This refers to conjunctivitis occurring within the first 28 days of life.

- It is most often due to a bacterial infection, which is typically acquired during vaginal delivery through exposure to bacteria in the birth canal.
- If left untreated, it can result in corneal ulceration and blindness.
- Neisseria gonorrhoeae gives a more acute onset whereas Chlamydia trachomatis is associated with a more delayed onset.

Symptoms

- Onset within 0–5 days (gonococcal) or 5–14 days (chlamydia)
- Red, swollen eyelids with purulent discharge
- Eye pain or tenderness
- Risk of corneal ulceration if untreated

Key tests

- Discharge should be swabbed for Gram-stain and culture

Management

- Prophylactic antibiotic ointment at birth to prevent gonococcal infection
- If conjunctivitis develops, treat with appropriate antibiotic eye drops

Birth Injuries

- **Hypoxic-ischaemic encephalopathy (HIE)**

This refers to a brain injury caused by a lack of oxygen supply to the brain.

- It is usually due to a significant hypoxic event occurring immediately before, during, or just after delivery.
- The damage is twofold: an initial phase of primary neuronal death due to oxygen deprivation, followed by a secondary phase of injury caused by reperfusion.
- It can occur due to any event that reduces oxygen delivery to the foetus, such as placental insufficiency, umbilical cord prolapse, and delayed resuscitation after birth.

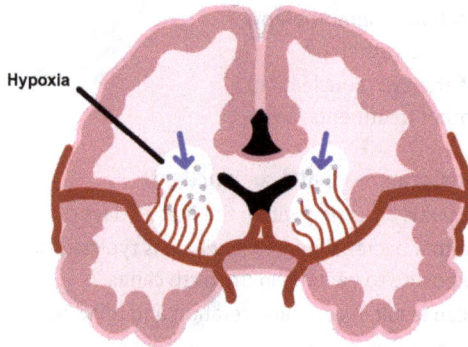

Symptoms

- Depressed level of consciousness
- Reduced muscle tone and weak or absent reflexes
- Seizures
- Delayed milestones, learning difficulties
- Respiratory distress and difficulty maintaining adequate oxygenation

Key tests

- Umbilical cord blood gas may show metabolic acidosis suggesting perinatal hypoxia
- MRI or CT brain may reveal signs of neonatal encephalopathy

Management

- Therapeutic hypothermia – infant is cooled to reduce temperature to 33–34°C
- Cooling starts within 6 hours of birth and continues for 72 hours
- This slows cellular metabolism, reduces brain injury, improves neurological outcomes, and enhances survival rates
- Manage complications such as seizures, feeding etc.

- **Soft-tissue injuries**

These include a variety of injuries that can occur during delivery, often as a result of mechanical trauma.
- The pressure exerted on the baby's head and body as it passes through the birth canal can cause bruising, swelling and other superficial injuries.
- Soft-tissue injuries are more common in difficult or prolonged deliveries.
- They can arise from the use of instruments such as forceps during assisted birth.

Key tests
- X-ray is used to check for skull fractures, which may accompany cephalohematoma
- CT head can help visualize the cephalohematoma and rule out other potential injuries like intracranial haemorrhage
- Ultrasound is useful for evaluating the cephalohaematoma and surrounding tissues

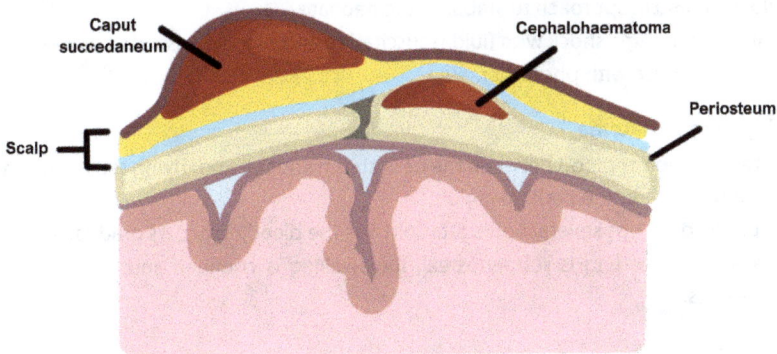

○ **Caput succedaneum**

This condition refers to a subcutaneous collection of oedematous fluid that forms on the presenting part of the scalp during delivery.
- The fluid accumulates external to the galea aponeurosis due to pressure from the cervix or vaginal walls
- It is a benign condition with no involvement of the brain or skull and does not cause long-term complications

Symptoms
- Soft, boggy swelling on the top of the baby's head
- The swelling has poorly defined edges and crosses cranial suture lines

Management
- No treatment required as the swelling usually resolves on its own within a few days

○ **Subgaleal haematoma**

This is a bleed into the potential space between the galea aponeurosis and the periosteum of the skull.

- It usually occurs following a ventouse-assisted delivery, where the negative pressure can rupture the small veins connecting the scalp to the dural venous sinuses.

Symptoms

- Fluctuant, boggy swelling over the scalp, often in the occipital region, developing hours or days after birth
- Overlying bruising of the skin
- May lead to haemorrhagic shock due to significant blood loss
- Jaundice can occur secondary to haemolysis of the accumulated blood

Management

- Follow an ABCDE approach to stabalise the neonate
- Treat haemorrhagic shock with fluid resuscitation and blood transfusion as needed
- Manage jaundice with phototherapy

○ **Cephalohaematoma**

This is a collection of blood between the periosteum and the underlying skull bone, most commonly affecting the parietal region.

- It typically develops several hours after birth as the bleeding occurs gradually.
- Because the bleeding is subperiosteal, the swelling is confined and does not cross suture lines.

Symptoms

- Soft, well-defined swelling on the scalp that does not cross suture lines
- May be associated with bruising
- In more severe cases, may lead to jaundice (due to breakdown of red blood cells), anaemia, or hypotension

Management

- Conservative management is appropriate in most cases
- The haematoma usually resolves spontaneously over several weeks to months
- Monitor and manage complications such as jaundice or anaemia

Neonatal Conditions

● **Hypoglycaemia**

This refers to a low blood glucose level, typically considered to be below 2.6 mM.

- A transient drop in blood glucose is common after birth as part of the neonate's adjustment to postnatal life.
- Even full-term babies can experience hypoglycaemia in the first 24 hours without significant complications.
- However, severe or prolonged hypoglycaemia may lead to long-term neurological damage if not addressed promptly.

Risk factors

- Prematurity, infection
- Gestational diabetes in mothers
- IUGR and macrosomia

Symptoms

- Can be asymptomatic
- Irritability, lethargy, apnoea, grunting, sweating and seizures

Management

- For mild cases, promote breastfeeding or bottle feeding to increase glucose levels
- For severe cases, administer IV glucose to raise blood glucose levels

● **Transient tachypnoea of the newborn (TTN)**

This is one of the most common causes of respiratory distress in newborns.

- In utero, the lungs are filled with fluid, which is typically squeezed out during vaginal delivery and absorbed into the bloodstream shortly after birth.
- TTN occurs when there is a delay in the reabsorption of this fluid, leading to temporary breathing difficulties.
- It is more common after Caesarean section, where the mechanical squeezing of the lungs as the baby passes through the vagina does not occur.

Symptoms

- Respiratory distress – tachypnoea, tachycardia, breathlessness

Key tests
- It is a diagnosis of exclusion after ruling out more serious causes (e.g. pneumonia)
- Chest X-ray may show hyperinflated lungs with fluid in the lung fissures

Management
- Supportive care with oxygen to maintain adequate oxygen saturations
- The condition is usually self-limiting and resolves within 24–72 hours as the lung fluid is gradually absorbed

- **Persistent pulmonary hypertension of the newborn (PPHN)**
This condition occurs when the pulmonary circulation fails to transition properly after birth, resulting in sustained high pulmonary vascular resistance.
- The elevated resistance leads to pulmonary hypertension and causes right-to-left shunting through persistent foetal circulatory pathways such as a patent foramen ovale (PFO) and patent ductus arteriosus (PDA), resulting in systemic hypoxia.

Causes
- Primary – idiopathic
- Secondary – associated with perinatal asphyxia, meconium aspiration syndrome, neonatal sepsis, or respiratory distress syndrome

Symptoms
- Central cyanosis shortly after birth
- Signs of respiratory distress and hypoxaemia
- Risk of developing chronic lung disease
- Increased susceptibility to hospital-acquired infections

Key tests
- Echocardiography confirms the diagnosis by showing elevated pulmonary artery pressures and right-to-left shunting

Management
- Oxygen therapy and mechanical ventilation as needed
- Pulmonary vasodilators (e.g. inhaled nitric oxide) to reduce pulmonary vascular resistance and improve oxygenation

- **Meconium aspiration syndrome**

This condition occurs when a newborn inhales meconium-stained amniotic fluid, typically during or shortly before delivery.

- Meconium acts as an irritant in the lungs, causing both mechanical obstruction and chemical pneumonitis.
- It causes inflammation which can give significant respiratory compromise.

Symptoms

- Respiratory distress – tachypnoea, breathlessness, coughing
- Increases the risk of persistent pulmonary hypertension of the newborn (PPHN)
- May also lead to pneumonia and sepsis

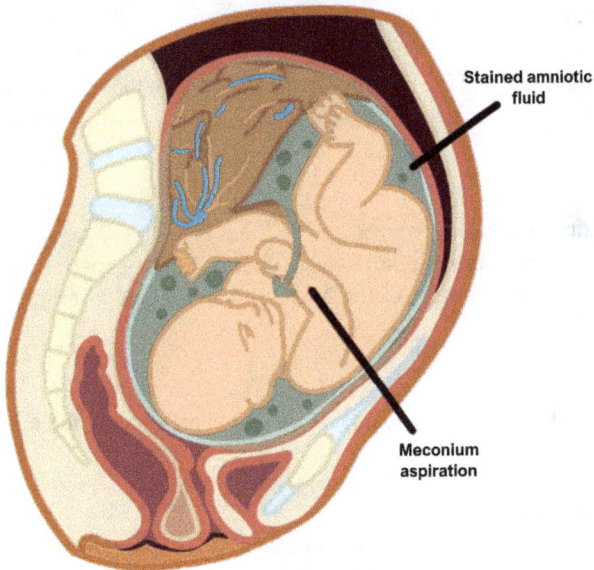

Stained amniotic fluid

Meconium aspiration

Key tests

- Bloods tests show raised inflammatory markers
- CXR can show patchy infiltrations in the lungs

Management

- Oxygen to support saturations, if severe may need invasive ventilation
- Use of anti-inflammatory agents and pulmonary vasodilators (e.g. inhaled nitric oxide) if pulmonary hypertension develops
- Antibiotics if evidence of infection

- **Sudden infant death syndrome (SIDS)**

This refers to the sudden, unexplained death of an infant under the age of one.
- It typically occurs during sleep and is commonly known as "cot death".
- It usually happens between midnight and 9 am.
- The exact cause remains unknown, but there are several risk factors that are thought to contribute to the syndrome.
- Certain factors, such as room-sharing and breastfeeding, are considered protective.

Risk factors
- These factors are additive and together can significantly increase the risk of death
- Infant-related – low birth weight, prematurity, male sex
- Parent-related – parental smoking, multiple births, maternal drug use, young mother under 21 years of age
- Environmental – sleeping the baby in a prone position (on their stomach), bed sharing, use of infant pillows, hyperthermia (over-wrapping) or covering the head

Key tests
- SIDS is a diagnosis of exclusion
- It is diagnosed if the cause of death remains unexplained after performing an autopsy, reviewing the medical history of the infant and family, and investigating the death scene

Management
- Following the death, families should receive emotional support and grief counselling to help them cope with their loss

- **Jaundice of the new-born**

Jaundice refers to yellowing of the skin and eyes.
- It is a common condition in neonates, affecting about half of all infants.
- Neonatal jaundice is usually due to the physiological breakdown of red blood cells as the infant has a high haemoglobin concentration at birth.
- The RBC lifespan in neonates is shorter than in adults (70 days vs 120 days), leading to increased breakdown.
- Additionally, the liver's ability to process bilirubin is immature during the first few days of life, contributing to jaundice.
- Breastfeeding can increase the risk of jaundice due to factors in breast milk that can reduce bilirubin excretion.

Jaundice, however, appearing within the first 24 hours of life is pathological.
- It occurs due to conditions that increase bilirubin production or release, such as:
- Haemolytic conditions – hereditary spherocytosis, G6PD deficiency
- Congenital infections – rubella, cytomegalovirus (CMV)
- Haematoma-related haemolysis
- Metabolic conditions – Crigler-Najjar syndrome

If untreated, jaundice can lead to **kernicterus**.
- Unconjugated bilirubin is fat-soluble and can cross the blood-brain barrier (BBB)
- It is neurotoxic, particularly damaging the basal ganglia, causing encephalopathy

Symptoms

- Muscle hypertonia or hypotonia with spasms, including torticollis
- Opisthotonos (hyperextension and arching of the back)
- "Sunsetting" sign (inability to move the eyes up and down)
- Seizures
- Lethargy and poor feeding

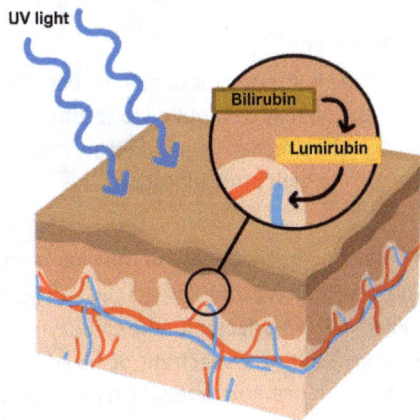

Key tests

- Measure serum bilirubin levels using blood tests or a transcutaneous bilirubinometer
- Plot bilirubin levels on a chart to determine if treatment is necessary

Management

- Treatment is guided by bilirubin levels, plotted on specific treatment charts
- If below the treatment line, encourage frequent feeding, ensure hydration, and support breastfeeding
- If above the treatment line, first line is phototherapy, which converts bilirubin to a water-soluble form, preventing it from crossing the BBB
- If this is unsuccessful, one can do exchange transfusion, which involves removing the infant's blood and replacing it with donor blood

- **Congenital diaphragmatic hernia**

A condition in which abdominal organs herniate through a defect in the diaphragm.
- Most cases occur on the left side and result in lung compression.
- It occurs as the pleuroperitoneal folds which form the diaphragm fail to seal properly.
- This leaves an opening through which the abdominal organs can enter the chest.

Symptoms

- Pulmonary hypoplasia, leading to respiratory distress (shortness of breath, cyanosis)
- Poor air entry on the left side of the chest
- Elevated blood pressure, displacement of the apex beat and heart sounds

Key tests

- Chest and abdominal X-ray reveals loops of bowel in the chest cavity

Management

- NG tube is inserted for suctioning bowel contents
- Intubation may be required to secure the airway
- Surgical correction is required to repair the diaphragm and return the abdominal organs to their proper location

- **Haemorrhagic disease of the new-born**

This condition is caused by vitamin K deficiency, leading to bleeding in neonates.
- Vitamin K is a cofactor for the carboxylation and maturation of clotting factors.
- It can result in a spectrum of bleeding disorders, ranging from minor bruising to significant haemorrhage, which may appear up to 8 weeks after birth.
- Risk factors include liver disease, breastfeeding as well as maternal use of anti-epileptics, which impair the synthesis of vitamin K-dependent clotting factors.

Symptoms

- Bleeding – bruising, haematemesis, malena and intracranial haemorrhage

Management

- If bleeding, administer intramuscular (IM) vitamin K and fresh frozen plasma
- Mainstay of treatment is preventative, as vitamin K is given to all infants immediately after birth, usually as a single IM injection
- Mothers on anti-epileptics should also receive oral vitamin K prophylaxis, which is usually given at 36 weeks' gestation

Prematurity Conditions

A premature infant is defined as one born before 37 weeks of gestation.
- Extremely preterm refers to gestational age < 28 weeks. These infants often require transfer to a tertiary centre for specialist management.
- Very preterm is 28–32 weeks.
- Moderate to late preterm is 32–37 weeks.

Premature infants have a higher likelihood of complications, as key organs have not had the chance to develop to support independent like outside of the uterus.
- Antenatal management for premature births typically includes the administration of magnesium sulphate (for neuroprotection) and steroids to aid lung maturation.

Premature infants often have delayed developmental milestones.
- To track their progress, a corrected age is used, which accounts for the number of weeks the baby was born prematurely.
- To calculate the corrected age, subtract the number of weeks the baby was premature from their actual age in weeks.
- For example, if a baby is 12 weeks old but was born 6 weeks prematurely, their corrected age would be 6 weeks.
- The corrected age is generally used until around 2 years of age, by which time premature infants are expected to catch up to their full-term peers.

- **Respiratory distress syndrome**
This condition is also known as surfactant deficient lung disease, as premature infants lack sufficient surfactant due to the immaturity of type II alveolar cells.
- It is a common condition in premature infants.
- Surfactant deficiency reduces lung compliance (making the lungs stiffer) and increases alveolar surface tension, leading to widespread alveolar collapse.
- This results in impaired gas exchange and an increased effort to breathe.

Symptoms
- Respiratory distress – tachypnoea, nasal flaring
- Sternal and subcostal recession (retractions of the chest wall)
- Expiratory grunting
- Cyanosis (in severe cases)

Key tests

- Blood gas (ABG) shows respiratory acidosis
- Chest X-ray typically shows a diffuse granular or "ground-glass" appearance with air bronchograms

Management

- Antenatally, steroids are given to the mother stimulate foetal surfactant production
- Postnatally, baby receives oxygen therapy and respiratory support with continuous positive airway pressure (CPAP) or high flow nasal cannula (HFNC)
- If still hypoxic, then consider invasive ventilation if needed
- Exogenous surfactant can be given to improve lung compliance and breathing

- **Bronchopulmonary dysplasia (BPD)**

This is a chronic lung disease seen in premature infants, particularly those who have been treated with oxygen.

- BPD is a result of delayed lung maturation and oxygen toxicity, which impair the development of the alveoli, preventing them from functioning normally.
- It is characterised by the need for long-term oxygen therapy in affected infants.

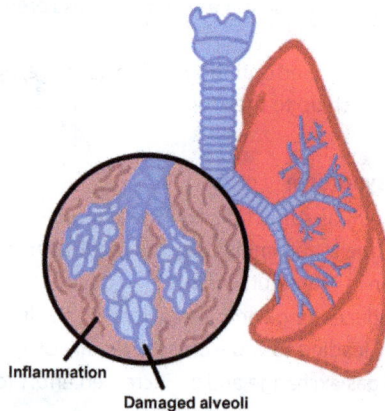

Inflammation

Damaged alveoli

Symptoms

- Respiratory – dyspnoea, tachypnoea, grunting, cyanosis
- Feeding difficulties and failure to thrive
- Increased risk of respiratory infections, particularly viral infections
- Increased risk of recurrent cough, wheezing, and lung hyperinflation
- Pulmonary hypertension, which can eventually lead to cor pulmonale (right-sided heart failure)

Key tests

- Chest X-ray shows hyperinflation, atelectasis (collapsed lung), and cystic changes
- To be diagnosed with BPD, the infant must meet the following criteria:
- A history of oxygen or mechanical ventilation treatment
- Abnormal respiratory function with findings consistent with BPD
- Requirement for long-term supplemental oxygen therapy

Management

- Supplemental oxygen and nutrition to support the infant's growth and development
- Antibiotics and vaccinations to prevent recurrent infections
- Steroids may be used to promote further lung development in some cases

- **Apnoea of prematurity**

This is a condition where premature infants experience episodes of absent breathing that last for more than 20 seconds.
- These apnoeic episodes can be accompanied by hypoxia or bradycardia.
- They are particularly common in infants born before 32 weeks of gestation.
- It is often caused by immaturity of the central respiratory drive, impaired coordination of respiratory muscles, and inappropriate triggering of the chemoreceptor response.
- It is frequently associated with underlying conditions, such as infection, meconium aspiration, or respiratory distress syndrome.

Symptoms

- Absence of airflow for 20 seconds or more, accompanied by bradycardia (heart rate < 100 bpm) or cyanosis/oxygen desaturation (SpO_2 drop)

Key tests

- Infant pneumogram or sleep study

Management

- Firstly, rule out other causes of apnoea, such as infection
- Avoiding triggers of the chemoreceptor response by careful positioning (e.g. avoiding excessive flexion)
- Caffeine is commonly used to stimulate the respiratory drive and reduce the frequency of apnoeic episodes
- If frequent or severe, respiratory support may be needed to assist with breathing

- **Necrotising enterocolitis (NEC)**

This refers to an acute inflammatory condition affecting the distal small bowel and proximal large intestine.

- It typically begins with feeding intolerance but can rapidly progress to bowel perforation and peritonitis.
- The exact cause is unknown, but it is believed to result from a combination of immature gut function, bacterial imbalance, and an exaggerated immune response.
- Breastfeeding is protective, with a higher incidence in formula fed infants.

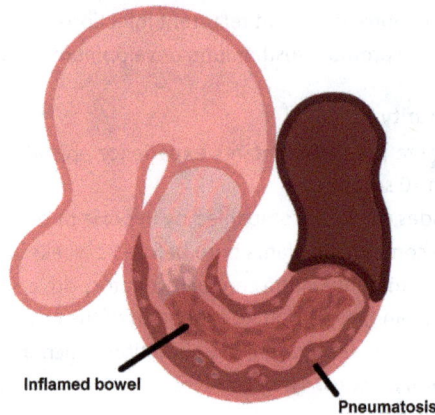

Inflamed bowel

Pneumatosis

Symptoms

- Early stages – feeding intolerance, vomiting (which may be bile-stained), and abdominal distension
- Late stages – shiny, distended abdomen, bloody stools, respiratory distress
- Can lead to bowel perforation, which may result in shock

Key tests

- Blood tests show raised inflammatory markers
- Abdominal X-ray shows air in the dilated bowel, pneumatosis (air within the bowel wall), or Rigler's sign (indicating bowel perforation)

Management

- Total gut rest with IV fluids and TPN (total parenteral nutrition)
- Administer antibiotics to reduce the risk of infection
- If bowel perforation occurs, surgical intervention (laparotomy) is required
- Once the condition stabilises, feeding is gradually reintroduced

- **Periventricular leukomalacia (PVL)**

This is a white-matter brain injury commonly seen in premature neonates.

- PVL is characterised by necrosis of the white matter near the lateral ventricles, often caused by a combination of ischaemia, inflammation and free-radical damage.
- After hypoxia, coagulation necrosis leads to tissue dissolution and the formation of cavities (holes) in the affected areas of the brain.

Symptoms

- Delayed motor milestones, difficulties with eye movement, squint and nystagmus
- Potential development of cerebral palsy, epilepsy and seizures

Key tests

- Cranial ultrasound may reveal multiple, bilateral cysts in the affected brain areas
- MRI can be used to confirm the diagnosis and provide more detailed imaging

Management

- Manage complications such as motor impairment and seizures

- **Germinal matrix and interventricular haemorrhage**

These are two related conditions characterised by bleeding in the brain.

- They typically occur within the first 3 days of life.
- The germinal matrix is an area in the brain above the caudate nucleus, with rapidly dividing neurons and fragile blood vessels sensitive to hypoxia and pressure changes.
- Premature infants are at high risk for rupturing these vessels because they lack the ability to autoregulate blood flow, leading to haemorrhage.
- A germinal matrix haemorrhage is confined to the germinal matrix.
- An intraventricular haemorrhage is more severe, with the bleed extending into the ventricles and potentially causing hydrocephalus.
- The symptoms depend on the size and location of the haemorrhage and can lead to long-term neurological problems.

Symptoms: Seizures, can lead to cerebral palsy and learning difficulties

Key tests: Cranial ultrasound

Management

- Steroids (dexamethasone) given to mother antenatally to reduce the risk
- If hydrocephalus develops, CSF drainage may be necessary
- Long-term involves managing complications such learning difficulties and epilepsy

Psychiatry

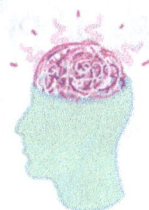

Basic Principles

A disease can be defined by the objective physical pathology and known aetiology.
- Conversely, an illness is the patient's subjective distress caused by a condition.

A major challenge in psychiatry is that many conditions have no known or understood pathophysiological cause. This makes it very difficult to diagnose diseases, since there is often no demonstrable pathology.
- Therefore, psychiatry talks about mental illness – this is a level of subjective distress which is greater in severity or duration than occurs in normal human experience.
- This allows us to diagnose patients regardless of our understanding of the pathophysiology of the condition and provide treatments.

A diagnosis in psychiatry involves the identification of a disease from its signs and symptoms. By giving a diagnosis to a set of symptoms, it allows us to do the following:
- Group a set of symptoms together
- Identify any underlying causes into a particular condition
- By recognising the symptoms as a condition, it permits the development of an evidence-based treatment plan
- After a diagnosis is made, we can estimate the outlook and prognosis for the patient based on cases seen before

A classification system provides a way of grouping together patients who are similar in their clinical features.
- There are two main classification systems used today in psychiatry.
- These systems are categorical systems, and the diagnosis is based on symptoms and descriptions rather than aetiology or typology.
- These include the international Classification of Diseases (ICD), which is made by the World Health Organisation (WHO).
- The second is the Diagnostic and Statistical Manual of Mental Disorders, which is produced by the American Psychiatric Association.

Mental Capacity

Mental Capacity can be defined as the ability to make your own decisions.
- The principle of individual autonomy in receiving healthcare is a cornerstone of modern medicine.
- The Mental Capacity Act (MCA) is an act of parliament which provides a legal framework for managing, empowering, and protecting individuals over the age of 16 who lack capacity.
- If the child is younger than 16, they only have capacity to make decisions provided that they are Gillick Competent.

There are 5 key principles of the MCA:
- A person is assumed to have capacity until it is established that the person lacks it.
- All practicable steps need to be taken in order to help a person make a specific decision.
- Individuals are allowed to make unwise decisions, and it should not be assumed they lack capacity if they do so.
- Decisions made on behalf of an incapable person must be made in their best interests.
- Any action taken must be the least restrictive of a person's rights and freedoms.

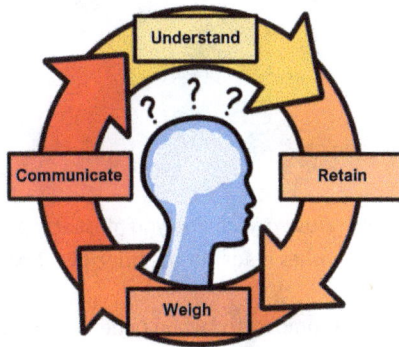

Mental capacity is assessed as a transient, time specific state which is decision specific. An adult lacks capacity if she/he:
a) has an impairment of, or disturbance in, the functioning of the mind or brain.
b) and are unable to (any one of):
   - understand the information relevant to the decision,
   - retain that information,
   - use or weigh that information in making the decision, or
   - communicate the decision made.

There are some important points regarding mental capacity.
- Capacity is decision-specific – the test should be reapplied for each new decision.
- Capacity can fluctuate – if appropriate, delay the decision until capacity improves.
- You have a duty to maximise the potential for competent consent by giving information in a form that the patient can understand and at a time when the patient is most able to understand.

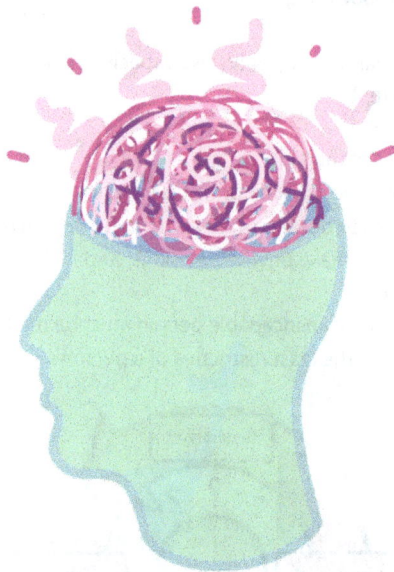

If a patient who has capacity refuses treatment, you must accept their decision.
- Treating them against their wishes is against the principle of patient autonomy.
- It can be deemed as assault.
- The situation becomes more complicated when patients lack capacity.

Under the MCA, there are 3 justifications for the provision of treatment for an adult who lacks capacity:
- If a valid advanced decision to refuse treatment (ADRT) exists.
- If a valid lasting power of attorney (LPA) for health and welfare exists.
- If neither exists, you should act in the patient's best interests.

- **Advanced decisions to refuse treatment (ADRT)**

An advance decision is made by an adult at a time when they have capacity to make such a decision (at time 1) to refuse medical treatment in the future (at time 2) in the event that they lose capacity.

- Advanced decisions to refuse treatment can be spoken rather than written.

Validity

An ADRT cannot be made when a patient does not have capacity.

- It is not valid if they have withdrawn the decision at a time when they had capacity.
- It is also invalid if the patient has granted an LPA to someone else that grants them the power to make decisions about the type of treatment.

Applicability

An ADRT is not applicable to the treatment in question if:

- That treatment is not the treatment specified in the ADRT.
- Any circumstances specified in the ADRT are absent.

Advanced decisions to refuse lifesaving/sustaining treatment carry extra conditions:

- They must be in writing.
- They must be signed, witnessed, countersigned and include a statement that the patient intends the AD to be respected even if their life is at risk.
- If unsure, doctors may apply to the Court of Protection for clarification of interpretation.

- **Lasting powers of attorney (LPA)**

This is a legal document where an adult who has capacity (the donor) may nominate an attorney (the donee), granting them the legal power to make decisions on the donor's behalf.

- There are 2 types of LPA, one for "health & welfare" and one for "property & finances".
- The LPA that covers health and welfare decisions includes giving or refusing consent to medical treatment. In addition, this can cover decisions ranging from how self-care is delivered through to where an individual lives.
- It can include decisions about life-saving treatment if express provision is made.

If a person without capacity did not grant an LPA, the Court of Protection can appoint a "personal welfare deputy" to make those decisions. They usually only do this if:
- There is doubt whether decisions will be made in someone's best interests (e.g. the family disagree about care).
- Someone needs to be appointed to make decisions about a specific issue over a period of time (e.g. where someone will live).

- **Best interests decision**

In the absence of a valid advance decision or LPA, the person providing treatment is responsible and must act in the best interests of the patient.
- When making a best interests decision, there are specific things to do and not do.

Do not
- Do not decide merely based on age or appearance, or assumptions.
- Do not make decisions about life-sustaining treatment that are motivated by a desire to bring about death.
- This means decisions about withdrawal of LST must not be made on the basis of whether continuing to live is in the best interest of the patient.

Do
- Favour the option that is least restrictive of the person's rights and freedom of action.
- Consider whether the person is likely to regain capacity. If this is the case, you may wish to delay the decision.
- Try to help/encourage the person to participate in the decision as much as possible.
- Consider the views and beliefs of the patient (cultural background, religion).
- Consult with those close to the patient (anyone named by the person as someone to be consulted on such matters).

For the treatment of mental disorders:
- Patients who are detained under S2/3 of the Mental Health Act may be given treatment for a mental disorder without their consent.
- This applies even if they have capacity to make decisions about their treatment.
- The justification here is that the treatment is necessary for the protection of others or for the patient.

Mental Health Act (MHA)

The main piece of mental health legislation in England is the Mental Health Act 1983.
- This was amended in 2007.

The Mental Health Act applies to patients with a "mental disorder" – this is any disorder or disability of the mind.
- Dependence on drugs or alcohol is excluded within this definition of mental disorder.
- However, individuals with a dependency can be included if they also suffer from a comorbid mental disorder.
- It also excludes patients with learning disability, unless their condition is associated with abnormally aggressive or seriously irresponsible conduct.
- It applies to people of any age, but children are usually treated under the framework of parental consent.

Sectioning

This part of the mental health act allows admission of a patient to a hospital using sections for assessment or treatment.
- For Sections 2, 3 and 4, the section is recommended by doctors but then needs approval by an Approved Mental Health Professional (AMHP) to complete the section.
- There are several safeguards available to patients including the power to apply for an independent review tribunal to scrutinise their section.
- This tribunal has the power of discharge.

To section for assessment the following statutory criteria must be met:
- The patient must be suffering from mental disorder.
- The disorder must be of a nature or degree warranting hospital detention for assessment.
- They need to be detained in the interests of their health, their safety or with a view to the protection of others.

To section for treatment:
- (In addition to previous 3 criteria)
- The treatment needed cannot be effectively provided unless the patient is detained.
- Appropriate medical treatment is available to them (medical treatment includes medications, nursing care, therapies etc.).

The main sections are summarised in the table below.
- Section 12 (S12) approved doctors have expertise in the diagnosis and treatment of mental disorder.

S	Purpose	Recommendation	Applicant	Duration
2	Assessment +/- treatment (this is non-renewable)	Two S12 approved doctors	AMHP	28 days
3	Treatment can be given for 3 months without consent - Then requires a second opinion doctor to certify - Renewable after 6 months	Two S12 approved doctors	AMHP	6 months

Emergency sections

S	Purpose	Recommendation	Length
4	Allows the patient to be admitted to a mental health unit and cared for whilst arrangements for detention under S2 or S3 are made	1 doctor who is S12 approved + AMPH approval is required	72 hours
135	Allows police to enter a private dwelling, remove an individual & convey to a place of safety	- Warrant is issued by a magistrate - The police officer executes the action	72 hours
136	Allows police to take someone to place of safety for assessment		72 hours
5(2)	A registered doctor can detain an inpatient for assessment (used when there is no time for S2) - Used on patients who withdraw consent (if they have capacity) or show objection (without capacity) - Cannot be used on patients in ED as they have not been formally admitted	1 registered doctor*	72 hours
5(4)	For patients in hospital, nurse detains inpatient for assessment when doctor comes	1 (NMC) registered nurse	6 hours

*Needs full GMC registration so F2 level and above.

Consent to treatment

As a general rule, once a patient is detained under S2, 3, 35, 36 or 37 of the MHA, consent is not required for the administration of psychiatric treatment.
- The justification for treatment is provided by S63.

Treatments which are covered by S63:
- Treatments for the disorder itself (e.g. antipsychotics for schizophrenia)
- Treatments for conditions causing the disorder (e.g. hypothyroidism causing depression)
- Treatments for physical consequences of the disorder (e.g. NG feeds in anorexia)
- Safe holds and physical control and restraint (when necessary)

To safeguard patients who are having compulsory treatment, some treatments require approval from an independent second opinion appointed doctor (SOAD).
- This usually occurs at the 3 month point of an admission for treatment if the patient is unable to consent. They are also mandated to be involved in special circumstances where treatment is restrictive (such as ECT).

Specific treatments mentioned in the MHA:

○ **Seclusion**

Confinement of a patient in a room with the sole aim of preventing harm to others.
- The patient needs review every 4 hours by doctor.

○ **Psychosurgery**

This is covered by section 57 and needs patient consent and SOAD authorization.

○ **ECT**

This is covered by section 58. It requires SOAD approval if the patient cannot consent. If the patient has capacity, then you must accept refusal.

Treatment of community patients

A community treatment order (CTO) may be used to facilitate discharge of a patient detained under S3.
- A CTO authorises a named consultant to exercise the "power of recall" if the patient requires treatment in hospital or there would be a risk of harm to the health/safety of the patient or to other persons if the patient were not recalled to hospital for treatment.

Psychotherapy

Psychotherapy works by helping people understand why they feel as they do.
- It uses a combination of reflecting about past events, altering unhelpful thinking patterns and building a relationship with a therapist.
- We can broadly split psychological therapies into 3 groups.

Supportive therapies

These represent the least intense level of psychotherapy which are typically used for mild depression and anxiety. They include counselling and supportive psychotherapy.
- The sessions are unstructured but allow the patient to establish a rapport with their therapist, reflect on experiences and get reassurance.
- It is a non-direct way of solving the problem and can be helpful in dealing with stress, bereavement and adjustment disorders.
- Patients usually have a course of about 6–10 sessions.

Psychodynamic therapies

These therapies arose from the work of Sigmund Freud who theorised that human behaviour is determined by unconscious forces derived from primitive emotional needs. These include psychoanalysis and psychodynamic psychotherapy.
- By looking at their current difficulties using psychoanalysis, patients can identify unconscious conflicts that have arisen from their past.
- These conflicts often explain the current difficulties being experienced.
- Psychodynamic sessions take place on a regular basis (at least weekly) and courses can last between 1–5 years.

Procedure
- The patient explores their subconscious by using free association (saying whatever is on their mind)
- The therapist interprets these statements to link the patient's past experiences with their current life and their relationship with the therapist
- This relies upon the recognition of 2 psychodynamic processes
- Transference – this is when the patient re-experiences strong emotions from early relationships with the therapist
- Counter-transference – when the therapist experiences strong emotions towards the patient

Disadvantages
- It takes a long time and often depends on the quality and training of the therapist
- Working through difficulties is often self-directed
- Patients can become dependent on the therapist

Cognitive and behavioural therapies

These therapies originate from the view that mental distress arises from abnormal thinking patterns and behaviours. These are addressed with therapies delivered in a structured, patient-centred approach.
- It is explicit and gives the patient clear strategies to improve their thinking and make a tangible difference.
- These therapies are intensive and usually time limited, with a course usually lasting about 6–12 sessions.

- **Cognitive behavioural therapy (CBT)**

This is a therapy that is structured around the interplay between thoughts, emotions and behaviours. Its aim is to tackle both the negative cognitive styles and unhelpful behaviours which lead to emotional difficulties in patients.

a) Cognitive aspects – the aim is to help people identify and challenge automatic negative thoughts and abnormal beliefs.

b) Behavioural techniques – this is based on the learning theory of operant conditioning (positive and negative reinforcement).
- It helps to identify habitual unhelpful behaviours (e.g. avoidance in anxiety) and to challenge these. This can include developing more helpful behaviours in times of stress (e.g. relaxation techniques).
- Graded exposure with positive reinforcement can also be used to incrementally change behaviour, which in turn has a positive effect on emotions.

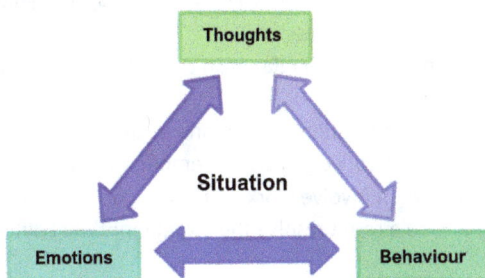

- **Cognitive analytic therapy (CAT)**

This is a short time-limited therapy which provides inexpensive psychological treatment drawing on cognitive therapy and analytical techniques.
- It looks at the ways an individual thinks and feels, exploring the past events and relationships that have shaped their current difficulties.

It focusses on 3 main phases:
- Reformulation phase – the therapist formulates the individual's difficulties in the context of their past experiences.
- Recognition phase – the individual uses diagrams to identify the role of the formulation in everyday difficulties.
- Revision phase – the individual then finds new and more adaptive ways of managing these situations by breaking harmful cycles and associations.

- **Dialectical behavioural therapy (DBT)**

This is a form of modified CBT which aims to change thinking styles and behaviours whilst also accepting oneself.
- It can be delivered individually or in a group.
- It involves moving towards a balance between "change techniques" and "acceptance techniques".
- This therapy is particularly useful in patients who repeatedly self-harm such as those with personality disorders.

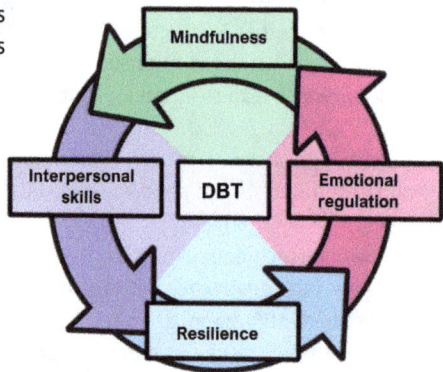

Other psychotherapies

- **Interpersonal therapy**

This is a type of psychological therapy which is based on psychodynamic therapies.
- It is used for moderate-severe depression.
- The patient explains who their close relationships are to the therapist who constructs an interpersonal network.
- The therapist formulates the patient's emotions in the context of problems arising within the interpersonal network e.g. a close member may have died causing grief.
- The rest of the sessions then involve work on how to cope and change their views of these relationships and as a result resolve the target emotional difficulty.

- **Family therapy**

This therapy uses the framework of the family as a unit where all individual difficulties have a significant impact on the function of the whole unit.
- The therapist asks questions and observes how the family interact with each other.
- The therapist then will give feedback and encourage positive engagement.
- In this way, changing one thing can lead to the whole system changing.
- It is especially beneficial for the treatment of children with eating disorders.

- **Eye movement desensitisation and reprogramming (EMDR)**

This is a type of psychotherapy that allows patients to access past traumatic memories, reprocess the trauma and as a result, experience less distress.
- It is mainly used for post-traumatic stress disorder (PTSD).

1. REVIEW	4. DESENSITIZE
- Identify issues - Treatment plan	- Conduct bilateral stimulation

2. PREPARE	3. IDENTIFY
- Create safe place - Renew bonds	- Identify events - Identify emotions

The therapist first takes a history from the patient to establish traumatic memories.
- The patient then recalls the disturbing events and the emotion they felt at the time (e.g. sexual abuse and feeling powerless).
- The patient and therapist then work together to create a positive belief about the event ("I am stronger now and not so powerless").
- The therapist then activates both sides of the patient's brain using dual activation stimulation (DAS) by making the patient perform eye movements.
- This allows the brain to reprocess the upsetting memories by removing the old emotions and associating them with the more positive, empowering emotion.
- This leads to the memory no longer being experienced as traumatic.

Physical Therapies

- **Electroconvulsive therapy (ECT)**

This uses electrodes to induce a modified cerebral seizure in the brain.

- This leads to massive amounts of neurotransmitter release, hormone secretion and a transient increase in blood brain barrier permeability.
- It is useful when requiring a rapid effective treatment after other treatment options have failed, in patients with severe depression and catatonia.

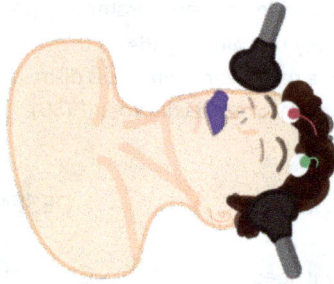

Patient should be nil-by-mouth for 4 hours before intervention.

- They are then given a short-acting anaesthetic and muscle relaxant.
- Preoxygenation is given to increase oxygen saturation.
- A shock is delivered to the scalp either bilaterally or unilaterally.
- This evokes a 20–60 s seizure within the brain.
- Typically, a course of ECT is delivered twice a week for between 3–6 weeks.

Side effects

- Headaches and arrythmias
- Short term memory impairment
- Retrograde amnesia
  (both short and long term)

Contraindications

- Raised intracranial pressure
  (absolute contraindication)
- Stroke and myocardial infarction
  (relative contraindication)

- **Deep brain stimulation (DBS)**

Deep brain stimulation (DBS) is a surgical procedure that implants a neurostimulator and electrodes in the brain to deliver impulses to specified targets in the brain.

- The exact mechanism of action of DBS is not known.
- It is used as a refractory treatment for movement disorders like Parkinson's disease, as well as treatment-resistant depression and obsessive-compulsive disorder.
- DBS carries the risks of major surgery (bleeding, infection) as well as neuropsychiatric side effects (hallucinations, depression, euphoria).

Mental State Examination

The mental state examination (MSE) is a way of observing and describing a patient's current state of mind to get a cross-sectional description of the patient's mental state.
- It is a time-specific snapshot of the patient's current mental state.
- This is combined with the psychiatric history, allowing clinicians to assess the overall state of the patient's condition. You can remember the components by the acronym.

A Brilliant **S**cientist **M**akes **A**ll **T**heories **T**oo **P**erfectly **C**omplicated "**In-it**"

Appearance

This is the first component of the mental state examination, which is a general description of the patient's appearance. It is important to include the following.
- An opening sentence summarising their gender build and ethnicity.
- A description of their clothes – is it appropriate for the setting?
- Are they well kempt or is their evidence of poor personal hygiene?
- Are there any distinctive features (e.g. adornments, tattoos, scars)?
- Are there any odd or repetitive movements? Do they appear suspicious or guarded?

Example: Mr. Bloggs is an obese Caucasian gentleman, dressed in a hospital gown on the ward. There was evidence of unkempt hair and poor dentition, and he had a large tattoo on his right wrist of a scorpion.

Behaviour

This describes the patient's ability to engage with you.
- What was their general manner – agitated, threatening, tearful?
- How was the eye contact – maintained, avoidant, intense?
- Rapport – could you establish a friendly rapport with them?

Example: He was polite, maintained good eye contact and was able to establish a friendly rapport during the interview.

Speech

The speech is important as it is correlated to mood and to the patient's thoughts.
- Describe the tone (variation in pitch), rate (speed) and volume (quantity).
- Normal speech can be described as "spontaneous, logical, relevant and coherent".
- In mania, patients may display "pressure of speech" (rate/volume are increased).
- In depression, the tone, rate and volume are usually decreased.

Example: Speech was normal in tone, rate and volume, spontaneous and coherent.

Describe if there are any specific patterns of abnormal speech.

Circumstantial	The patient cannot answer a question without giving excess unnecessary detail. However, they will still be able to answer the question in the end
Tangential	The patient goes off on a tangent and will not answer the question
Perseveration	Repeating ideas or words despite an attempt to change the topic
Clanging	A speech pattern where sounds rather than the meaning govern the use of words
Neologisms	The use of made-up words e.g. saying "head-shoe" instead of "hat" (seen in schizophrenia)
Echolalia	Repetition of someone else's speech, including the question that was asked

Mood

This describes the patient's underlying emotion, which is steady and prevailing:
- First describe subjective mood – this is how the patient describes their own mood.
- Then describe objective mood – this is your assessment of the patient's mood.
- This can be anxious, depressed, dysthymic, euthymic (normal) or elated.

Example: He was subjectively "low"; objectively depressed.

Affect

This is the observed, short-term external demonstration of emotion.
- Whereas mood is like the generate climate, the affect is used to describe the current transient state which incorporates responses to external stimuli.
- A normal affect can be described as reactive, where the patients demonstrates appropriate emotional responses to external stimuli and matters.

Abnormal affects include the following:
- Blunted (lacking emotional response)
- Labile (excessively changeable)
- Suspicious
- Incongruous (out of tune with subject matter e.g. laughing about bereavement)

Example: Blunted at times, but overall reactive to content of discussion.

Thought form

This refers to how the patient structures their thoughts and whether they are connected to each other:
- Assess whether their thoughts are logical, relevant and coherent or disordered.
- Assess for any specific abnormalities in thought form.

i) Flight of ideas – this is where patients leap from one topic to another without an obvious links between the ideas.

ii) Derailment/loosening of associations – here there is little to no logical link between words or statements. There are specific terms to learn.
- Word salad – this is a complete jumble of words Example: Blunted at times, but overall reactive to content of discussion
- Verbigeration – sounds/words repeated in a senseless way
- Knights move thinking – unexpected and illogical leaps from one topic to another

iii) Thought block – this is where patient's thought processes suddenly halt.

Example: The patient had relevant and coherent thoughts with no evidence of any formal thought disorder.

Thought content

This refers to the actual content of the patient's thoughts, including delusions.
- This is important as various mental illnesses usually give specific types of beliefs.

Overvalued ideas
These are understandable thoughts, but they are pursued by the patient beyond bounds of reason to the point that it causes distress (e.g. an intense belief that they are responsible for a death).

Delusion
This is a false belief out of keeping with the patient's sociocultural background held with unshakeable conviction even in the face of contradictory evidence.

Obsessions
Persistent and intrusive thoughts, impulses and mental images which cause distress.

Ideas of reference
This is a belief that innocuous events are of specific significance to the individual.
- For example, a casual conversation amongst others being interpreted as others talking negatively about that individual.

Negative cognitions
This includes low self-esteem, guilt, worthlessness, hopelessness etc.
- Depersonalisation – the feeling that the patient is disconnected from their body/mind.
- Derealisation – feeling as if the outside world is in some way unreal and disconnected.

Suicidal ideation
Always check for thoughts, plans and intent to end their life, as this will form a critical part of assessing their risk to themselves and others.

Example: The patient had no delusions. He described low self-esteem, guilt and had suicidal thoughts daily, but had no plans or intent to end his life.

Perception

This section addresses whether the patient experiences phenomena which are not present in reality.

Illusion
This is a misinterpretation of a normal perception (e.g. mistaking a rope for a snake).
- It can occur in healthy people but is more frequent in psychotic illness.

Hallucinations
These are perceptions which occur in the absence of an external stimulus. They are experienced as coming from the outside world, rather than a product of the mind.
- They occur in any sensory modality but auditory and visual are the most common.
- You can experience hallucinations in the normal human experience when falling asleep (hypnagogic hallucinations) or on waking (hypnopompic hallucinations).
- If auditory hallucinations are present, make sure you characterise them further according to whether they are command type, second person (directly talking to the individual) or third person (talking about the individual).
- The latter commonly occurs in schizophrenia as a running commentary.

Pseudo-hallucinations
These are experienced as mentally internal perceptions with some preserved insight e.g. "I hear a voice in my head saying, 'I'm wrong' but I know it's in not real."

Example: He said that he could smell rotting flesh, and he heard the voice of his dead mother blaming him for her death.

Cognition

This involves testing the 5 basic aspects of brain function to see if the patient has functional impairment. If any of these are impaired, then do a formal assessment of cognition using either MOCA or ACE-R. Check for:
- Level of consciousness – is the patient alert and responsive?
- Orientation – are they aware of the time (day, date, time), place and who they are?
- Attention and concentration – can the patient count backwards in 3 s/7 s or spell WORLD backwards?
- Memory – can the patient repeat a list of >3 objects or remember an address immediately and after 5 minutes?
- Executive functioning – can the patient understand/interpret proverbs or perform approximations (e.g. height of landmark)?

Example: Alert and well orientated. However, the patient could not concentrate and had poor working memory.

Insight

This section is about the patient's understanding of their condition and its cause as well as their willingness to accept treatment. Address the following:
- Does the patient realise they are ill – do they acknowledge their experiences are abnormal and symptomatic of an illness?
- Treatment – are they willing to accept types of treatment offered after counselling?
- Can they appreciate the complexity of their care plan when aspects of risk management are incorporated?
- Treatment – are they happy to stay in hospital? Will they consent to treatment?

Example: Patient is aware that he has psychotic depression. He understands the need for treatment. Consenting to take medication and for psychological therapy.

Antidepressants

- **Selective serotonin reuptake inhibitors (SSRIs)** – Fluoxetine, sertraline, citalopram, escitalopram, paroxetine

These are inhibitors of the serotonin transporter (SERT), which prevent the reuptake of serotonin (5-HT) from the synaptic cleft, potentiating its action.

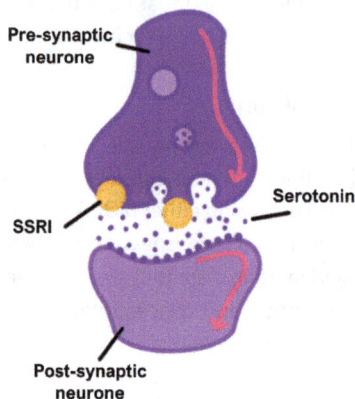

Pre-synaptic neurone

Serotonin

SSRI

Post-synaptic neurone

- They are first-line in the treatment of depression but can take a few weeks to work.
- When starting patients on SSRIs, review them after 2 weeks.
- If young (< 30) or at a higher risk of suicide then it is suggested to review them after 1 week, as a side effect is increased suicidal thoughts in the early phase of treatment.

Side effects

- Gastric irritation
- Hyponatraemia (due to SIADH)
- Anxiety
- Suicidal thoughts (more in young)
- Weight gain
- Sexual dysfunction
- Headaches
- Prolongation of the QTc interval

There is also a small risk of bleeding platelets store high concentrations of 5-HT.
- Caution should be given when SSRIs are used with NSAIDs as there is a potentiation of the effect on 5HT activity increasing the risk of GI bleeding.
- You can mitigate this risk by prescribing a proton pump inhibitor.

Pregnancy	Fluoxetine is usually the SSRI of choice in pregnancy
	Paroxetine (< 20 weeks) can lead to heart defects
	Sertraline (> 20 weeks) is associated with persistent pulmonary hypertension of the newborn
Breastfeeding	Sertraline is the SSRI of choice
Children	Fluoxetine is the SSRI of choice, and it has the longest half-life

- **Serotonin noradrenaline reuptake inhibitors (SNRIs) –** Duloxetine, venlafaxine

These drugs inhibit both serotonin and noradrenaline (NA) reuptake.
- This potentiates 5-HT and NA transmission at the synaptic cleft.
- They act as SSRIs at low doses, whereas a higher dose is needed to achieve the nor-
  adrenergic effects.

Side effects

- Hypertension, tachycardia, SSRI side effects

- **Noradrenaline re-uptake inhibitors (NARIs) –** Reboxetine, atomoxetine

These drugs help to boost noradrenergic and dopaminergic activity in the prefrontal
cortex but are less effective for depression than SSRIs and SNRIs.

Side effects

- Insomnia, postural hypotension, sweating

- **5-HT$_2$ antagonists –** Trazodone, nefazodone

These can cause substantial drowsiness at low doses so are often used off label to treat
insomnia as well as anxiety and depression.

Side effects

- Sedation, GI disturbances and priapism (erection for hours)

- **Tricyclic antidepressants –** Amitriptyline, nortriptyline, dosulepin

These drugs inhibit the NET (NA transporter) and SERT (5-HT reuptake protein) but not
the dopamine (DA) transporter.
- They have many side effects as they are antagonists of α-adrenoceptors, muscarinic
  acetylcholine and histamine H$_1$-receptors.

Side effects

- Anticholinergic – memory dysfunction, dry mouth, blurred vision, constipation, urinary
  retention
- Antihistaminergic – weight gain, sedation
- α-receptor inhibition – postural hypotension, reflex tachycardia, arrhythmias
- Lengthening of the QTc interval
- Inhibition of Na$^+$ channels in heart/brain – seizures, coma, arrhythmias, delirium
- SIADH – leads to hyponatraemia

- **Mirtazapine**

This drug inhibits negative feedback α_2-receptors on 5-HT neurones, which is thought to lead to enhanced noradrenergic and serotonergic activity in the brain.
- It is a strong antagonist of serotonin 5-HT$_{2A}$ and 5-HT$_3$.
- It is also a potent antagonist of histamine H$_1$ receptors, a property that may explain its prominent sedative effects.
- However, it also blocks the 5-HT receptors in other pathways leading to the side effects of sexual dysfunction.

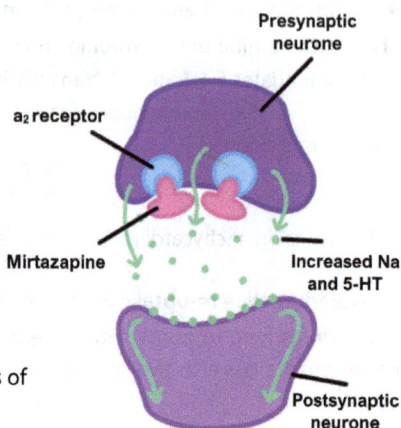

Presynaptic neurone

a₂ receptor

Mirtazapine

Increased Na and 5-HT

Postsynaptic neurone

Side effects
- Increased appetite, weight gain, sedation

- **Monoamine oxidase inhibitors** – Phenelzine, tranylcypromine, moclobemide

These drugs inhibit the activity of the enzyme monoamine oxidase (MAO-A and MAO-B) which normally degrades noradrenaline and serotonin, prolonging their action.
- There are associated with a high risk of discontinuation syndrome on cessation.

Side effects
- Postural hypotension
- In the presence of indirectly acting sympathomimetics (e.g. tyramine in food, amphetamines) they can lead to excessive neurotransmission giving rise to arrhythmias and hypertension
- Can also cause serotonin syndrome when given together with SSRIs

- **Agomelatine**

This is a melatonin agonist at MT$_1$ and MT$_2$ receptors but also blocks the 5-HT$_{2C}$ receptor. It has been shown to resynchronise circadian rhythms in animal models.
- It is also thought to boost DA and NA in the pre-frontal cortex which gives it an antidepressant effect.

Side effects
- Sedation (so taken at night), elevated liver enzymes, weight gain, fatigue

The anti-depressants drugs are associated with a few complications.

○ **Discontinuation syndrome**

This is a syndrome which can occur when antidepressants are stopped suddenly.
- The underlying mechanism is unclear, but it can affect up to half of patients who stop their medication abruptly.
- It is seen in greater incidence in patients who have taken medicines for more than a month as well as the antidepressants with a shorter half-life.
- To prevent it, patients should stay on SSRIs for 6 months after remission from their symptoms and the dose should be gradually reduced over at least a 4-week period.

Symptoms

- Flu-like symptoms – nausea, vomiting, diarrhoea, headaches, sweating
- Sleep disturbances – insomnia, nightmares, constant sleepiness
- Sensory and movement disturbances – imbalance, tremors, vertigo, dizziness
- Brain "zaps" – shock sensations starting in the head and moving through the body
- Mood disturbances – anxiety, dysphoria

Management

- Consider restarting the anti-depressant and then weaning off slowly
- Consider switching to an anti-depressant with a longer half-life (e.g. fluoxetine)

○ **Serotonin syndrome**

This is when excessive serotonin transmission leads to hyperstimulation of the CNS causing autonomic and neuromuscular excitation with an altered mental state.
- Symptoms usually have a fast onset, occurring within a matter of hours.
- It is associated with recreational drug use (ecstasy and amphetamines) as well as MAO-inhibitors and SSRIs at high doses or combining serotonergic drugs.

Symptoms

- Cognitive effects – headache, agitation, hypomania, confusion, hallucinations
- Autonomic effects – dilated eyes, hyperthermia, hypertension, tachycardia, nausea
- Somatic effects – myoclonus (muscle twitching), hyperreflexia, tremor

Management

- Supportive management with IV fluids and benzodiazepines
- If severe, 5-HT antagonists (cyproheptadine) can be used

Antipsychotics

These drugs primarily work by blocking the dopamine D_2 receptors in the mesolimbic and mesocortical areas of the brain.

- The greater the dopamine receptor binding affinity, the better the clinical potency and efficacy of the drug.
- They are classically divided into two major groups: 1st generation (typical antipsychotics) and 2nd generation (atypical).
- Although many side effects are seen in both typical and atypical antipsychotics, some are more likely to be experienced by one group over the other.

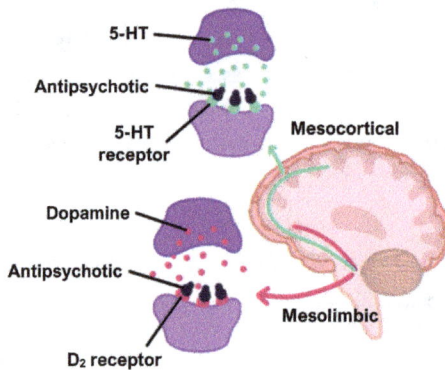

Common side effects

- Anticholinergic – diplopia, dry mouth, confusion
- Sedation
- Prolongation of the QT interval
- Hyperprolactinaemia – galactorrhoea, amenorrhea, sexual dysfunction
- SIADH – hyponatraemia
- Postural hypotension
- Cardiovascular disease – increased risk of stroke and venous thromboembolism

General monitoring

- As the anti-psychotics have so many side effects, regular monitoring FBC, U&E, LFT, blood glucose, BMI and prolactin is important
- These parameters are assessed on a variable schedule (e.g. baseline, at 3 months and then on an annual basis)
- As many affect the QTc interval, it is important to conduct a baseline ECG and carry out an annual cardiovascular risk assessment

- **1st generation** – Haloperidol, chlorpromazine, fluphenazine, trifluoperazine

These drugs principally antagonise dopamine D_2 receptors. They give an immediate quietening action and have a greater effect on alleviating positive symptoms.
- "Typical" refers to their propensity to cause extrapyramidal side effects, which are seen in greater incidence in this group compared to the atypical antipsychotics.

Extrapyramidal side effects (EPSEs)
- These refer to symptoms that are archetypically associated with the extrapyramidal system of the brain's cerebral cortex. They include:
- Acute dystonia – sustained muscle contraction e.g. torticollis, oculogyric crisis
- Akathisia – severe restlessness
- Parkinsonism – tremor and bradykinesia
- Tardive dyskinesia – slow abnormal, involuntary movements that usually have a late onset. They typically involve chewing or pouting movements

Management
- In the acute phase, can use anticholinergic medications e.g. procyclidine
- Consider reducing the dose of antipsychotic or switching to an atypical antipsychotic

- **2nd generation** – Olanzapine, risperidone, quetiapine

These drugs have lower D_2 receptor affinity but also cause an additional block of 5-HT receptors. They have an effect of alleviating both positive and negative symptoms.
- These have replaced the typical drugs as first-line for several conditions.
- They are less associated with causing EPSEs but have other effects.

Side effects
- Reduced seizure threshold
- Metabolic syndrome – weight gain, poor glucose control (diabetes)
- Risperidone is particularly associated hyperprolactinaemia
- Olanzapine is associated with significant weight gain

- **Aripiprazole**

Unlike the other drugs, this is a dopaminergic partial agonist rather than antagonist.
- It has the most tolerable side effect profile.
- It is a good choice if patients have experienced or are at high risk of hyperprolactin-aemia, metabolic syndrome or QTc prolongation.

- **Clozapine**

This is a 3rd line treatment, only used in patients who are "treatment resistant".
- This is defined as continuous symptoms after at least 2 trials of other antipsychotics.
- It has a unique receptor profile acting on dopamine and serotonin receptors.
- It is very effective as an antipsychotic but has some serious adverse effects in addition to the ones above.

Side effects
- Risk of agranulocytosis (neutropenia), particularly in the first year – this requires weekly FBC monitoring for the first 18 weeks
- Myocarditis and seizures – these are common on initiation
- CYP enzyme metabolism – the clozapine plasma level is increased when smokers stop smoking as smoking is a CYP enzyme inducer
- Constipation, paralytic ileus and toxic megacolon
- Hypersalivation

Neuroleptic Malignant Syndrome
This is one of the most dangerous complications of the anti-psychotics.
- The dopamine blockade triggers massive amounts of glutamate release which causes sympathetic hyperactivity and muscle damage.
- Risk factors include high doses of typical antipsychotics, rapid dose increases and underlying organic brain disease.
- Symptoms usually occur within hours to days of starting the antipsychotic.
- Blood tests typically show an acute kidney injury, raised CK (muscle damage), leucocytosis (raised WCC) and a metabolic acidosis.

Symptoms

- High fever (hyperthermia)
- Muscle "lead pipe" rigidity
- Reduced reflexes
- Agitated delirium with confusion
- Hypertension and tachycardia
- Pupils are usually normal

Management

- Stop the antipsychotic and treat the hyperthermia aggressively
- May require supportive care in ICU with circulatory and ventilatory support
- Dantrolene – this inhibits ryanodine receptors to stop Ca^{2+} release and relax muscle
- Bromocriptine – this is a dopamine agonist which can also be used

Mood Stabilisers

These drugs are used in the management of mania as they help to stabilise mood.
- They can also be used as adjuncts in the management of affective disorders.

- **Lithium**

This is a drug that is thought to influence multiple neurotransmitter systems.
- It inhibits phospholipid recycling, decreasing activity of messengers DAG and IP_3.
- It comes in many preparations (carbonate/citrate) with different bio-availabilities.
- It is used as a first-line maintenance treatment in bipolar disorder.
- It has a very narrow therapeutic range is excreted by the kidneys.

Side effects
- Nausea and vomiting
- Weight gain
- Fine tremor
- Idiopathic intracranial hypertension
- Slower activity on EEG
- Raised WCC (leucocytosis)
- T wave flattening and inversion on an ECG
- Not used in first trimester of pregnancy due to association with Ebstein's foetal anomaly

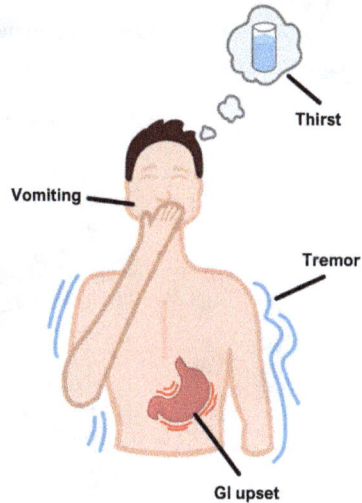

Thirst

Vomiting

Tremor

GI upset

Lithium also affects many hormonal systems giving additional side effects:
- ADH – leads to nephrogenic diabetes insipidus and nephrotoxicity
- Thyroid – causes thyroid enlargement and potential hypothyroidism
- PTH – can cause hyperparathyroidism increasing serum calcium levels

Monitoring
- Due to its narrow therapeutic index, lithium levels should initially be checked weekly then every 3 months once the level is stable
- It is also important to check thyroid and renal function every 6 months

Toxicity
- This is associated with serum lithium concentrations > 1.5 mM
- It is triggered frequently by dehydration, renal failure or nephrotoxic drugs

- These cause renal dysfunction which results in lithium accumulation in the body
- Toxicity presents with motor signs (coarse tremor and hyperreflexia) and neurological symptoms (confusion, seizures)
- There is no specific antidote to lithium toxicity and treatment is generally supportive
- In severe toxicity, peritoneal or haemodialysis may be required

- **Anti-epileptics – Sodium valproate, carbamazepine**

These drugs inhibit voltage gated sodium channels.
- They are typically used to treat epilepsy, but have an additional effect of mood stabalisation, thought to be due to their ability to boost cortical GABA activity.

Side effects
- Valproate is known to be teratogenic so it is avoided in females of childbearing age
- Carbamazepine is a cytochrome P450 inducer

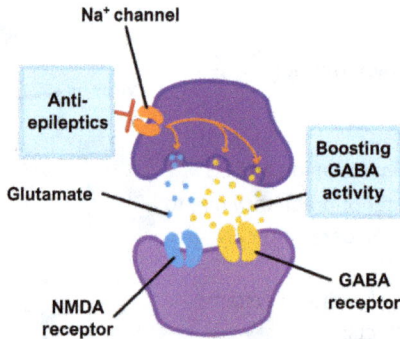

- **Lamotrigine**

Lamotrigine inhibits voltage-gated sodium channels, stabilises presynaptic neuronal membranes and inhibits presynaptic glutamate and aspartate release.
- It is a good choice during pregnancy.

Side effects
- Associated with Steven-Johnsons syndrome and should be titrated slowly

- **Second generation antipsychotics – Olanzapine, quetiapine, risperidone**

In addition to their efficacy in treating psychosis, these drugs have mood stabilising properties and so are often used in conjunction with mood stabilisers.

Affective Disorders

Affective (mood disorders) are characterised by persistent emotional disturbances resulting in functional impairment. The aetiology of affective disorders can be formulated using the biopsychosocial model.

Biological
- 5-HT – low levels of endogenous 5-HT and Na are thought to decrease mood
- Cortisol – overactivation of the hypothalamic-pituitary-adrenal (HPA) axis precipitates the onset of and maintenance of low mood

Psychological
- Beck's triad – negative views about the self, the world and the future precipitate and maintain depression
- Attributional style of thinking – there is a higher incidence of depression in people who blame themselves for life events

Social
- Stressful events and childhood adversity – these factors are associated with pre-disposing, precipitating and maintaining depression

- **Depression**

This is a mental health condition, which is a leading cause of disability worldwide.
- According to the World Health Organisation (WHO), about 280 million people world-wide have depression, including 5% of the world's adults.
- It is characterised by periods of low mood which leads to functional impairment and emotional distress.

Core symptoms

- Low mood (often worse in the morning – diurnal variation)
- Anhedonia – this refers to the inability to experience joy or pleasure
- Reduced energy (fatigue)

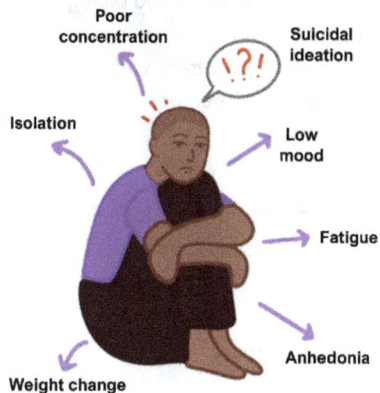

Poor concentration
Suicidal ideation
Isolation
Low mood
Fatigue
Anhedonia
Weight change

Other symptoms

- Reduced concentration/attention
- Guilt and worthlessness
- Changes in appetite with associated weight change
- Sleep disturbances (early morning waking)
- Suicidal ideation
- Psychomotor disturbances

Diagnosis

- To be diagnosed, patients require ≥ 2 core symptoms which last at least 2 weeks
- Mild = 2 core symptoms + ≥ 2 other symptoms
- Moderate = 2 core symptoms + ≥ 4 other symptoms
- Severe = 3 core symptoms + ≥ 5 other symptoms

Special cases

Severe depression
- This can lead to psychotic symptoms e.g. delusions and hallucinations
- Delusions are typically mood-congruent and include delusions of guilt, poverty or nihilism. Hallucinations will also usually be of critical voices or the smell of rotting/decomposing flesh

Children
- In children, the core symptom can be either low mood or irritable mood

Elderly
- Depression can present with cognitive symptoms (a depressive pseudodementia)
- Unlike dementia, the onset of memory loss will have been acute or sub-acute
- There are often associated biological symptoms of depression e.g. weight loss
- Patients can have preserved awareness of their memory loss
- Patients usually present with global memory loss whereas dementia usually presents with short term memory impairment first

Key tests

- The Patient health questionnaire-9 (scored out of 27) is used to grade depression
- It asks patients to report over the last 2 weeks how often they have been experiencing symptoms. It composes of 9 items, each of which is rated from 0–3

- Mild = 5–9
- Moderate = 10–14
- Moderate/severe = 15–19
- Severe is > 19

Management

Mild/moderate
- The patient should be involved in treatment decisions as much as possible
- Options include various therapies, both group and individual
- This includes guided self-help, CBT, behavioural activation, exercise programmes, IPT, counselling, short term psychodynamic psychotherapy and SSRIs
- Medication should not be offered 1st line unless this is a patient preference

Severe
- 1st line is individual CBT and an antidepressant (SSRI)
- In children, it is advised to not use SSRIs if avoidable
- However, if required, the first choice is usually fluoxetine

When starting someone on SSRIs, review them after 2 weeks.
- If they are young (< 30) or at a higher risk of suicide then review < 1 week as activation symptoms as side effects can include new or worsening suicidal ideation.
- Treatment with antidepressants should continue for 6 months after treatment response is achieved.
- If multiple treatments of differing classes of antidepressants have failed, ECT or deep brain stimulation of subgenual cingulate cortex can be considered.

- **Schizoaffective disorder**
This is a mental disorder which is characterised by having psychotic and mood symptoms within the same episode.
- A diagnosis is made when person has symptoms of schizophrenia and a depression or mania but does not meet the diagnostic criteria for either condition individually.
- It can either be bipolar type (manic with schizophrenic symptoms) or depressive type (depressive with schizophrenic symptoms).

Diagnosis
- Main criterion is the presence of psychotic symptoms for at least two weeks with mood (manic/depressive/mixed) symptoms

Management
- Antipsychotics +/- mood-stabiliser (if manic) +/- anti-depressant (if depressed)
- Psychotherapy e.g. CBT which can individualised or with the family

- **Anxiety disorders**

Anxiety is an unpleasant emotional state involving subjective fear, discomfort and physical symptoms mediated through autonomic arousal.
- The disorder occurs when anxiety is persistent or situational, is associated with distress and impairs function.
- It is common and the incidence in women is double that of men.
- The causes can similarly be viewed from a biopsychosocial model.
- It is important to also rule out any organic causes of anxiety – these include hyperthyroidism, heart disease, drugs (salbutamol, SSRIs, caffeine, steroids).

○ **Generalised anxiety disorder**

This is an anxiety disorder which characterised by persistent "free floating" anxiety that is not focused on any one subject or situation.
- Symptoms need to be present for at least 6 months (ICD-11) to get a diagnosis.

Symptoms

- Physical – insomnia, autonomic hyperactivity
- Emotional – subjective worry, increased vigilance
- Social impairment and dysfunction

Diagnosis

- The generalised anxiety disorder scale (GAD-7) is a questionnaire consisting of 7 elements (scored 0–3) which provides a total cumulative score out of 21
- It is used as a screening tool for generalised anxiety and asks patients to rate how often they experience anxiety-type symptoms
- Mild anxiety = 6–10   - Moderate = 11–15   - Severe = 16–21

Management

Mild
- Low intensity interventions – individual guided self-help, group therapy

Moderate/severe
- CBT or SSRI (sertraline is the first-line SSRI)
- Be careful in young people as SSRIs increase anxiety initially after commencing treatment and can lead to suicidal thoughts
- If acutely anxious with associated risks, may consider a short course of benzodiazepines (used with caution as high risk of dependence)

○ **Panic disorder**

This is a disorder which is characterised by short episodes of intense anxiety which occur unpredictably.

Symptoms
- Brief attacks of intense terror and apprehension
- Marked by trembling, shaking, confusion, dizziness, nausea, and difficulty breathing
- Attacks last a few minutes and patients have an "anticipatory fear" of getting attacks

Management
- 1st line is CBT or SSRI
- If SSRI not tolerated or no response in 3 months, can try imipramine or clomipramine

● **Phobias**

This refers to an excessively disproportionate fear of specific stimuli which is characterised by avoidance of the stimulus.

○ **Agoraphobia**

This refers to fear of a crowded situation from which escape is difficult (public places, shops, transport etc.). It is often associated with panic disorder.

Management: 1st line is CBT or SSRI

○ **Simple phobia**

This refers to a single isolated phobia (e.g. injections/spiders).

Management: 1st line is graded exposure therapy and response prevention

○ **Separation anxiety disorder**

This refers to fear of being apart from a caregiver, which is seen in children.

○ **Social phobia**

A persistent fear of social situations due to fear that they will be embarrassed.

Management: 1st line is CBT, if treatment refractory add on an SSRI

● **Obsessive-compulsive disorder (OCD)**

This disorder is characterised by the presence of distressing obsessions and compulsions, which results in emotional disturbance or functional impairment.
- It is associated with parental overprotection, childhood streptococcal infection and Tourette's syndrome.

There are subtypes that include either predominantly obsessive rumination, predominantly compulsive behaviour or both obsession and compulsions together.

Symptoms

- The 2 main symptoms are having obsessions and compulsions leading to distress
- Obsession – an intrusive idea, image or impulse which is intrusive and hard to resist. Patients are aware that this is a product of their own mind despite the thoughts often being repugnant e.g. feeling contaminated, sexualised images
- Compulsion – a repetitive action that a patient performs with reluctance in order to neutralise an obsession e.g. handwashing, arranging objects in a certain way

Diagnosis

- Presence of obsessions and/or compulsions > 1 hour a day for > 2 weeks
- Must cause emotional distress or interfere with activities of daily living

Management

- If mild – 1st line is CBT and exposure and response prevention (ERP)
- If moderate/severe – combined treatment with CBT with ERP and SSRI

- **Bipolar disorder**

This is a disorder which is characterised by recurrent episodes of altered mood including both elevations and depressions.
- The peak age of onset is in the early 20s and it is seen equally in males and females.
- The majority of patients have a recurrence of manic or depressive episodes.
- Patients will have episodes of depression interspersed with mania/hypomania.

Symptoms

Depression
- Low mood, anhedonia and low energy for > 2 weeks

Mania
- This refers to a period of elevated or irritable mood which meets 5 criteria:
i)   Elevated/irritable mood lasting 7 days or more
ii) At least 3 of: less sleep, flight of ideas, disinhibition, high energy levels, grandiosity
iii) Marked impairment of social functioning
iv) No psychotic symptoms in the absence of mood disturbance
v)   No organic factors causing the mania (e.g. stimulant drugs or brain tumour)

Hypomania
- This is a less severe form of mania which lasts for 4 days or more
- In comparison to mania, there are no psychotic symptoms
- There is a noticeable mood change but limited impact on work and social function

Types
- Bipolar disorder I – episodes of mania and depression (most common)
- Bipolar disorder II – episodes of hypomania and depression

Management
- Involves maintenance treatment and acutely treating depressive/manic episodes
- If the patient has symptoms of mania, they need an urgent referral to the community mental health team given the potential associated risks (e.g. of suicide)

Maintenance therapy
- Offer psychological interventions (e.g. CBT) and a mood stabilising drug
- 1st line is lithium, 2nd line is sodium valproate, olanzapine or quetiapine
- Avoid sodium valproate in women of childbearing age given risk of teratogenesis

For mania
- First ensure that the patient stops taking any antidepressant which may precipitate the manic episode, then treat with antipsychotics
- 1st line is an antipsychotic e.g. olanzapine, quetiapine, risperidone, haloperidol
- It resistant, switch antipsychotic and then consider adding lithium
- Third-line refractory treatments include ECT

For depression
- Treat with antipsychotics alone or in combination with SSRIs
- Avoid prescribing SSRIs by themselves as they can precipitate mania
- 1st line is quetiapine or olanzapine +/- fluoxetine
- 2nd line includes anti-epileptics with mood stabilising effects such as lamotrigine

Psychotic Disorders

Psychosis is the misrepresentation of thoughts and perceptions that originate from a patient's own mind, which they experience as reality.
- It describes a constellation of symptoms and is not a diagnosis in itself.

As with all psychiatric conditions, the aetiology of psychosis can be looked at using a biopsychosocial model.

Biological
- Genetics – twin studies show schizophrenia has 50% concordance rate in MZ twins
- Dopamine – psychosis is associated with high levels of dopaminergic transmission in the brain. Antipsychotics block D_2 receptors whereas L-Dopa induces psychosis
- Neurodevelopmental factors – rates are higher in people with low birth weight, developmental delay etc.
- Physical illness – structural brain disease or neuroinflammation can lead to psychotic symptoms

Psychological
- Mental illness – conditions associated with psychosis include schizophrenia, depression, bipolar affective disorder and insomnia
- A history of abuse, trauma and childhood adversity are strongly associated

Social
- Stress – social deprivation, urbanisation and stressful live events are associated with the development and persistence of psychosis

Phases of illness
- Functional illnesses (disorders not directly attributable to a physical illness/substances), are often early indicators in a prodromal phase
- This precedes the more acute onset of illness
- A prodrome can include anxiety, depression, social withdrawal, reduced performance in work/employment, ideas of reference or holding unusual beliefs

● **Schizophrenia**

This is the most famous psychotic condition, which is more frequent in men.
- It typically arises before the age of 40 and is linked with the risk factors before.
- In the 19th century it was known as "Dementia praecox".

Patients with schizophrenia face distressing symptoms of schizophrenia and also find it difficult to tolerate side effects of treatment.
- Both symptoms and side effects can be understood through looking at the dopamine pathways in the brain. There are 4 main dopaminergic pathways in the brain.

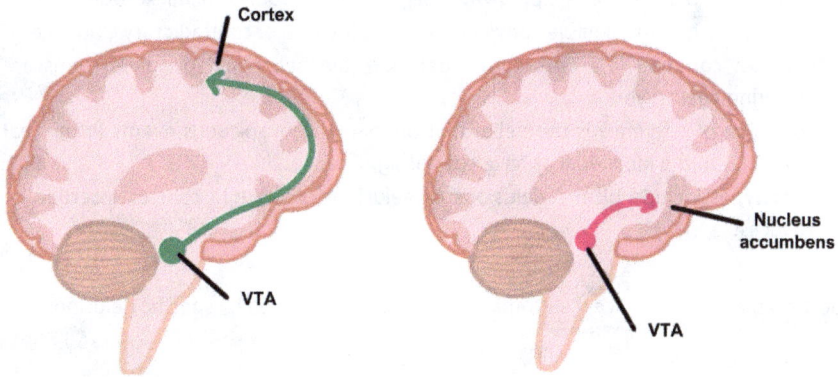

Mesolimbic (ventral tegmental area to nucleus accumbens)
- This is involved in the reward pathway and attributing salience to a stimulus
- Excessive dopaminergic activity in this pathway is thought to produce positive symptoms such as delusions and hallucinations

Mesocortical (pre-frontal cortex)
- Dopamine mediates pathways involved in executive function, emotion and speech
- Underactive dopamine in this pathway is associated with the negative symptoms of schizophrenia such as alogia, anhedonia and blunted affect

Nigrostriatal (substantia nigra to basal ganglia)
- Dopamine here increases voluntary motor movements
- Anti-psychotic (D_2-blockers) action here can lead to extrapyramidal symptoms

Tuberoinfundibular (to anterior pituitary)
- Dopamine neurones in this pathway inhibit prolactin secretion
- This explains why anti-psychotics (D_2-blockers) elevate prolactin release giving hyper-prolactinaemia, leading to amenorrhoea and loss of libido

Positive symptoms
- These are defined as symptoms that manifest through their presence

Hallucinations
- This is a perception which the patient experiences as coming from the outside world
- However, it occurs in the absence of an external stimulus. The most common are 3rd person auditory hallucinations or voices a giving running commentary

Delusion
- This is a false belief out of keeping with the patient's sociocultural background
- This is held with unshakeable conviction even in the face of contradictory evidence
- The most common is a persecutory delusion, the belief that people/systems are conspiring against you
- A delusion of reference is the belief that ordinarily inconspicuous events in the real world refer to the individual or have special significance
- Other types include bizarre delusions or delusions of thought control, insertion or broadcast

Some patients experience syndromes which are characterised by specific delusions.

○ **Cotard's syndrome**
This a delusion which is characterised by a false belief of death.
- The patient believes that they or part of their body is dead or non-existent.
- It is associated with psychotic depression and can lead to extreme neglect as patients believe they no longer need to eat or drink.

○ **De Clerambault's syndrome (erotomania)**
This centres on a delusion about love which is usually seen in young women.
- Individuals will falsely believe that a famous person has fallen in love with them.
- There will often be a complex delusional narrative as to how this occurred.

○ **Othello's delusion**
The patient believes that their spouse is being unfaithful without any sufficient proof.

○ **Folie à deux (shared delusional disorder)**
This is a rare condition when a delusion from a psychotic primary individual is induced in another secondary individual.

Catatonia
- This refers to a complex neuropsychiatric behavioral syndrome that is characterised by abnormal movements, immobility, abnormal behaviors, and withdrawal
- The most common signs of catatonia are immobility, mutism, withdrawal and refusal to eat, staring

Thought disorder
- This is a positive symptom of schizophrenia which describes an impaired capacity to sustain coherent discourse, in written or spoken language

Passivity phenomena
- This is the sense that the individual is no longer able to control their own thoughts, actions, emotions or impulses
- It is often associated with delusions that explain the sense e.g. delusions of persecution by another individual who is in control of the patient

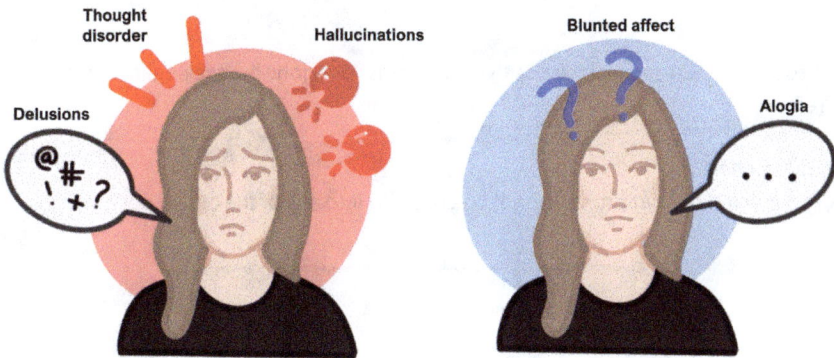

Negative symptoms
- These are defined as symptoms that are present through their absence
- They can be remembered by the 5 A's
- **A**ffect blunted – restricted emotion with poor emotional display
- **A**logia – paucity of speech
- **A**sociality – social isolation
- **A**nhedonia – lack of pleasure
- **A**volition – lack of motivation

Subtypes

Paranoid
- This is the most common type of schizophrenia which is characterised by prominent hallucinations and delusions but mostly normal intellectual functioning and emotion
- The patient feels very suspicious and persecuted

Catatonic
- An uncommon type which is characterised by prominent psychomotor disturbances
- Patient display rigidity, posturing, and abnormalities of voluntary movement

Hebephrenic/disorganised
- This has an early onset, with unpredictable behaviour and speech
- The affect and mood can be inappropriate (e.g. giggling inappropriately)
- Patients can also have fleeting hallucinations and delusions
- Disorganised thoughts and behaviour are prominent

Residual
- A subtype where most of the positive symptoms have gone but the negative symptoms remain

Undifferentiated
- This is when the symptoms cannot be classified into any of the other subtypes

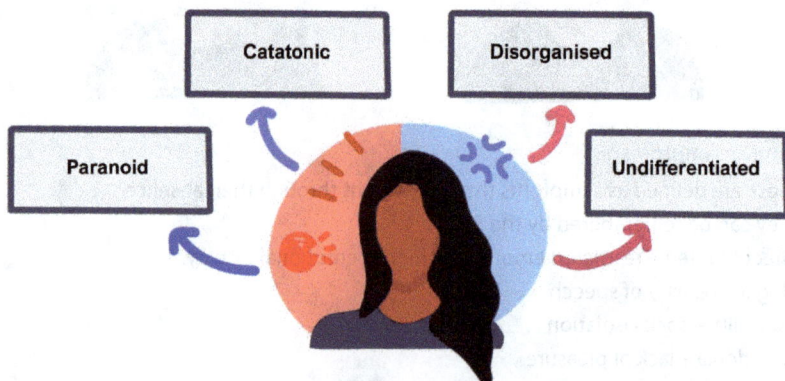

Diagnosis

- The DSM-5 needs > 2 of the following experienced for 1 month. At least 1 should include 1–3. In addition to the symptoms above, there must be a significant impact on social/occupational functioning.
1. Delusions
2. Hallucinations
3. Disorganised speech
4. Disorganised/catatonic behaviour
5. Negative symptoms

Management

Antipsychotics
- The primary management is oral antipsychotics in a staged approach
- 1st line is an oral atypical anti-psychotic (quetiapine, olanzapine, risperidone)
- 2nd line is oral typical anti-psychotic (haloperidol, chlorpromazine etc.)
- 3rd line is clozapine – used for psychosis refractory to other treatments

When prescribing antipsychotics, monitor weight, lipids, glucose and the QTc interval at baseline as well as regular intervals post commencement
- Start at the minimum dose with monotherapy and then titrate up the medication
- Efficacy of a treatment is assessed at 4–6 weeks of a tolerated dose before considering switching to an alternative antipsychotic
- For single episode of psychosis medicate for 6–24 months
- After 2nd episode advise 5 years, if > 2 episodes, life-long medication is advised

Psychotherapy
- CBT – offered to all and helps to challenge delusions and develop coping strategies
- Therapy also includes family therapy to support carers
- Counselling includes psychoeducation to build insight and prevent relapses

Social support
- This includes support around housing, vocation and finances

Prognosis

- The suicide risk peaks in the initial years post diagnosis and is higher in young men
- Good prognostic indicators include female sex, patients with fewer negative symptoms, acute onset and remission and those with good social support

Stress Reactions

- **Acute stress reaction**

This is an acute reaction which occurs rapidly (minutes to hours) after a sudden and stressful event, such as sexual assault, near-death experience, physical illness etc.
- Symptoms can arise and terminate very quickly. Most cases resolve rapidly within 3 days. If symptoms persist > 1 month, it can lead to post-traumatic stress disorder.

Symptoms

- Initial state of being dazed and confused
- Purposeless overactivity, agitation or withdrawal
- Intense brief anxiety
- Autonomic arousal – sweating, dry mouth, vomiting

Management

- Counselling and trauma-focused CBT can help the patient to process the event

- **Post-traumatic stress disorder (PTSD)**

This is a chronic condition that occurs following a traumatic event e.g. sexual assault, near death experience. These events get stored as emotionally charged memories which the patient re-experiences.
- To receive a diagnosis, symptoms must be present > 1 month with an onset < 6 months after the traumatic experience.
- It is associated with a higher risk of depression, substance misuse and unexplained physical symptoms.

Symptoms

- Persistent intrusive thoughts
- Re-experiencing of the event – flashbacks, nightmares and intrusive images
- Autonomic hyperarousal – startle, hypervigilance, insomnia
- Avoidance – patient avoids situations and stimuli associated with the event
- Feeling emotionally detached from people and a lack of ability to experience feelings

Management

- 1st line is trauma-focused CBT (CBT) or eye movement desensitisation and reprocessing (EMDR) therapy
- SSRIs can help to treat the autonomic arousal symptoms and co-morbid depression

- **Adjustment disorder**

This is a condition which encompasses the abnormal psychological symptoms which occur in response to life adversity (e.g. job loss, divorce, physical illness etc).
- Symptoms occur within weeks of a stressful life events and last < 6 months.
- The symptoms mimic those of anxiety and depression, but they are of lower severity, and the patient will typically overcome them within 6 months.

Symptoms
- Anxiety – autonomic arousal, insomnia, hypervigilance
- Depression – sadness, tearfulness, anhedonia, fatigue

Diagnosis
- A diagnosis is only made when symptoms are not sufficient to meet criteria for diagnosing anxiety or depression

Management
- 1st line is counselling, allowing catharsis, problem solving and support to address the stressor
- 2nd line is CBT

- **Abnormal grief reaction**

This is an adjustment disorder which specifically occurs after a bereavement and is characterised by prolonged grief of greater intensity than would occur in other people.
- People are left feeling numb and confused about their role in their life.

Normal grief occurs in 5 stages: denial, anger, bargaining, depression, acceptance.
- These last < 2 years and do not require specific management other than support.
- Stages often overlap and mix and are not necessarily persistent.

In an abnormal grief reaction, the grief is delayed and there is a greater intensity of expression of the stages of normal grief lasting > 2 years.
- It is more likely if the death was unexpected, there was a difficult relationship with the deceased individual or normal grieving was constrained (e.g. putting on a brave face for the children).

Management
- CBT is the mainstay of treatment

Delirium

This refers to an acute confusional state which is characterised by a rapid onset, fluctuant course of global dysfunction of the brain due to a variety of insults.
- It is more commonly seen in people aged > 65 and those with a background of cognitive decline, in particular dementia.
- However, it can be experienced by anyone, especially in hospital environments.

Causes

- The main causes can be remembered using the acronym PINCH-MEE

Pain   **H**ydration
Infection (often a UTI in elderly)   **M**edication (drugs)
Nutrition   **E**lectrolytes (e.g. hyponatraemia)
Constipation   **E**nvironment

Delirium is usually divided into 3 main subtypes.

○ **Hypoactive**

This is a type of delirium where the patient will be withdrawn, drowsy and excessively sleepy. They might display inactive or reduced motor activities and when awake, appear to be in a daze.

○ **Hyperactive**

This is a type where patients will be restless, agitated and may display aggressive behaviour. They may exhibit strong emotions with fear, paranoia and hallucinations.

○ **Mixed**

In this situation, the patient will display signs of both hypo- and hyperactive delirium.

Other symptoms

- Simple, transient delusions – often persecutory with associated ideas of reference
- Autonomic overactivity – sweating, tachycardia and dilated pupils
- Disturbance of the sleep-wake cycle – patients can be more alert during the evening (sun-downing) and drowsy during the day

Key tests

- Full history and physical examination (to identify any causative factors)
- Mental state examination to confirm diagnosis
- Blood tests – FBC, U&E, inflammatory markers, thyroid tests, folate, Vit B_{12}, calcium
- Septic screen to assess for infection – urine culture, blood cultures, CXR
- Brain imaging – CT head or MRI

Diagnosis

- To be diagnosed with delirium, patients should satisfy different the following criteria
- Impaired attention and awareness with perceptual disturbances (visual illusions, hallucinations) or cognitive disturbances (memory/speech/orientation deficit)
- The symptoms must develop over short period of time (hours/days)
- The symptoms should be fluctuating in nature
- Evidence of an underlying physical cause (not a pre-existing psychiatric disorder)

Management

- Treat the underlying cause and correct any electrolyte and fluid imbalances
- Aim for conservative measures first before introducing pharmacological agents
- Conservative measures – aim to make the environment as comfortable as possible, reducing changeover of staff, avoiding over stimulation, optimizing hearing/vision and orientating to time with a clock
- Medical management involves sedatives, including benzodiazepines (lorazepam) or haloperidol (caution is needed in Parkinson's or Lewy body dementia)

It is important to be able to distinguish between delirium and dementia.

	Delirium	Dementia
Onset	Rapid	Slow and chronic
Progression	Fluctuating during day	Slow decline over years
Duration	Short but can lag	Months to years
Cognition	Impaired	Intact early, impaired late
Sleep-wake cycle	Disrupted	Normal
Speech	Confused	Word-finding problems
Thoughts	Disorganised/delusional	Lack of thoughts
Perceptions	Disturbances/hallucinations	Intact early on
Behaviour	Hypo or hyperactive	Normal but forgetful

Dementia

Dementia is not a specific disease but is rather a general term for the impaired ability to remember, think, or make decisions, that interferes with doing everyday activities.
- It is defined by a progressive deterioration in cognitive ability.
- Memory is commonly affected but it can include pure language disorders.
- The most common type of dementia is Alzheimer's disease, which is followed by vascular dementia, Lewy body dementia and frontotemporal dementia.
- Risk factors include age, low educational achievement, vascular risk factors, genetic factors and a positive family history.

Dementia can be difficult to diagnose and there are many assessment tools.
- An abbreviated mental test score (AMTS) can be performed as a screening tool.
- More extensive tests include the mini-mental state examination (MMSE), General Practitioner Assessment of Cognition (GPCOG), Montreal Cognitive Assessment (MOCA) and the Addenbrooke's Cognitive Exam (ACE).

Management
- Exclude reversible causes including infection, electrolyte imbalances etc.
- Blood tests – FBC, U&E, ESR, LFTs, bone profile, glucose, TFT, Vit B_{12} and folate
- Refer to old-age psychiatrists or neurologists (memory clinic)
- Neuroimaging – MRI can exclude structural causes (e.g. subdural haematoma) and identify features of each dementia

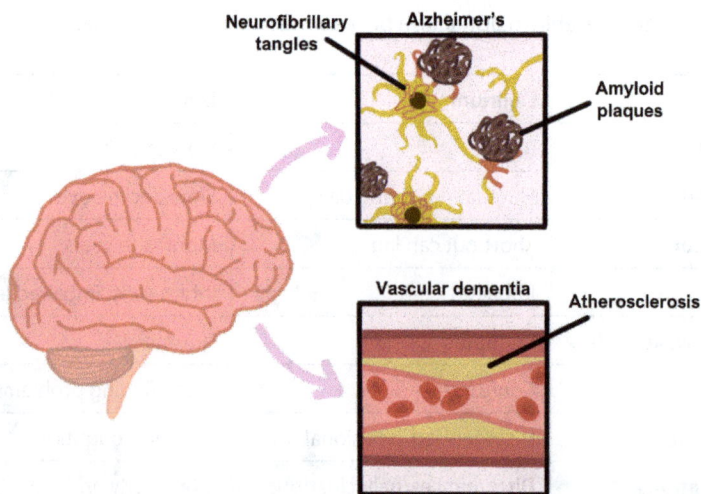

● **Alzheimer's disease**

This is the most common cause of dementia worldwide.

- The disease is characterised by progressive degeneration of the cortex and subcortical areas, and typically occurs sporadically with advancing age.
- Early onset Alzheimer's disease can be familial (e.g. autosomal dominant mutation in presenilin) as well as in Down's syndrome.
- Pathogenesis of the disease is still not fully understood, however it is known that the degradation product of amyloid precursor protein (B-amyloid peptide) accumulates, giving rise to amyloid plaques.
- In addition, tau proteins are known to coalesce, forming neurofibrillary tangles.

Symptoms

- Memory loss – this is progressive, initially affecting short-term memory and later affecting long term episodic memory
- Learned motor and language skills are lost over time
- Changes in behaviour (aggression) and personality

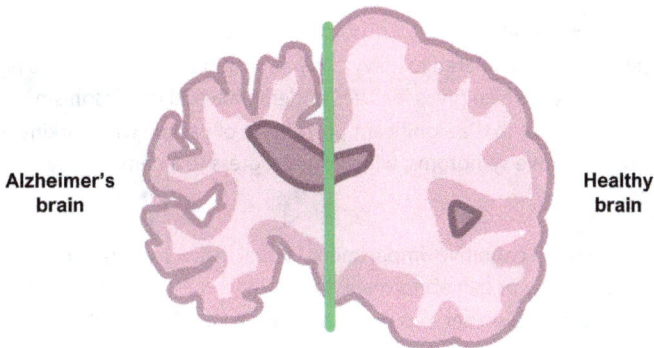

Alzheimer's brain   Healthy brain

Diagnosis

- This is based on clinical features and excluding other diseases
- There is increased usage of imaging and fluid biomarkers, but a definitive diagnosis is only possible at post-mortem

Management

- MDT approach – social support, occupational therapists
- Acetylcholinesterase inhibitors – donepezil, rivastigmine, galantamine
- NMDA antagonists (memantine) can be used in late-stage disease
- Antipsychotics/antidepressants can be used for non-cognitive dementia symptoms

- **Vascular dementia**

This is a very common cause of dementia, which occurs due to brain ischaemia secondary to large vessel infarcts and small vessel disease.
- Risk factors include ischaemic heart disease, hypertension and diabetes mellitus.

Symptoms

- Sudden-onset and stepwise deterioration in memory (after every brain infarction)
- Gait abnormalities, may have focal neurological deficits

Diagnosis

- This is based on clinical features and the exclusion of other causes
- CT/MRI scan will show evidence of strokes and small vessel disease

Management

- Control vascular risk factors (diabetes, hypertension)
- There is no specific pharmacologic therapy
- Behavioural and psychotropic medication if needed for symptomatic management

- **Lewy body dementia**

This is a type of dementia related to Lewy body deposition in the substantia nigra, limbic and neocortical areas, which gives features of dementia and parkinsonism.
- It is important to note that a significant proportion of people with Parkinson's disease also develop cognitive symptoms, which can progress to a dementia syndrome.

Symptoms

- Triad of fluctuating cognitive impartment, visual hallucinations and parkinsonism (bradykinesia, rigidity or gait abnormality)
- REM sleep behaviour disorder also commonly occurs
- Dysautonomia

Diagnosis

- This is based on clinical features
- SPECT (DaT scan) shows reduced dopamine transporter uptake

Management

- This involves acetylcholinesterase inhibitors (donepezil) and memantine
- Antipsychotics are avoided as they can cause irreversible Parkinsonism

- **Frontotemporal dementia (FTD)**

This is a type of dementia which classically affects the frontal and temporal lobes, which causes classic symptoms and is associated with early-onset dementia.

- A behavioural variant FTD (Pick disease) is the most common subtype, which is characterised by the presence of Pick bodies, intracytoplasmic round aggregates of tau protein, which cause destruction of neurones.
- The age of onset is typically before 65 and it progresses slowly.
- Progressive non-fluent aphasia and semantic dementia variants are language pre-dominant phenotypes of frontotemporal dementia.

Symptoms

- Early personality changes – impaired social conduct, disinhibition
- Changes to appetite
- Impairments in executive function

- **Hydrocephalus**

This refers to increased CSF volume in the brain, due to an imbalance between production and absorption. Causes are divided into obstructive (non-communicating) and non-obstructive (communicating).

Causes

Obstructive
- This refers to a mechanical blockage of the flow of CSF between the ventricles
- This causes dilation of the ventricles above the structural block
- In these cases, lumbar puncture is dangerous as it may cause a brain herniation
- Common causes include tumours and developmental abnormalities

Non-obstructive
- This refers to an imbalance between production and absorption of CSF
- Common causes include Increased production (choroid plexus tumour) or a failure to reabsorb the CSF (SAH, meningitis)

Symptoms

- If acute, causes symptoms of raised intracranial pressure – early morning headache, worse on lying down, nausea/vomiting, blurry/double vision etc.
- If chronic, it can be asymptomatic or give insidious symptoms

- **Normal pressure hydrocephalus**

This is a non-obstructive subtype of hydrocephalus.
- It produces large ventricles without an increase in intracranial pressure.
- It is largely idiopathic, can be a secondary to a stroke, bleed or infection.
- It is classically associated with producing a triad of symptoms, including dementia.

Symptoms

- Slow onset triad of urinary incontinence, gait instability and dementia

Key tests

- Cognitive tests – MMSE
- 1st line brain imaging is CT head
- Lumbar puncture is used for diagnosis and therapy, a pre- and post-LP timed walk

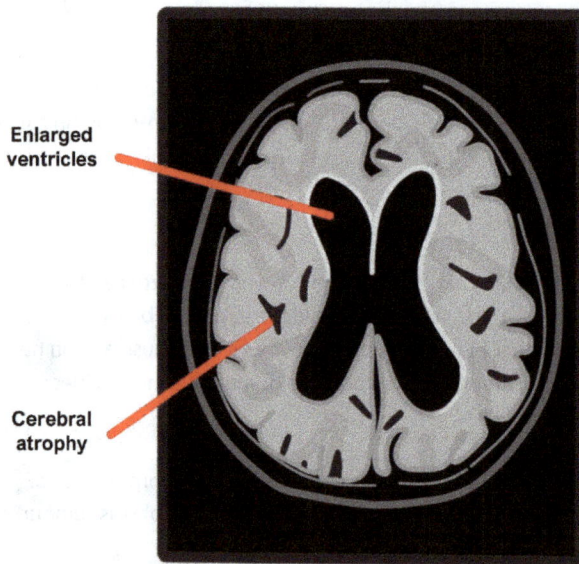

Management

- If acute, external ventricular drain (EVD)
- Long-term treatment is ventriculoperitoneal shunting, which diverts CSF from the ventricles to the peritoneum

Eating Disorders

Eating disorders are a group of conditions which are characterised by a disorganised pattern of food consumption with associated physical and emotional distress.
- They are more common in females than males with an onset around age 15–30.
- The two most common conditions are anorexia nervosa and bulimia nervosa, which share similar features.

As with most psychiatric conditions, the aetiology can be considered using the bio-psychosocial model.

Biological
- Genetics – twin studies show that eating disorders share a large genetic component
- 5-HT – altered brain serotonin contributes to dysregulation of appetite, mood, and impulsivity

Psychological
- Personality – association with anxious, obsessive-compulsive, and depressive traits
- Self-esteem – associated with low self-esteem and body image disturbances

Social
- Childhood – sexual and emotional abuse, overprotective environment, dysfunctional family dynamics
- Media – exposure to media coverage of underweight individuals, dietary fads etc.

Common symptoms
- These can be split into tissue-specific and metabolic

Metabolic
- Bradycardia, hypotension, fatigue, lethargy (low levels of T_3)
- Weight loss, poor glucose tolerance
- Hypercholesterolaemia, low K
- Low libido (low FSH, LH, oestrogen and testosterone)
- High cortisol and growth hormone

Tissue
- Bone – osteoporosis
- Muscle breakdown and weakness
- Enlarged salivary glands
- Lanugo hair – soft, unpigmented furry hair
- Russell's sign (hand callouses) as a result of self-induced vomiting

- **Anorexia nervosa**

This is a disorder which is characterised by restrictive eating, due to a morbid fear of weight gain. Patients lose weight either by dieting, purging (vomiting), laxative/diuretic abuse or exercise. It carries about a 10% mortality risk.

Diagnosis (3 key features)

- Low body weight (< 85% expected body mass)
- Distorted body image
- Morbid fear of weight gain
- In addition, patients may also experience amenorrhea and loss of sexual interest

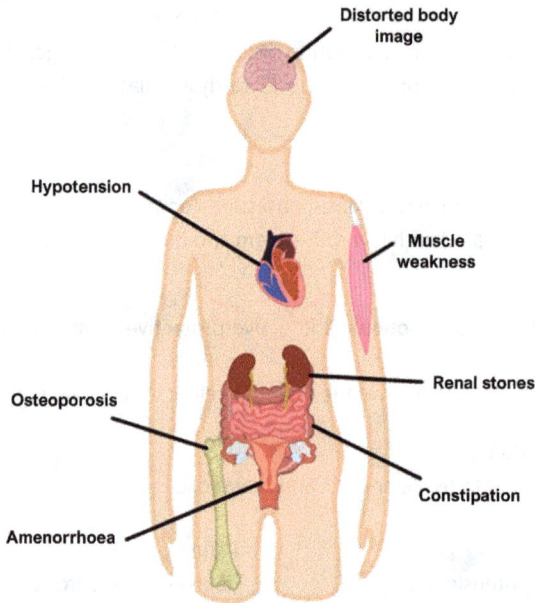

Management

Acute

- Consider nasogastric feeding tube if BMI < 13, bradycardic, K^+ < 3 mM or if patients are clearly dehydrated

Chronic

- Referral for specialist care
- In children, 1st line is anorexia-focused family therapy, 2nd line is CBT
- In adults, 1st line is eating-disorder focused CBT or specialist supportive clinical management (SSCM)

- **Bulimia nervosa**

This disorder is characterised by episodes of binge eating followed by intentional purgative behaviours in order to lose weight. However, the weight is typically normal.
- Purging behaviours include intentional vomiting, laxative/diuretic abuse or excessive exercise.
- With CBT, 30–40% of patients manage to achieve remission.
- It has a much lower mortality risk than anorexia.

Diagnosis (5 key features)
- Preoccupation with body shape and weight
- Recurrent binge eating (an amount that is clearly more than people would eat and with a clear loss of control)
- Inappropriate compensatory behaviours to stop weight gain
- These occur at least once/week for at least 3 months
- Episodes do not occur during an episode of anorexia nervosa

Management

Acute
- Consider nasogastric feeding tube if BMI < 13, bradycardic, K^+ < 3 mM or patients are clearly dehydrated

Chronic
- In children, 1st line is bulimia-focused family therapy, 2nd line is CBT
- In adults, 1st line is eating-disorder focused CBT or interpersonal therapy (IPT)
- Fluoxetine is licensed in bulimia only, not anorexia

- **Binge eating disorder**

This is an eating disorder characterised by recurrent episodes of binge-eating without the purging behaviours.
- Binge eating disorder has 2 key aspects: eating much more than normal and with a clear loss of control.

Symptoms
- Recurrent episodes of binge eating
- Emotional distress/anxiety
- Typically co-occurs with obesity (BMI > 30)

Management
- 1st line is guided self-help, then group CBT
- If severe or previous approaches not successful, consider individual CBT

Substance Abuse

- **Alcohol**

Alcohol abuse is defined as the regular or binge consumption of alcohol leading to an inadvertent impact on an individuals' physical health, mental health or social function.

- 1 unit (10 mL) of alcohol is about equivalent to a small glass of wine, or a single measure of spirits.
- Units = volume (L) × alcohol by volume (ABV) (%)
- e.g. a 750 ml bottle of 12% strength wine has 750/1000 × 12 = 9 units
- Both men and women should drink no more than 14 units a week and their alcohol consumption over the week should be spread evenly over 3 days or more.

There are several complications that can arise from problematic alcohol use.

○ **Acute intoxication**

This is a state caused by excess alcohol consumption. It gives the symptoms of being "drunk" and can resemble other causes of acute confusion, especially head trauma.

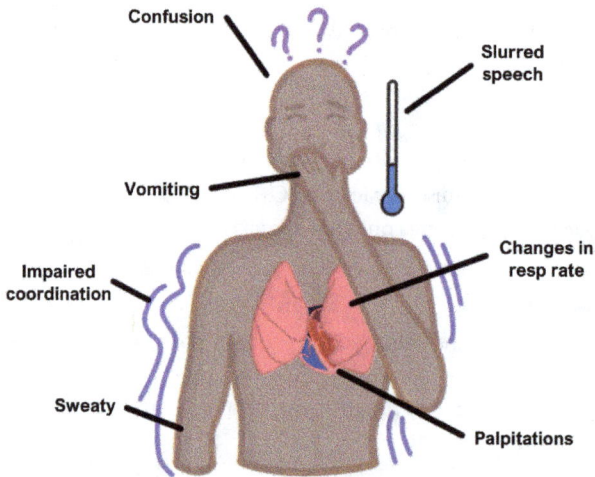

Confusion · Slurred speech · Vomiting · Changes in resp rate · Impaired coordination · Sweaty · Palpitations

Symptoms
- Slurred speech, impaired coordination and judgement
- These symptoms may mask underlying neurological symptoms or hypoglycaemia

Management
- Supportive management as effects usually wear off in 24 hours

○ **Alcoholic ketoacidosis**

This is a complication of alcoholism which leads to raised ketone levels in the blood causing an acidosis, without a hyperglycaemia.

- When alcoholics miss meals or vomit, this can lead to episodes of starvation, and so the body switches from carbohydrate to fat metabolism generating ketone bodies.

Symptoms

- Nausea, vomiting and abdominal pain
- May be signs of hypovolaemia – tachycardia and hypotension
- In contrast to diabetic ketoacidosis, patients are usually more alert and lucid

Key tests

- Blood gas – metabolic acidosis with a raised anion gap and elevated ketones
- In contrast to DKA the glucose levels will be normal/low

Management

- IV fluids with dextrose and thiamine (to prevent Wernicke's encephalopathy)

○ **Alcohol dependence**

This is a compulsion to drink alcohol with associated physical and psychological harm.

- ICD 10 criteria for diagnosis include a strong desire to drink alcohol, difficulty in controlling use, persistent use despite harm and prioritizing use over other activity.
- It also includes tolerance to alcohol as well as withdrawal states.

Key tests

- The CAGE questionnaire is a screening tool used to identify problematic drinkers
- Have you tried to **C**ut down drinking?
- Have people **A**nnoyed you by suggesting you do so?
- Have you felt **G**uilty about drinking?
- Have you needed an **E**ye-opener (early morning drink)?

Management

- Patients are referred to an alcohol dependence programme to help them quit
- Behavioural interventions – group therapy, CBT
- Pharmacological measures include disulfiram, which inhibits acetaldehyde dehydrogenase, so people feel hungover as soon as they drink alcohol
- Acamprosate is a weak NMDA antagonist which is used to reduce alcohol cravings

In addition to affecting the liver, one of the main neurological problems is that it leads to thiamine (vitamin B_1) deficiency. This leads to haemorrhage in the mammillary bodies and ventricle walls leading to 2 conditions.

- **Wernicke's encephalopathy**

This is characterised by an acute peripheral neuropathy and central dysfunction which can lead to cerebellar degeneration.
- This condition is often triggered by infection in those with thiamine deficiency or carbohydrate/glucose loading in those with thiamine deficiency.

Symptoms

- Classic triad of ataxia, ophthalmoplegia/nystagmus and acute confusion

Key tests

- It is largely a clinical diagnosis based on the clinical history and examination
- MRI can show hyperintense signals in the periventricular thalamus, mammillary bodies and the periaqueductal grey matter
- Decreased red cell transketolase – this is an enzyme that catalyses transfer of alcohol group between sugars

Management

- Alcohol cessation and IV Pabrinex, this contains high doses of vitamin B_1

- **Korsakoff's syndrome**

This is the consequence of untreated Wernicke's encephalopathy which leads to a non-progressive dementia (memory loss).
- It can also be associated with AIDS, cancers that have spread throughout the body, chronic infections and poor nutrition.

Symptoms

- Both anterograde and retrograde amnesia
- Confabulation – a symptom of memory dysfunction where patients make up accounts to fill in gaps in their memory

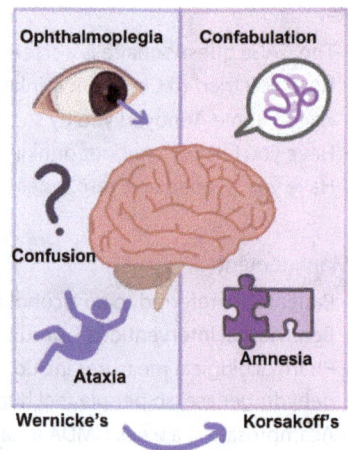

○ **Alcohol withdrawal**

Alcohol consumption enhances GABA-inhibition in the CNS and inhibits NMDA glutamate receptors. In withdrawal is thought that the opposite occurs (less GABA and more NMDA transmission).

Symptoms

- Early symptoms – increased anxiety, with sweating and agitation
- Seizures with visual hallucinations
- Delirium tremens (from 48–72 hours) – Course tremors, agitation, delusions, confusion and visual hallucinations

Management

- 1st line are benzodiazepines e.g. oxazepam/chlordiazepoxide on a weaning protocol

In addition to alcohol, it is important to know the symptoms of overdosing on other common recreational drugs.

● **Cocaine**

This drug blocks the reuptake of dopamine and noradrenaline (and 5-HT) increasing transmission at synapses.
- Cocaine is usually snorted excepted crack cocaine which is smoked.
- It is a stimulant as it resembles a state of increased sympathetic activity.
- It can cause increased energy and concentration, euphoria and hyperactivity.

Side effects

- Cardiovascular – increased HR/BP, hyperthermia, can lead to aortic dissection
- Heart – QRS widening and QT prolongation
- GI – reduced appetite and increased risk of ischaemic colitis
- Psychological – insomnia, agitation and hallucinations e.g. formication, a sensation of insects under the skin
- They can trigger psychotic episodes with more persistent hallucinations/delusions than seen in intoxication states

Management

- Benzodiazepines are usually first line in acute overdose
- Treat complications (e.g. myocardial infarction, aortic dissections)
- Consider antipsychotics if there is evidence of psychosis

- **Cannabinoids**

Cannabis is extracted from the plants Cannabis Sativa and Cannabis Indica.

- The active stimulatory ingredient is tetrahydrocannabinol (THC) which binds to CB1 receptors. On the other hand, the other component is cannabidiol (CBD) which is known to dampen the THC effects.
- It causes euphoria and relaxation, with a distortion of sense of time and place.

Side effects

- Respiratory – red eyes, dry mouth and coughing
- Psychological – can lead to paranoid thinking, anxiety and an increased risk of developing psychosis (schizophrenia)
- GI – increased appetite after the high

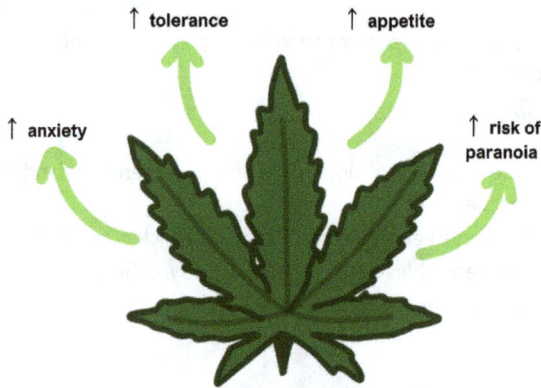

- **MDMA (ecstasy)**

A psychoactive drug which blocks the reuptake of monoamines, particularly serotonin and noradrenaline. It is commonly used as a "club drug" and induces a euphoric state.

- It causes increased energy, empathy, as well as pleasure (mild hallucinogen).

Side effects

- Cardiovascular – hyperthermia causing sweating, tachycardia, hypertension
- Water intoxication – patients can subsequently drink excessive water to rehydrate (compounded by ecstasy's effect of increasing ADH levels), causing hyponatraemia and death
- Psychological – insomnia, increased psychomotor activity, trismus (locked jaw)

Personality Disorders

Personality can be defined as the pattern and range of emotional, cognitive and behavioural characteristics that make up an individual.
- It is composed of 4 main domains: cognition, impulse control, social communication and affect/emotion.
- As these components exist on a spectrum, it can be challenging to determine whether traits are normal or disordered.

A personality is disordered when one or more of these personality components crosses a threshold and leads to psychosocial distress, harm or functional deficit.
- The trait should be pathological, pervasive and persistent (3 P's).
- It must lead to stereotyped responses which can be traced to childhood.
- The trait should be quantitatively significantly different from others of a similar background (beyond a cut off).
- It should lead to distress or impair social function for the patient.
- It should not be due to another mental disorder or medical condition.

With most psychiatric conditions, the aetiology can be considered using a biopsycho-social model and is most relevant in childhood.

Biological
- Genetics – twin studies show personality disorders share a large genetic component

Psychological
- Early life experiences – adverse events including neglect and abuse are highly associated with the development of personality disorders

Social
- Society – chaotic home environments, disconnection with society and dysfunctional peer group interactions predispose to the development of personality disorder

- **Emotionally unstable personality disorder (EUPD)**
This is the one of the most common personality disorders which is characterised by a dysregulated emotional state at its core.
- It is also referred to as borderline personality disorder (BPD).

The aetiology can be considered by looking at disruptions to the normal psychological development milestones a child passes through.

Secure attachment
- From early childhood, secure attachments (usually to a parent figure) form
- This attachment later forms the basis of adult relationships
- Disruption to secure attachment formation in childhood can lead to adult relationships being volatile or dominated by extremes of emotion
- Relationships can become intense in onset but also fragile in terms of longevity

Distress tolerance
- Children as they develop learn how to manage their emotions to distressing events.
- Difficulties in achieving distress tolerance in childhood can lead in adulthood to problems in controlling emotions in adulthood with pronounced anger/frustration
- They also predispose the development of maladaptive coping mechanisms to manage distress later in life

Emotional literacy
- Adolescents learn to be aware of their emotions and control them in social situations
- Disruption in childhood to literacy can lead in adulthood to reduced awareness of emotions and inappropriate reactions in social situations

Self-identity
- By the end of adolescence, we have a stable sense of who we are as individuals
- Disruptions to identity formation can lead to an unstable sense of self in adulthood

Symptoms
- Intense interpersonal relationships alternating between love and hate
- Fear of abandonment
- Unstable self-image/identity
- Difficulty controlling emotions
- Unstable mood
- Impulsive behaviour in ≥ 2 different domains (e.g. sex, gambling, drugs)
- Recurrent suicidal behaviour (often as a poor coping response to stressful events)
- Persistent feeling of emptiness and low mood
- Quasi psychotic symptoms

Emotionally unstable PD is split into the borderline type and impulsive type.
- The borderline subtype has prominent emotional instability with repeated acts of self-harm (as shown above).
- The impulsive subtype has prominent impulsive behaviour without the repeated acts of self-harm.

Emotionally unstable PD clinically resemble bipolar disorder, but there are some key differences.

Emotionally unstable PD	Bipolar disorder
Usually a history of childhood abuse	Is not always linked to child abuse
Emotions associated with life events	Depression/mania are unrelated to life events
Impulsivity is a chronic complaint in these patients	Impulsivity only seen during the manic or depressive phase
Mood changes occur suddenly, from low to agitated and vice versa amidst pervasive low mood	Distinct phases of depression and mania with euthymia in between

The other personality disorders share the same core features but differ in which component of personality is abnormal.
- By conceptualising the disorders like this, it can help to remember the key features, rather than learning all the individual diagnostic criteria for each type of PD.

- **Antisocial/dissocial personality disorder**

Trait: Impaired impulse control, leading to high levels of aggression and insensitivity

Origin: Stems from a disregard of others or societal norms

Symptoms
- The patient has no regard for rights or safety of others
- They are irresponsible (e.g. cannot keep a job)
- Highly aggressive and impulsive behaviour, and often break the law and get arrested
- Very deceitful and untrustworthy blaming others for their actions, with an accompanied lack of remorse

- **Avoidant/anxious personality disorder**

Trait: Impaired emotional confidence, giving anxiety and tension in relationships

Origin: Stems from a fear of criticism or rejection by others

Symptoms
- Patient avoids activities which involve social contact due to a fear of not being liked
- They are restrained in relationships and can't go "all-in" in case they get rejected
- Patients isolate themselves socially but still have a craving for social contact
- Can have an inferiority complex and will put themselves down in front of others

- **Dependent personality disorder**

Trait: Impaired emotional confidence resulting in submissive and clingy behaviour

Origin: Stems from fear of criticism or rejection from others

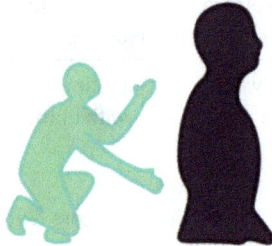

Symptoms
- Excessive need to be taken care off
- A need for others to take responsibility for their life decisions
- Patients will cling to their partners due to the fear of being left alone
- Wanting their partner to have a substantial role in their lives, making decisions for them and giving them constant care
- Will go out of their way to get support

- **Histrionic personality disorder**

Trait: Impaired self-confidence leading to extroverted behaviour to gain attention

Origin: Stems from a need to be the centre of attention

Symptoms
- Very attention seeking in behaviour and appearance
- Excessively dramatic, impressionist speech and narcissistic
- Provocative behaviour with exaggerated but superficial emotional expression
- Influenced easily by others or circumstances

- **Narcissistic personality disorder (DSM only)**

Trait: Disrupted sense of self which leads to an over-inflated sense of self-importance

Origin: It stems from a constant need for admiration from others

Symptoms
- Constant fantasies of success and power
- Feel self-entitled and that they can only be understood by high status people
- Actively takes advantage of others to achieve their own goals, with a lack of remorse
- Very envious of others with an arrogant attitude

- **Obsessive-compulsive/anankastic personality disorder**

Trait: Excessive perfectionism producing very stereotyped behaviours and inflexibility

Origin: Stems from a pervasive pursuit of efficiency at the expense of other activities

Symptoms
- Excessive obsession with rules, lists, schedules and order
- Devote themselves to work and productivity at the expense of interpersonal relationships and recreation
- They have obsessional thoughts (but unlike OCD these are not unwanted but instead are accepted)
- Little affection and warmth; their relationships and speech have a formal and professional approach
- Obsessed with controlling their environments thus satisfying their need for control

- **Paranoid personality disorder**

Trait: Impaired ability to form relationships/confide in others

Origin: It stems from impaired trust in relationships leading to constant suspicion

Symptoms
- Recurrent suspicion without proof about others' loyalty
- Preoccupied with conspiracy theories
- Hypersensitivity with an unforgiving attitude when insulted

- **Schizotypal personality disorder**

Trait: Impaired cognition causing odd thinking patterns and perceptual abnormalities

Origin: Stems from disorganised thinking (akin to a quasi-psychosis)

Symptoms
- Patient has strange beliefs and displays magical thinking e.g. telepathy
- They express odd thoughts and display odd speech patterns
- Patients may have ideas of references (some insight retained) and unusual perceptual disturbances
- Lack of close friends and excessive social anxiety
- Inappropriate affect (react abnormally to external stimuli)

- **Schizoid personality disorder**

Trait: Impaired social communication leading to insensitivity to social norms

Origin: Stems from emotional coldness

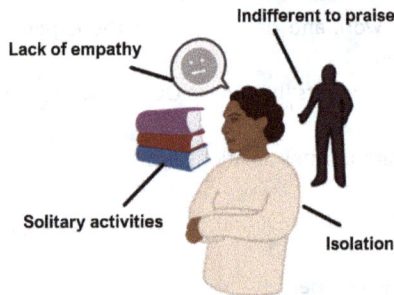

Symptoms
- Acts aloof, cold and indifferent leading to interpersonal problems
- They are indifferent to praise or criticism
- They prefer isolation and stay away from social activities
- Lack desire for companionship and sexual interactions

Common management
- MDT approach, using mixture of psychotherapy and encouraging self-awareness
- Psychotherapy – CBT/DBT instils effective interpersonal communication, distress tolerance and emotional regulation
- Medication – there is limited evidence for psychotropics as a primary treatment of personality disorder. However, you can use anti-depressants or anti-psychotics to treat comorbidities as an adjunctive treatment

Medically Unexplained Symptoms

- **Somatic symptom disorder**

A disorder where patients experience physical symptoms without an organic explanation. The most common symptoms mentioned usually involve the GI tract (abdominal pain) or the skin.

- Patients do not accept negative test results as reassuring. Individuals become disproportionately preoccupied with their symptoms and anxious as a result.
- It is more common in young women and can lead to multiple investigations and procedures despite the absence of disease.

- **Hypochondrial disorder**

This is a disorder where patients are convinced that they have a serious underlying disease e.g. cancer or HIV. As before, there is no physical or organic explanation.

- Patients cannot accept negative test results and instead feel distress and worry.
- It is more common in men and people who have more contact with disease (e.g. health workers).

- **Conversion disorder**

This is a condition in which a patient exhibits physical symptoms such as paralysis or numbness where the primary aetiology is psychological.

- The patient doesn't consciously fake the symptoms or try to exaggerate them but functions as if they exist.
- Investigations and examination will likely be normal or inconsistent.
- Patients are typically aloof to their disorder and do not appear concerned (called "la belle indifference"). This indifference is key in distinguishing between conversion and somatoform disorders.

Management

- First it is important to exclude an organic cause
- Once excluded, psychotherapy and social interventions are used

- **Dissociative disorders**

This is a group of conditions which are more common in women.

- They involve psychiatric symptoms which occur in the absence of organic pathology such as disruptions or breakdowns in memory, awareness, identity or perception.

Psychoanalytical theory proposes that painful memories are "cut-off" from the conscious self and "converted" into more bearable physical symptoms.

○ **Dissociative amnesia**

A condition where the patient has disruption to recollection of traumatic or personal information. It is seen as a way to cope with previous emotional trauma.

○ **Dissociative fugue**

This is a form of dissociative amnesia in which the patient flees away from their home.
- Patients display amnesia over their identity, memories and personality.
- This can last from a few hours to a number of weeks.

○ **Dissociative identity disorder**

The most severe form of dissociative disorder in which the patient develops alternate, multiple personalities. It is strongly linked to early childhood trauma (sexual abuse).
- Patient has amnesia for when the different personalities manifest but may be aware of their existence.

Management

- After excluding organic causes, psychotherapy is the main management strategy

● **Factitious disorder (Munchausen's syndrome)**

This is a condition where patients will produce physical or psychological symptoms in order to enter a sick role. The sick role offers compassion, shifts inter-personal dynamics and absolution of certain roles or responsibility.
- Patients can feign the symptoms, exaggerate them or deliberately hurt themselves to produce symptoms e.g. patients can take hallucinogens, inject faeces to induce sepsis or intentional misuse prescription drugs.

Management

- Psychotherapy, can include family therapy plus addressing any social stressors

● **Malingering**

This is when a patient feigns/exaggerates symptom primarily for financial/other gain.
- Unlike before, it is not done to enter a sick role but instead to receive compensation, personal damages or get off work.
- It is not a medical diagnosis but can create a large burden on health care systems.

Paediatric Psych Conditions

- **Attention deficit hyperactivity disorder (ADHD)**

This is a disorder which is characterised by inattention, hyperactivity and impulsivity.

- It is much more common in boys than girls and is usually diagnosed in the primary school years.
- In order to distinguish this condition from extremes of "normal behaviour", there are 3 key features that must be present in order to satisfy the diagnostic criteria.

i) Persistent – the disruptive behaviour must be present most of the time.
- If the behaviours fluctuate, then they could simply be a responsive reaction to a change in the environment.

ii) Pervasive – the disruptive behaviour must be seen across multiple environments.
- If the behaviour was only seen at home, parental and family factors are more likely to be the underlying cause. Similarly, if the behaviour solely exists at school, an alternative cause such as bullying may explain features such as inattention.

iii) Developmental delay – similar to many paediatric conditions, ADHD leads to delays in motor, cognitive and language development.

Symptoms

- Inattention – easily distracted, forgets activities, loses possessions, does not listen attentively
- Hyperactivity – unable to play quietly, restlessness
- Impulsive – cannot wait their turn, interruptive in class

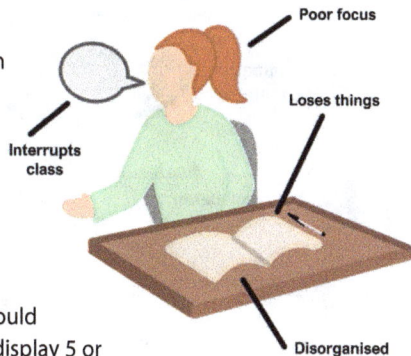

Poor focus

Loses things

Interrupts class

Disorganised

Diagnosis

- Clinical history – for children < 16, they should display 6 symptoms. For those > 17, must display 5 or more symptoms.
- School observation – this is needed to show that the behaviour is pervasive across different environments
- Formal tests e.g. QB test – measures impulsivity, attention and concentration

Management

- First is a 10-week watch and wait period to see if symptoms resolve
- If symptoms persist, refer to child and adolescent mental health
- 1st line is a parent education and training programme
- Pharmacological treatment is methylphenidate for a 6-week trial. It is important to monitor the BP after dose adjustments and BP, height and weight every 6 months
- If this is unsuccessful, subsequent pharmacological options include lisdexamphetamine and dexamphetamine
- If these are not tolerated or the patient has social anxiety, trial atomoxetine (SNRI)

In adults, methylphenidate and lisdexamfetamine can both be used 1st line.
- These medications can be cardiotoxic so perform a baseline ECG prior to treatment.

- **Autism spectrum disorder (ASD)**

This is a developmental disorder which is more common in males.
- It has an onset before the age of 3.
- It represents a spectrum ranging from mild impairment to severe disability.
- It is thought that children exhibit extreme "male" brains with higher level of systemising over empathising.

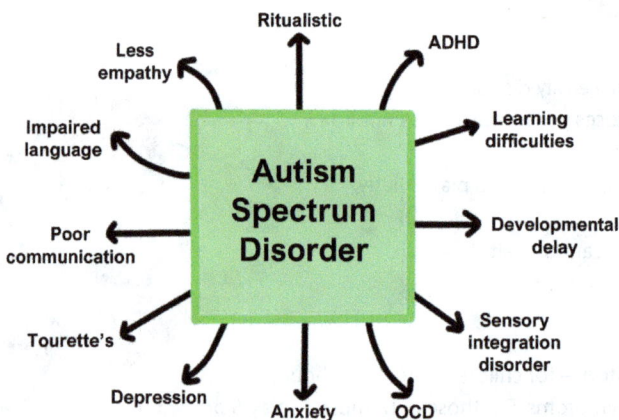

Symptoms

- All 3 should be present for a diagnosis to be made
- Global impairment of language and communication
- Impairment of social relationships
- Ritualistic and compulsive behaviour

- In addition, most patients have a low IQ
- It is also associated with ADHD, epilepsy and other neurological abnormalities
- Some may have isolated skills e.g. (memory, computation) but this is the minority

Management

- MDT supports education, promotes independence and improves social skills
- Mixture of behavioural therapy, special education and family counselling
- Medication may be used to treat comorbidities (e.g. methylphenidate for ADHD) but has no specific primary role

- **Asperger's syndrome**

This is thought to be a less severe form than autism which is characterised by more minor functional impairment. The diagnosis is only in the ICD-10 and not the DSM-5.
- It is typically diagnosed after the age of 3, whereas autism is diagnosed earlier on.
- Delays in social communication become evident at this age.

Symptoms

- The main feature is a schizoid personality trait
- Individuals are more indifferent to praise or criticism and can act in an aloof manner
- They prefer solitary activities and have few interests
- Lack desire for companionship and sexual interactions, with few friends
- They have pedantic speech and pre-occupation with obscure facts
- However, they will usually have normal intelligence and language development

- **Conduct disorder**

This is a type of personality disorder (PD) which occurs in children and is similar to antisocial PD. About one third will develop adult antisocial personality disorder.
- It is characterised by persistent disruptive, deceptive and aggressive behaviour.
- Associated with low self-esteem, ADHD and developmental disorders.
- It is associated with family conflict, violent parents and alcoholic parents.

Symptoms

- Child shows disobedience and no remorse for behaviour
- Engages in crimes like stealing, arson, fighting and damage to property

Management

- Mixture of parental training, school interventions and behavioural interventions

Bonus - Electrolytes

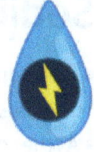

MEDICAL CONDITIONS

Sodium

- **Hyponatraemia**

This refers to a low concentration of plasma sodium ions.

- As the concentration depends on both sodium levels and water volume, hyponatraemia can either be due to a lack of sodium ions or too much water.
- The causes for hyponatraemia can be subdivided by the fluid status of the patient.

Causes

- Hypervolaemic – heart failure, renal failure, liver failure
- Hypovolaemic – diuretic use, poor oral intake, diarrhoea, vomiting, burns, Addison's
- Euvolaemic – SIADH, psychogenic polydipsia
- Pseudohyponatraemia – due to high lipid, glucose or protein levels

Symptoms

- Low serum osmolality makes the brain swell giving symptoms of raised ICP
- Can cause headache, confusion, reduced consciousness and seizures
- Increased risk of falls, particularly in the elderly

Key tests

- Hyponatraemia screen, which includes paired serum and urine osmolalities as well as a urinary sodium – this is very helpful in determining whether there is excessive sodium loss from the kidneys or whether they can retain sodium ions
- Thyroid function tests should be sent to rule out hypothyroidism
- Check cortisol level to exclude Addison's disease

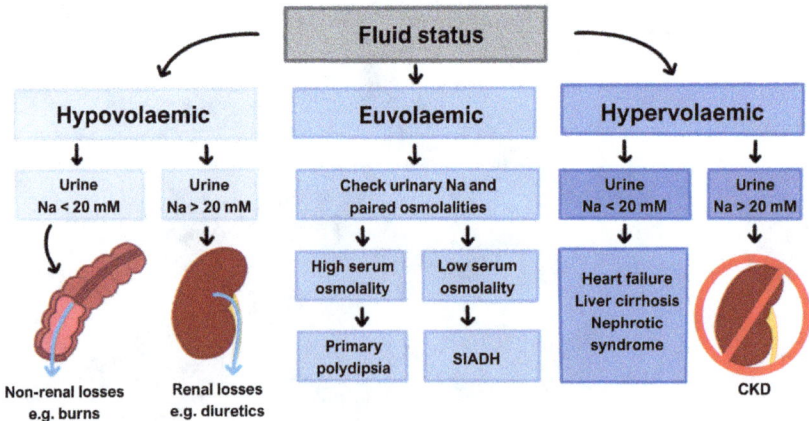

Management

- Correct the underlying cause rather than just treat Na^+ concentration alone
- For hypovolaemic hyponatraemia – IV fluids (e.g. 0.9% saline)
- For euvolaemic hyponatraemia – first line is fluid restriction. If due to SIADH, can also treat with demeclocycline or vaptans
- For hypervolaemic hyponatraemia – first line is fluid restriction, then diuretics
- If the patient is very symptomatic (e.g. seizures), they can be given hypertonic (3%) saline to correct the sodium. This should ideally be done in a high dependency unit

Central pontine myelinolysis
This is a complication which arises from correcting the sodium level too quickly.
- It can cause rapid demyelination of the neurons in the pons.
- This can present with lethargy and confusion and give rise to seizures as well as paralysis of limbs (locked in syndrome).
- Therefore, one should aim to correct sodium ions by about 4–6 mM per 24 hours.

- **Hypernatraemia**

This refers to a high concentration of sodium ions, which usually occurs due to water loss, resulting in an increased concentration of sodium ions.

Causes

- Dehydration – poor oral intake, vomiting, burns, diarrhoea
- Diabetes insipidus – reduced action of ADH causing poor water reabsorption
- Excessive diuretic use
- Iatrogenic – excessive IV fluids with saline

Symptoms

- Weakness, dry mucous membranes, increased thirst
- If very severe, can cause reduced consciousness and seizures

Management

- Address the underlying cause – stop offending drugs, encourage oral fluid intake
- IV fluids – 0.9% saline can still be given as this is more dilute than the patient's blood
- Alternatively, 5% dextrose is a good choice of fluid for gentle rehydration
- Avoid correcting too quickly as rapidly reducing the sodium can lead to fluid shifts causing cerebral oedema raising intracerebral pressure

Potassium

- **Hypokalaemia**

Low potassium causes hyperpolarisation of cells and reduces the excitability of nerve and muscles, leading to symptoms such as muscular weakness and arrythmias.

Causes

- Secondary to low magnesium
- Poor oral intake
- Losses – diarrhoea/vomiting
- Refeeding syndrome
- Drugs e.g. diuretics

Symptoms

- Muscle weakness
- Light-headedness
- Palpitations

Key tests

- Blood tests show low potassium (important to check magnesium levels too)
- ECG shows small/inverted T waves, long PR interval and prominent U wave

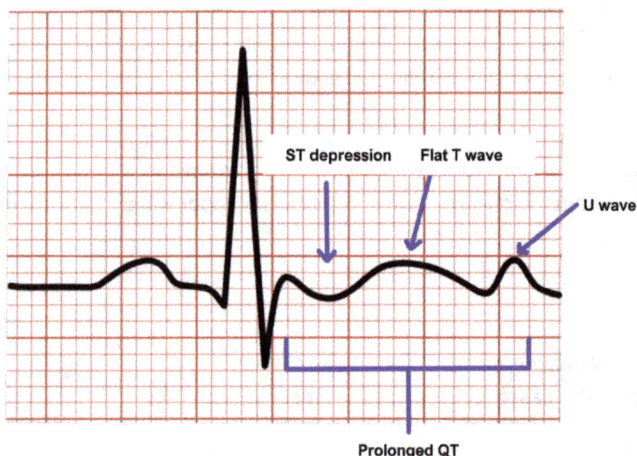

Management

- Correct underlying causes e.g. stop diuretics
- Ensure magnesium levels are replete
- Oral K replacement (or IV potassium if severe/oral not suitable)
- In severe deficiency, concentrated KCl can be given but this should be given through a central line with cardiac monitoring due to risk of precipitating arrythmias

- **Hyperkalaemia**

High potassium levels are very dangerous as they cause depolarisation of cells increasing excitability of nerve and muscle, increasing risk of cardiac arrhythmias.
- If patient is well but has a high $[K^+]$ this may be due to artefact, caused by K^+ ions leaking out of RBCs due to haemolysis, contamination or delayed analysis.

Causes

- Renal failure (acute and chronic)
- Drugs – ACEi, MRA
- Addison's disease
- Tumour lysis syndrome

Symptoms

- Palpitations and chest pain
- Risk of arrythmias and sudden death

Key tests

- Blood test to check potassium. If the result is unexpected, send a repeat sample to ensure the first is not an artefact (e.g. raised potassium due to haemolysis)
- ECG shows tall, tented T waves, wide QRS (can lead to VF)

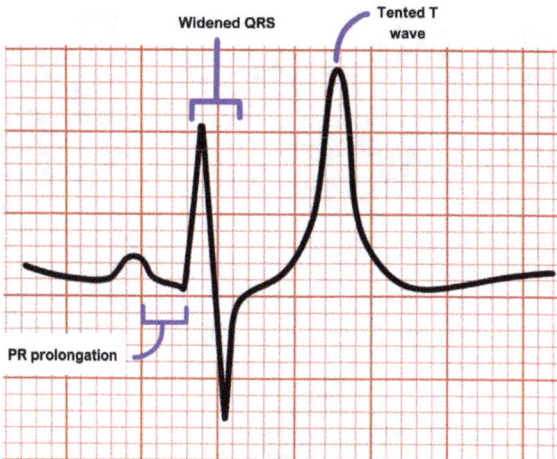

Management

- Treat if K^+ > 6.5 mM or if there are visible ECG changes
- IV calcium gluconate (this stabilises the cell membrane to reduce arrythmia risk)
- IV insulin in dextrose solution and nebulised salbutamol (pushes potassium into cells)
- Potassium binders such as Lokelma or calcium resonium (reduces GI absorption)
- Stop any offending drugs and treat the underlying cause

Calcium

The majority of calcium in the body is stored in the bones. Calcium ions in the plasma are bound to negative glycoproteins on the membrane and stabilise sodium channels.

- **Hypocalcaemia**

This refers to a low serum concentration of calcium ions.
- A decrease in calcium ion concentration reduces the threshold for action potentials and increases the excitability of motor neurones.

Causes

- Associated with raised phosphate – CKD, hypoparathyroidism, rhabdomyolysis
- Associated with low phosphate – vitamin D deficiency, pancreatitis, osteomalacia

Key tests

- Check PTH, phosphate, Mg and vitamin D levels

Symptoms

- These can be remembered by the acronym SPASMODIC

Spasm	**S**eizures	**D**ermatitis
Perioral paraesthesia	**M**uscle tone up	**I**mpetigo herpetiformis
Anxious	**O**rientation impaired	**C**hvostek sign

Management

- If mild deficiency, oral calcium supplements. Give IV if severe
- Ensure vitamin D and magnesium levels are replete

- **Hypercalcaemia**

This refers to a high concentration of serum calcium ions. This decreases the excitability of nerve and muscle leading to symptoms including lethargy.
- The most common reasons are malignancy (paraneoplastic, bone metastases, myeloma) and primary hyperparathyroidism.

Symptoms

- Bones – ectopic calcification (e.g. cornea) and bone pain
- Stones – renal stones and renal failure
- Groans – abdominal pain, vomiting, constipation
- Moans – confusion, irritability, depression
- Other – polyuria, polydipsia, weakness, fatigue

Key tests

- The main distinction to make is malignancy vs primary hyperparathyroidism
- The most important investigation to send first is parathyroid hormone
- If PTH is raised, this suggests primary hyperparathyroidism (or tertiary)
- If PTH low, this suggests that it is low to compensate for a high calcium level
- Check phosphate levels, renal function, ALP to guide diagnosis

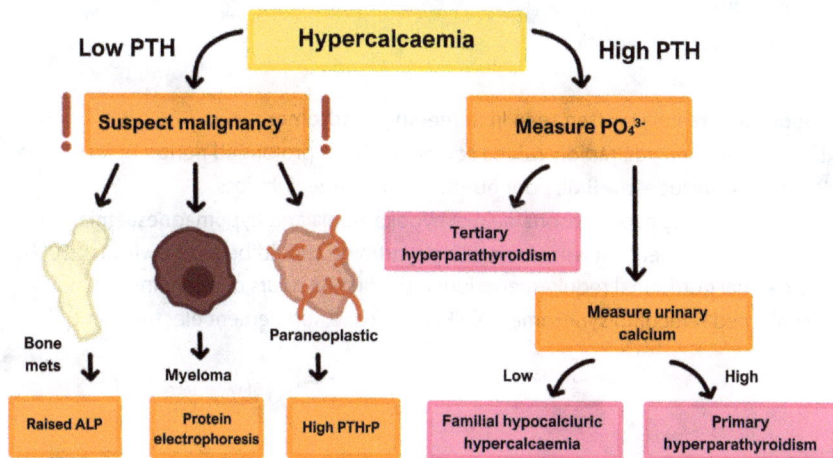

Management

- 1st line is fluids (e.g. 0.9% saline)
- If calcium level is still elevated, bisphosphonates (e.g. zoledronate) are used to reduce osteoclast resorption of bone
- Additional options include steroids, cinacalcet and denosumab
- It is important to treat the underlying cause e.g. surgery for primary hyperparathyroidism, chemotherapy if due to malignancy

Phosphate

Phosphate is a key anion which is needed for the synthesis of DNA, proteins and membranes as well as acting as a buffer for H^+ ions in the body.

- **Hypophosphataemia**

This refers to a low phosphate concentration. It is relatively common and usually carries little clinical significance unless phosphate levels become very low.

Causes

- Vitamin D deficiency
- Primary hyperparathyroidism
- Low oral intake, refeeding syndrome

Symptoms

- Muscle weakness, rhabdomyolysis
- Arrhythmias
- White cell dysfunction

Management

- Phosphate supplementation

Hypophosphataemia is often seen in **Refeeding syndrome**.
- This occurs when you rapidly refeed someone after a prolonged period of starvation.
- Risk factors include low BMI, poor nutritional intake, weight loss.
- It classically gives hypophosphataemia, hypokalaemia and hypomagnesaemia.
- To prevent it, patients at risk of refeeding syndrome should be fed slowly at < 50% of their actual nutritional requirement during the first 48 hours of refeeding.
- If confirmed refeeding syndrome, give Pabrinex and supplement electrolytes.

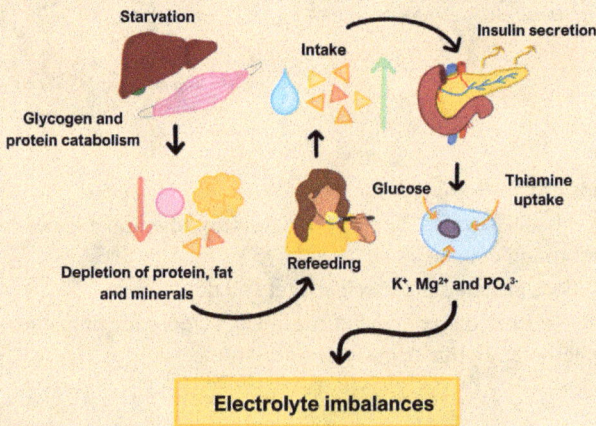

Magnesium

This is a key intracellular ion which has a host of roles within the body.
- It prevents calcium ion entry into smooth muscle and enhances Ca^{2+} uptake into the sarcoplasmic reticulum, resulting in muscle relaxation.
- It inhibits acetylcholine release whilst giving B_2 agonism, increasing cAMP levels.
- Plasma concentration tends to follow that of Ca^{2+} and K^+.

● **Hypomagnesaemia**

This refers to a low concentration of magnesium ions in the body. Similarly to hypocalcaemia, this raises the excitability of nerve and muscle as there is less Ca^{2+} reuptake into the sarcoplasmic reticulum (SR).

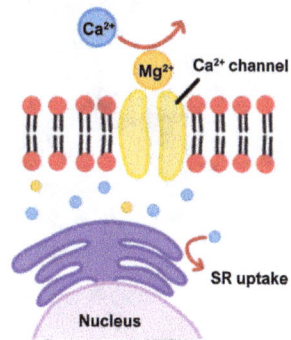

Causes

- Drugs – loop and thiazide diuretics, PPI's
- Poor supply – total parenteral nutrition, refeeding syndrome
- Excessive loss – diarrhoea (natural or due to IBD)
- Secondary to low Ca^{2+}, low K^+ and low PO_4^{3-}

Symptoms

- Increased nerve and muscle excitability – seizures, tetany
- Secondary hypoparathyroidism, as magnesium is needed for PTH secretion
- Cardiac arrythmias (torsades de pointes), due to prolongation of the QTc interval

Key tests

- ECG shows small or inverted T waves, long PR interval and a prolonged QTc interval

Management

- Oral of IV (if severe) magnesium replacement

● **Hypermagnesaemia**

This refers to a high concentration of magnesium. In clinical practice, it is less commonly seen than hypomagnesaemia.

Causes: Renal failure or iatrogenic (excessive antacids)

Symptoms: Neuromuscular depression, hypotension and respiratory depression

Management: Rarely requires treatment unless very severe

Further Reading

This section contains resources that students can consult for additional information.

Cox, M.M. and Nelson, D.L. (2008). *Principles of Biochemistry*. W H Freeman & Co.

Dinulos, J.G.H., *Habif's Clinical Dermatology: A Color Guide to Diagnosis and Therapy*. 7th ed. Edinburgh: Elsevier; 2021.

Drake, R.L., Vogl, W. and Mitchell, A.W.M. (2020). *Gray's Anatomy for Students*. 4th ed. Philadelphia: Elsevier.

Hoffbrand, A.V. and Moss, P.A.H., *Hoffbrand's Essential Haematology*. 7th ed. Chichester, West Sussex Hoboken, NJ: John Wiley & Sons; 2016. 369 p. (Essentials).

Joint Formulary Committee (2023). *British National Formulary (BNF)*. 85th ed. London: Pharmaceutical Press.

Layden, E.A., *Clinical Obstetrics and Gynaecology - E-Book*. 5th ed. Philadelphia: Elsevier; 2022. 1 p.

Lerchenfeldt, S. and Rosenfield, G. (2019). *BRS Pharmacology*. Lippincott Williams & Wilkins.

Marcdante, K.J., Kliegman, R.M., Schuh, A.M., Nelson, W.E., editors. *Nelson Essentials of Pediatrics*. 9th ed. Philadelphia, PA: Elsevier; 2023. 829 p.

National Institute for Health and Care Excellence (2023). Find Guidance | NICE. [online] NICE. Available at: https://www.nice.org.uk/guidance.

Ritter, J., Flower, R.J., Henderson, G., Yoon Kong Loke and Rang, H.P. (2020). *Rang and Dale's Pharmacology*. 9th ed. Endinburgh: Elsevier.

Wilkinson, I.B., Raine, T., Wiles, K., Goodhart, A., Hall, C. and O'Neill, H. (2017). *Oxford Handbook of Clinical Medicine*. 10th ed. Oxford: Oxford University Press.

Index

www.ingramcontent.com/pod-product-compliance
Lightning Source LLC
Chambersburg PA
CBHW052116230326
41598CB00079B/3729